TREATMENT FOR CHRONIC DEPRESSION

TREATMENT FOR CHRONIC DEPRESSION

Cognitive Behavioral Analysis System of Psychotherapy (CBASP)

James P. McCullough, Jr., PhD

Foreword by Marvin R. Goldfried, PhD

THE GUILFORD PRESS
New York   London

© 2000 by James P. McCullough, Jr.
Published by The Guilford Press
A Division of Guilford Publications, Inc.
72 Spring Street, New York, NY 10012
http://www.guilford.com

Printed in the United States of America

This book is printed on acid-free paper.

Last digit is print number: 9 8 7 6 5 4 3 2

Library of Congress Cataloging-in-Publication Data
McCullough, James P.
   Treatment for chronic depression: cognitive behavioral analysis system of
psychotherapy (CBASP) / James P. McCullough, Jr.; foreword by Marvin R.
Goldfried.
      p. ; cm.
Includes bibliographical references and index.
ISBN 1-57230-527-4 (hard : alk. paper)
   1. Depression, Mental—Treatment.   2. Cognitive therapy.   I. Title.
   [DNLM: 1. Depressive Disorder—diagnosis.   2. Cognitive Therapy.
3. Depressive Disorder—therapy.   WM 171 M477t 2000]
RC537 .M394 2000
616.85′270651—dc21
                                                                99-050333

*To Rosemary, whose consequences
for my expressions of love to her
have been endearing, sustaining,
and an awakening for me.*

About the Author

I never thought about being a university professor until I took my clinical internship at the old Georgia Mental Health Institute in Atlanta. The time was 1968–1969, the height of the behavior therapy revolution in psychology. My clinical program at the University of Georgia espoused the Boulder Model approach to training; however, no one ever explained to my satisfaction how one integrates research and practice in a professional role. In those days (and perhaps today), PhD graduates had to make a choice: either one became a researcher and gravitated toward the university or medical school setting or one became a private practitioner.

Internship training exposed me to behavior therapy for the first time. My internship supervisor, Dr. Douglas Slavin, required me to select one psychological learning theory (the choice was mine) and to conceptualize all my cases adhering to the principles of the theory. In addition, I was required to administer psychotherapy to both in- and outpatients applying learning theory principles.

Not surprisingly, I chose B. F. Skinner's operant model and proceeded to immerse myself in Skinnerian psychology. Over time, I realized that the operant program offered a way to integrate research and practice. Now I could operationalize treatment formulations with patients using operant procedures as well as collect data and measure patient change using single-case methodology. In short, operant psychology provided me with a means to conduct research with my clinical patients. Research and practice "merged" in the conduct of my clinical duties.

I also realized that (for me) the most important clinical research must be research that "emerges out of practice"—that is, patient issues must become the focus of my clinical research. It was at this juncture that I decided to enter the university and try to establish a research career *centered around clinical practice*. I entered academia in 1970 and became a member of the clinical psychology training faculty at the University of Southern Mississippi. In 1972, I moved to Virginia Commonwealth University as an Assistant Professor of Psychology. For 30 years, my patients have continued to pose the research questions that I seek to answer. Over time, treating chronically depressed patients and studying their diagnostic characteristics have consumed most of my research efforts and energies.

I am no longer the strict behavior therapist I once was, but readers will find my operant leanings obvious throughout the book. Being a Boulder Model psychologist is still as exciting to me today as it was 30 years ago in Atlanta. I hope I have passed some of this scientist-practitioner excitement on to my clinical students.

Foreword

The treatment of depression continues to remain a challenge to clinicians and researchers alike, especially when the depression is chronic in nature. Different psychosocial interventions have been developed—such as cognitive therapy or interpersonal psychotherapy—but there is no clear evidence that one is better than the other. Still, positions have been taken on preferred treatments, depending on whether one believes that depression is the result of distorted thinking or problematic interpersonal relations. My own sense is that such "either-or" thinking is more of a reflection of political and ideological battles within the field than it is of good clinical judgment. Indeed, I once asked two well-known cognitive therapists whether they would use cognitive therapy with a patient who was depressed because of a failure to grieve for a loss. Without hesitation, each responded: "Of course not!" When then asked what they would do, each indicated that he would help the patient to grieve—an intervention that is included within the interpersonal psychotherapy manual!

In our book *Clinical Behavior Therapy* (1976), Davison and I acknowledge the multiple roots of depression, suggesting that depression can be characterized by patients' beliefs that they do not have the ability to make an impact on their world—including their relationships with others. This may be due to faulty beliefs, lack of ability, or both. That chronic depression is not simply due to faulty thinking, but also to an undeveloped behavioral and affective style that prevents individuals from getting what

they want from others, is a major theme of this very exciting book by
Dr. James P. McCullough. Complicated problems cannot readily be
resolved by simple solutions, and our currently available interventions,
which are theoretically pure, may not have the conceptual and procedural breadth to provide what chronically depressed patients need.
McCullough's approach does. It focuses on the depressed patient's problems in living and, while acknowledging the influence of biological factors, offers a creative integration of the contributions to our understanding of human behavior made by such seemingly diverse individuals as
Sullivan, Piaget, and Skinner.

There are several aspects of McCullough's treatment approach that I
find particularly attractive. One in particular is the emphasis placed on
facilitating assertiveness, a clinical focus that was quite popular in the
1970s. For various reasons, the topic of assertiveness disappeared from the
cognitive behavioral literature in recent years. One reason might be
because clinical research funded by the National Institute of Mental
Health since the 1980s has required a DSM diagnosis, thereby causing a
gradual extinction of research efforts on such undiagnosable (and non-
fundable) problems as unassertiveness. Another reason that the topic of
assertiveness has not been written about in recent years is that Beck's now
popular cognitive therapy—which unfortunately was mislabeled "cognitive behavior therapy" in the large-scale collaborative treatment study of
depression (Elkin et al., 1989)—focuses mostly on distorted cognitions
rather than on patients' inability to get what they want from others. However, depressed patients who do not read the literature continue to have
problems with assertiveness. Furthermore, open-minded and perceptive
cognitive behavior therapists have continued to recognize difficulties
in self-assertion as an important issue in patients' lives. Fortunately,
McCullough is such a therapist.

McCullough's clinical description of how a shift from a submissive to
an assertive mode can produce a dramatic—if only temporary—shift in
mood is an *exact parallel* to what I have observed clinically. In contrast to
seeing themselves as passive and helpless victims of uncontrollable life
events, patients now feel empowered, often describing themselves as "centered," "strong," and "confident." McCullough cites this phenomenon as
an example of "negative reinforcement," in that patients' assertive interactions reduce the distressed emotional state typically associated with
their submissiveness. While the behavior therapist in me can well understand this conceptualization, the transtheoretical part of me would rather
view this as an example of the "corrective experience."

It is beyond the scope of this foreword to document fully why I believe that the corrective experience is at the very heart of the therapeutic change process. However, a description of the corrective experience, and the historical context of the patient's life in which it occurs, may make it clear why I believe it is so important. On the basis of early social learning experiences, individuals develop cognitive, affective, and interpersonal patterns that serve as prototypes for how they will deal with others. To the extent that these early experiences did not provide them with the ability to get their needs met interpersonally, they confront current life circumstances resigned to the belief that they are unable to obtain what they want from others. And while this cognitive-affective and behavioral stance may have been an appropriate reaction to interpersonal events earlier in their lives, it may no longer be adaptive in their current life situations. It is within this historical context that assertiveness can facilitate a corrective experience, which involves the following progression: (1) an expectation and fear that it is dangerous to express one's needs to others; (2) an intellectual awareness that this anticipatory fear is a remnant of one's past; (3) a desire to take the risk by expressing oneself; (4) actually taking that risk and behaving differently; (5) experiencing surprise and relief upon realizing that one's worst fears, in fact, did not materialize; (6) feeling a sense of personal empowerment, rather than the self-recrimination typically associated with one's submissive response; and (7) using this experience as a platform from which to reevaluate one's past maladaptive cognitive, affective, and behavioral patterns.

As one may expect, it is not always easy for a person to make a shift in a lifelong pattern of submissiveness, and to do so often requires the support and encouragement of an understanding and caring therapist. Indeed, there is general agreement in the field that the therapeutic relationship is an indispensable aspect of the therapeutic change process. In publications considering the role of the therapy relationship, the concept of the "alliance" has been used to describe the importance of the personal bond between therapist and patient, their agreement on the goals of treatment, and their agreement on how these goals will be achieved in therapy. In this regard, I have traditionally viewed the therapeutic alliance as the context within which therapy techniques can be applied, in much the way anesthesia provides the context in which surgical procedures may be effectively employed.

Although there may be some merit to this view of the therapy relationship as the contextual background against which the real work—the foreground—of therapy can take place, I have more recently begun to appreciate how something that is in the background can have more importance than one realizes. This greater appreciation of the therapeutic role of the patient-therapist relationship has gradually become evident to me through my ongoing discussions with psychodynamic and experiential colleagues at meetings of the Society for the Exploration of Psychotherapy Integration (SEPI), and through my own personal experiences with a particularly nurturing therapist.

Unlike traditional cognitive behavior therapy, McCullough's approach places the therapeutic relationship very much in the foreground of the intervention. Indeed, it is part and parcel of the corrective experience. By becoming personally involved in a disciplined way with chronically depressed patients, by providing caring feedback on the negative impact made by patients within the therapy relationship, and by modeling empathy and intimacy, therapists are able to offer patients an interpersonal experience that is different from what they have been accustomed to. McCullough refers to this as "interpersonal discrimination learning." My psychodynamic colleagues call it "reparenting."

In alerting cognitive behavior therapists to the potentially corrective nature of the relationship, McCullough cautions against maintaining too didactic and directive a therapeutic stance. It is all too easy to allow the helpless submissiveness of the depressed patient to "pull" for therapeutic dominance. If the goal is to facilitate interpersonal assertiveness, argues McCullough, then it makes sense to work toward facilitating within the therapeutic relationship as well. Not to do so may work against the development of self-assertiveness, in much the same way that a personal trainer's efforts in physically assisting his/her trainee in lifting weights would be counterproductive. As McCullough words it, "Let the patient do the work of therapy."

The integration of a cognitive behavior approach with an interpersonal focus adds to an ongoing movement in the field to blend these complementary orientations. Thus McCullough's contribution joins a list of such related works as Kohlenberg and Tsai's (1991) *Functional Analytic Psychotherapy*, Linehan's (1993) *Cognitive-Behavioral Treatment of Borderline Personality Disorder*, Safran and Segal's (1990) *Interpersonal Process in Cognitive Therapy*, and Wachtel's (1977) *Psychoanalysis and Behavior Therapy*.

In his creative integration of cognitive behavioral and interpersonal concepts and procedures, McCullough has given us a clinically sound and empirically grounded approach to the treatment of chronic depression. However, his contribution has relevance beyond that, such as in working

with distressed couples. As you read the clinical insights contained in this
book, it will become evident that the focus on the patient's role in contributing to a problematic interaction; the monologue-like, noncooperative use of language in an interpersonal situation; problems in achieving authentic empathy with others; and the difficulty in maintaining
emotional control all have relevance for intervening with couples. In
short, you are about to read not only a description of a clinically innova-
tive and empirically grounded approach to treating chronically depressed
patients, but a presentation of an intervention that has the potential for
widespread application.

MARVIN R. GOLDFRIED, PHD
State University of New York at Stony Brook

Acknowledgments

Many people, both indirectly and directly, have had a hand in the writing of this book. My graduate students, many of whom are named in the text, were my first inspiration with their myriad questions about psychotherapy and its efficacy. Together we lived through the behavioral revolution in the 1970s, then the cognitive and interpersonal revolutions in the 1980s, all the while trying to determine the best way to modify the behavior of chronically depressed adults. My chronically depressed private patients, all 225 of them, have kept me aware that the stakes are high for finding an effective treatment for their disorder and that improving the quality of their lives is worth all my time and effort.

This book could not have been written without the relationship I shared for many years with "Mr. Interpersonal Psychotherapy" himself, Dr. Donald J. Kiesler. The relationship with Don was especially sustaining for me during the 1980s, when finding an outlet to publish my single-case psychotherapy research was difficult. During this period, our discussions helped me see how the therapist-patient relationship could be used as a vehicle to modify patient behavior.

In the late 1980s, two events occurred that had a significant impact on my clinical research and practice. In 1988 Dr. Hagop S. Akiskal invited me to present my chronic depression data to the psychiatry Grand Rounds at the University of Tennessee Medical School in Memphis. Hagop's encouragement of my work has remained consistent over the years, and he continues to challenge my ideas as well as fuel my interest in the chronic depressions, particularly dysthymia. His biopsychosocial view of depression plays a prominent role in my conceptualization of the psychopathology of chronic depresssion. The next year, Dr. James H. Kocsis, at the Department of Psychiatry, Cornell University, and Dr. Martin B. Keller, chairperson of the Department of Psychiatry, Brown University, invited me to be a field site coordinator and a member of the DSM-IV Mood Disorders Field Trial Committee studying dysthymia, major depression, and two minor depression categories. The Field Trial Committee consisted of a group of mood disorder investigators who shared similar research interests in the chronic depressions. Marty Keller has always been our "leader"—beginning with the DSM-IV Field Trial, continuing through a national chronic depression study sponsored by Pfizer Pharmaceuticals, Inc., and then leading us through the Bristol-Myers Squibb (B-MS) National Chronic Depression Study (Bristol-Myers Squibb, 1996). Throughout the 1980s and 1990s, Marty's work has significantly influenced the direction chronic depression research has taken. His long-term research focus on the chronic depressions and his intense commitment to science have been a personal model of excellence for me.

I continue to collaborate with the original field trial committee members (Drs. M. B. Keller, D. N. Klein, J. H. Kocsis, and R. M. A. Hirschfeld), as well as others—Drs. Bruce Arnow, Steve Bishop, Janice A. Blalock, John E. Carr, David C. Clark, David L. Dunner, Greg Eaves, Jan Fawcett, Baruch Fishman, Alan J. Gelenberg, Robert H. Howland, Gabor Keitner, Lorrin M. Koran, Rachel Manber, John C. Markowitz, Ivan W. Miller, Philip T. Ninan, Larry Pacoe, Barbara O. Rothbaum, James R. Russell, Alan F. Schatzberg, Michael E. Thase, Madhukar Trivedi, Dina Vivian, and John Zajecka, and Ms. M. Paige Young—who have since been pulled into the original Field Trial circle. Taken together, these collaborative experiences have deepened my understanding of chronic depression as well as provided me with the opportunity to test my CBASP model in a large randomized clinical trial. This book describes these events and underscores the contribution that my colleagues have made to my work.

Several individuals have directly contributed to this writing. Dr. Daniel N. Klein, Professor of Psychology at the State University of New York at Stony Brook, read several chapters and made many insightful comments; Dan and I enjoy a warm and productive relationship. Dr. Michael E. Thase, whose clinical research savvy always plays a prominent role in our research group, is a Professor of Psychiatry on the faculty of Western Psychiatric Institute and Clinic, University of Pittsburgh; Mike has been a good friend and colleague and has contributed in a number of ways to my views of chronic depression. I am particularly indebted to Dr. A. John Rush, without whose support CBASP might never have been selected for the B-MS National Chronic Depression Study; John is a Professor of Psychiatry and a member of the Department of Psychiatry at the University of Texas Southwestern Medical Center at Dallas. I also want to thank Dr. John C. Markowitz, my fellow psychotherapy colleague and a Gerald Klerman interpersonal psychotherapy maven. He is currently an Associate Professor of Psychiatry at Cornell University. John continues to assist and support my work, and he is one of the few contemporary psychotherapy researchers who studies the efficacy of psychotherapy with chronic depressives.

I want to acknowledge the direct contributions of my department chairperson, Dr. Steven B. Robbins, and express the gratitude I feel for his energetic support of my work and research since the early 1990s which has been nothing short of incredible. Steve keeps asking me when the book will be completed, but he has been patient with my tardiness. I thank Dr. Janice A. Blalock, an excellent researcher and clinician, and Dr. James A. Schmidt for reading Chapter 8 and then for giving me their helpful feedback. Jim Schmidt is Associate Professor of psychology at Western Illinois University and a former doctoral student of Don Kiesler. His suggestions prevented me from making several statements about the Interpersonal Circle that I would have regretted.

I also want to thank my daughter, Kristin R. McCullough, a creative computer expert, who used her knowledge of graphics to design most of my figures and tables. Similar gratitude must be expressed to Ms. Patricia E. Johnson, the administrative coordinator of the Virginia Commonwealth University (VCU) Unipolar Mood Disorders Institute. Trish has been helpful to me throughout the writing period. My colleague and associate director/medical director of the Unipolar Mood Disorders Institute, Dr. Susan G. Kornstein, has been a wonderful friend for years. Susan is also an Associate Professor in the Department of Psychiatry at VCU. She and I founded the Unipolar Mood Disorders Institute in 1992 and have worked together ever since. We led the Institute staff through two national chronic depression research projects, and I hope there will be more. I must also mention that Susan's research on the relation between gender and depression has acquired a national reputation.

Dr. Marvin R. Goldfried, Professor of Psychology at the State University of New York at Stony Brook, graciously consented to write the foreword. I wanted Marv to write it because of his integrative work in the psychotherapy field. He is a visionary, and I like his visions. My work herein is an integrative enterprise, and he quickly recognized what I have tried to do. I am grateful for his kind words.

I must also thank my colleague at B-MS Company, Fran Borian, the assistant director of the neuroscience clinical trials in medical operations. Fran worked closely with me in my role as psychotherapy coordinator for the B-MS National Chronic Depression Study. Her strong support of the "psychotherapy arm" of this large 5-year 12-site study, which included 70 certified CBASP psychotherapists, was unwavering and intense. We literally could not have acomplished what we did without Fran.

Finally, I must thank The Guilford Press and Senior Editor Kitty Moore for their willingness to help me publish the book. Last but not least, I feel very grateful to my editor, Margaret O. Ryan, who has labored under my tedious writing and produced a very nice product. Margaret, a master of the written word, probably knows the CBASP program better than I. I hope that she is pleased with the final outcome.

JAMES P. McCULLOUGH, JR., PhD
Virginia Commonwealth University

Contents

4.   Course Patterns, Comorbidity,   51
      and Psychological Characteristics

PART II. CBASP METHOD AND PROCEDURES

5.   Strategies to Enhance Motivation for Change   69

6.   Elicitation Phase of Situational Analysis   105

PART III. HISTORY AND OTHER ASPECTS OF CBASP

APPENDICES

TREATMENT FOR CHRONIC DEPRESSION

*Treating the chronically depressed adult—
dislodging the refractory cognitive-emotional
and behavioral armor that is the disorder—
is analogous to breaking through a granite
wall using a 10-pound sledgehammer. One
hits the wall repeatedly in the same area
with little or no effect until, almost
imperceptibly, a slight hairline crack appears.
Under continuous pounding, the crack
gradually enlarges until, finally, the wall
breaks and crumbles.*

PART ONE

CBASP AND THE PSYCHOPATHOLOGY OF THE PATIENT

CHAPTER ONE

A Therapist's Problems with a Chronically Depressed Patient

"Bill" is a skilled cognitive behavioral therapist who has been in practice for over 10 years. Over lunch, he told me about a psychotherapy patient he had been seeing for the past six months. The patient, "Ken," was very bright, a 43-year-old male who earned an MBA degree from Harvard University some years ago. Ken was a sales representative for a local firm; Bill felt that Ken was grossly underemployed.

Bill said that Ken's lifelong depression had begun with early-onset dysthymia during adolescence. He had had four major depressive episodes over the years, returning to the dysthymia baseline following each episode. When he first began treatment, he met criteria for major depression and was diagnosed with recurrent major depression with antecedent dysthymia (double depression).

Bill said that Ken was not improving. In addition to psychotherapy, Ken had been taking imipramine, but following his lack of response, he was switched to a selective serotonin reuptake inhibitor (SSRI) 16 weeks later. He was currently taking 200 mg daily of sertraline and was still not responding. His Beck Depression Inventory scores had remained in the 25–30 range for six months, indicating clinical depression.

Bill wanted to talk more about the case, so I continued to listen. He said that working with Ken had left him feeling helpless, professionally incompetent, frustrated by the patient's lack of response, and angry at both himself and Ken. Nothing he tried had worked. The patient remained depressed, unmotivated to change, and interpersonally detached and submissive. Bill said that Ken also complained regularly of an overwhelming feeling of hopelessness. Not infrequently, he would miss therapy appointments, then call in later to say, "I just forgot." Ken's wife had recently moved out of the bedroom because she was disgusted by his lack of progress in therapy.

"Tell me what you have tried to do so far," I asked.

Bill's answer sounded like a litany of cognitive behavioral techniques. False-belief hypotheses had been challenged, but the patient maintained a passive facade in the face of the disputational tactics. Identifying dysfunctional beliefs in Ken's worldview was not difficult. The problem was that Ken remained impervious to attacks on his illogical way of thinking. The patient never completed homework assignments and trying to motivate him to work outside the session was not successful. Bill attempted to demonstrate the connection between Ken's thoughts, behaviors, and affect in sessions, but it was difficult keeping him focused. Ken often complained, "This therapy stuff is not helping my depression." Use of active disputation; homework assignments; role playing in the session to improve assertive behavior skills; increasing the delivery of empathy, support, and encouragement—nothing had worked. It was also obvious to me that Bill was doing most of the work in the therapy, and it was easy to understand his frustration and anger with the patient's lack of progress. Bill's sense of helplessness with the case was summed up nicely with the patient's frequent protests: "It's no use, I'll always be depressed!"

Listening to therapists talk about chronically depressed patients always evokes the same reactions in me. I feel a vague sense of helplessness; then I begin to feel incompetent; and at about that point I have a knee-jerk impulse to say, "Why don't you try this or that . . . or assume more of an active, take-charge role?" Today was no exception. I felt helpless and incompetent, and then felt the urge to suggest that Bill try yet another strategy. Just as all my colleague's energy and efforts had been sucked into the bottomless pit of chronic depression, additional treatment suggestions from me would be likely to suffer the same fate.

Treating the chronically depressed patient is one of the most demanding challenges psychotherapists face. The task is compounded by the fact that most of these patients feel hopeless and therefore are unmotivated to change, making it interpersonally difficult to work with them (approximately 50% will meet criteria for a comorbid Axis II disorder). In a chronically depressed adult, a therapist typically encounters an individual who tenaciously maintains a destructive lifestyle.

My reaction to Bill was supportive. "I understand your frustration with Ken. Patients like him were once labeled 'neurotic crocks' (Lipsett, 1970) because physicians could not molify their complaints either with medicine or with other therapeutic procedures. How much time do you have to talk about the case?"

"I've got a couple of hours. My next appointment is not until 4 P.M."

"It will take us more time than that."

"What do you mean?"

"I've been trying for years to figure out the best way to treat patients like Ken, and I think I can give you a hand. But it's going to take us more than two hours. We can start, though, by talking about a new way to treat chronically depressed patients." Then I began to describe the Cognitive Behavioral Analysis System of Psychotherapy (CBASP). I explained to my colleague that encountering similar difficulties with other patients like Ken had been the reason I developed CBASP.

The CBASP method addresses the exhausting problems that Bill faced with Ken and other patients like him. I hope that what you read in the following pages will help you become more effective in your work with chronically depressed patients.

CHAPTER 2

Introduction to Chronically Depressed Patients and the CBASP Program

PATIENT: I don't know what to say about myself except that I have failed at everything. My marriage is really messed up, I can't seem to hold a job, I don't have many friends, and those I do have are not very close, things just keep getting worse and worse. I wake up depressed, I go to sleep depressed, nothing will ever work out for me. I've thought about taking my life, but I'd probably screw that up and be a vegetable the rest of my life. I'm a hopeless case and not really sure why I'm sitting here telling you this stuff.

THERAPIST: How long have you felt this way?

PATIENT: I've felt this way all my life. Started feeling bad when I was in middle school, about 22 years ago, and have felt bad ever since.

CRUCIAL BEGINNINGS

Chronically depressed patients share several prominent characteristics. In the initial encounter with such a patient during the first session, a clinician will typically observe the following:

- Repeated expressions of misery and helplessness
- A submissive and defeated demeanor

- Wariness of interpersonal involvement that extends to interactions with the clinician
- An entrenched conviction that nothing can be done to control his/her depression
- Rigidly stable behavior patterns that do not appear to be affected by either positive or negative events

The clinician is likely to experience several interpersonal reactions toward the patient during this first session:

- A general feeling that the patient expects the therapist to "fix" him/her
- A powerful urge to assume a dominant, take-charge role to "fix" the patient or show the individual the error of his/her ways
- A sense of helplessness and futility in being able to help the patient change his/her behavior
- A feeling of apprehension about working with an individual who is so detached

The first meeting is a crucial encounter for both the psychotherapist and the patient. If clinicians want to be successful with chronically depressed patients, they need two assets: *an understanding of these patients' psychopathology, and a disciplined plan for assisting these individuals in overthrowing the depressive predicament.* In my own work with these patients, I have found it helpful to frame the salient motivational and behavioral issues in terms of several questions I ask myself:

- How can I effectively treat a patient who is not motivated to change?
- What can I do to mitigate the patient's overwhelming feelings of helplessness and hopelessness which tend to neutralize every therapeutic strategy?
- Why do I keep having these inadequate and helpless feelings when I am with this patient?
- Why do I keep feeling that nothing I do will make a difference?
- Why is it so easy to feel that changing the patient's behavior is up to me?
- Are chronically depressed adults appropriate candidates for psychotherapy?

Over the years I have designed the CBASP treatment model to answer all of these questions, which are the topics of this and subsequent chapters.

Why Yet Another Psychotherapy Model?

I am aware that I am contributing to an already bloated array of psychotherapy techniques currently available to practitioners. Mahoney (1991) noted that more than 400 therapy programs had been proposed by psychologists and psychiatrists up to and including the year 1990—and, of course, even more have been developed during the 1990s (Chambless et al., 1998). The reason I am proposing CBASP at this time is that, as far as I can determine, no therapy model is currently available that addresses the unique problems chronically depressed patients present to psychotherapists.

THE CHRONIC DEPRESSIONS: NEW *DSM* CATEGORIES

The chronic depressions have only recently begun to receive the attention they deserve. Prior to 1980, chronic depression was considered to be a personality disorder in both *DSM-I* (American Psychiatric Association, [APA], 1952) and *DSM-II* (APA, 1968). This perspective began to change with the publication of *DSM-III* (APA, 1980), wherein dysthymia was introduced on Axis I as a chronic affective disorder. Chronic major depression did not emerge as a formal diagnostic category until 1987, when *DSM-III-R* (APA, 1987) was published.

The *DSM-IV* (APA, 1994) Mood Disorders Field Trial (Keller, Klein, et al., 1995) reported that one of the chronic disorders—recurrent major depression with antecedent dysthymia without full interepisode recovery (double depression)—was the modal diagnostic category (26%) for 349 subjects diagnosed with a current major depressive episode. Diagnostic developments in *DSM-III*, *DSM-III-R*, and *DSM-IV* have increasingly highlighted the group of chronic mood disorders that constitute the target population for CBASP. The field is slowly recognizing that until very recently, the chronic depressions have been grossly misdiagnosed, understudied, and undertreated (Harrison & Stewart, 1993; Keller & Hanks, 1994; McCullough et al., 1996).

TREATMENT PROGNOSIS

Some years ago, Akiskal et al. (1980) noted the general belief among clinicians that chronic depression does not respond favorably to either pharmacotherapy or psychotherapy. In the same vein, Keller (1990) described the chronic disorders as "treatment resistant." Considerable data in the recent past have supported these viewpoints. For example, prognosis is not generally favorable among patients with a preexisting dysthymia condition (Keller & Shapiro, 1982, 1984; Keller, Lavori, Endicott, Coryell, & Klerman, 1983; Keller, Lavori, Lewis, & Klerman, 1983); in fact, dysthymia patients run a 90% lifetime risk of having one or more major depressive episodes (Keller, 1988). Poor response to treatment has also been reported (Keller, Lavori, Klerman, et al., 1986; Keller, Shapiro, Lavori, & Wolfe, 1982b) among chronic patients who report a history of recurrent major depressive episodes. Moreover, an unfavorable prognosis also characterizes persons whose depression remains untreated for long durations (Keller & Hanks, 1994; Keller et al., 1992).

Even when response to treatment occurs, recovery rates are usually moderate. For example, in a recently completed double-blind randomized trial of sertraline (an SSRI) and imipramine (a tricyclic antidepressant, or TCA), 635 chronic major and double depression patients (mean lifetime depression duration = 16 years) were treated (Keller et al., 1998). The outpatients were recruited at 12 research sites located throughout the United States in a study sponsored by Pfizer Pharmaceuticals. In an intent-to-treat analysis of response rates (where all completing subjects as well as noncompleters were counted) following 12 weeks of treatment with either sertraline or imipramine, only 17% (105 out of 623 subjects) achieved full recovery status while 35% (217 out of 623 subjects) reported a partial response to treatment. Forty-eight percent (299 out of 623 subjects) did not respond to either the SSRI or the TCA.

Not only does chronicity complicate response to treatment; it also seems to increase the probability for relapse and recurrence (Keller, Lavori, Rice, Coryell, & Hirschfeld, 1986; Keller & Hanks, 1994; Keller, Lavori, Lewis, et al., 1983; Keller, Shapiro, Lavori, & Wolfe, 1982a, 1982b; Keller, Lavori, Klerman, et al., 1986). While treatment outcomes among the population with chronic unipolar depression have reflected some success, much work remains to be done to enhance existing recovery rates.

Regarding psychotherapy with the chronic disorders, Markowitz

(1994) notes that very few data are available. Most of the existing studies in the area (e.g., de Jong, Treiber, & Henrich, 1986; Fennell & Teasdale, 1982; Harpin, Liberman, Marks, Stern, & Bohannon, 1982; Markowitz, 1993a, 1993b, 1994; Mason, Markowitz, & Klerman, 1993; McCullough, 1984a, 1991) suffer from small sample size and methodological problems. Recently Thase and colleagues (Thase et al., 1994, 1992) treated 62 chronically depressed males with cognitive behavioral therapy (CBT) for 16 weeks. The authors reported that the effectiveness of CBT was limited, writing that "chronically depressed patients had slower [and] less complete responses to CBT ... " (Thase et al., 1994, p. 204). From the above-cited reports concerning the use of traditional psychotherapeutic methods (i.e., cognitive therapy [CT; Beck, 1963, 1964, 1976; Beck, Rush, Shaw, & Emery, 1979]; interpersonal psychotherapy [IPT; Klerman, Weissman, Rounsaville, & Chevron, 1984]), no firm conclusions can be drawn about the efficacy of the interventions. However, in studies utilizing an adequate sample size and investigating the efficacy of CBT with chronically depressed adults (Thase et al., 1992, 1994), the outcome data were not promising.

A psychotherapy study was undertaken with a quasi-chronic sample at the Western Psychiatric Institute and Clinic, University of Pittsburgh (Frank et al., 1990). The study was conducted on subjects with "recurrent major depression," so a percentage of the patients did not meet current criteria for chronic depression. IPT (Klerman et al., 1984) was combined with imipramine in the acute phase. Approximately 68% (157 of 230 subjects) responded to the combination treatment and entered a 17-week continuation phase.

At the end of the continuation phase, 128 patients were randomized into one of five three-year maintenance protocols (imipramine alone; IPT constructed for maintenance delivery alone [IPT-M]; and IPT-M plus imipramine; IPT-M plus placebo; and placebo alone). While the drug patients were maintained on a "full dose" of imipramine during maintenance, patients randomized into the IPT-M conditions received only a "low dose" of one IPT-M session per month. Therefore, the survival rates among the three IPT-M cells may unduly reflect this design bias. Imipramine alone was found to be as effective as combination treatment in preventing relapse. IPT-M alone and IPT-M plus placebo were more effective than placebo alone in relapse prevention but less effective than imipramine alone. Unfortunately, we don't know what the survival rates would have been had the psychotherapy patients been allowed to see their therapists on an "as needed" basis (full dose) during the maintenance period. I also don't know how CBASP, developed specifically for the treatment of the chronic depressive disorders, will fare in comparison with programs such as CT and IPT.

MEDICAL COMPLAINTS, COMORBIDITY, AND SPONTANEOUS REMISSION

Chronically depressed adults are among the highest utilizers of general medical services (Howland, 1993b). In a recent observational study of general health (Wells, Burnam, Rogers, Hays, & Camp, 1992), the authors compared patients with dysthymia and double depression patients to those with acute major depression, subthreshold depression, and past histories of depression. Wells et al. found that patients in the two chronic categories reported poorer general health scores, lower energy, more bodily pain, and greater impaired general functioning than did patients in either the subthreshold group or the depression-in-the-past group. Interestingly, few differences in these health variables were obtained when the groups with the chronic depressive disorders were compared to the group with acute major depression.

Because comorbidity contributes to poor treatment outcome (Farmer & Nelson-Gray, 1990; Keitner, Ryan, Miller, Kohn, & Epstein, 1991; Rohde, Lewinsohn, & Seeley, 1991), it is important to note that approximately 50% of chronically depressed adults, when assessed via structured clinical interviews, have also received a comorbid personality disorder diagnosis from Clusters B and C in DSM-III-R (Kaye et al., 1994; McCullough, 1996a; Pepper et al., 1995; Sanderson, Wetzler, Beck, & Betz, 1992). These data underscore the fact that interpersonal problems are prominent variables that clinicians face when treating this population. The chronic depressions are also not likely to remit spontaneously without treatment (McCullough et al., 1988, 1994a). Not only are spontaneous remission rates low among the untreated (< 13%), but when remission does occur, an individual is likely to report a recurrence of the disorder within two to four years.

The chronically depressed patient is one of the most difficult outpatients we see in psychotherapy. The diagnostic nomenclature has only recently described the population, and continued misdiagnosis and undertreatment are still disturbingly common. The chronic disorders continue to have a poor reputation when it comes to treatment response, and the survival rates following treatment are not particularly good. It is in this rather bleak and discouraging context that I introduce the CBASP psychotherapy program.

UNIQUE FEATURES OF CBASP

CBASP incorporates eight unique features that distinguish it from other psychotherapy programs:

1. CBASP is the only psychotherapy program designed *specifically* to treat the chronic depressive disorders.
2. Arrested maturational development is viewed as the etiological basis of chronic depression.
3. CBASP conceptualizes depression and its modification in terms of a "person × environment" perspective, which educates patients regarding their "stimulus value" within their living context.
4. The treatment goals include fostering the ability to engage in Piagetian formal operations social problem solving and empathic responsivity in the conduct of social interaction.
5. Therapists are encouraged to become personally involved with patients in a disciplined way in order to modify their behavior.
6. Patient transference issues are conceptualized following an in-session transference hypothesis generation technique (Significant-Other History) and are proactively challenged throughout the process of treatment.
7. A therapy technique called "Situational Analysis" (SA) is used to exacerbate the psychopathology of the patient in the therapy session.
8. Negative reinforcement methods are utilized as essential motivational strategies in order to modify behavior.

1. *The CBASP program is designed specifically to treat the chronic depressive disorders.* In 1974 one of my early clinical psychology graduate students, Dr. William F. Doverspike, and I began work on constructing a program to treat chronically depressed patients. In 1983 another student, Dr. Matthew D. Kasnetz, produced a patient manual (Kasnetz, McCullough, & Kaye, 1995)—as part of his master's thesis—(*Patient Manual for Cognitive Behavioral Analysis System of Psychotherapy* [CBASP]). This manual is still distributed to all CBASP patients at the end of the second treatment hour. Various procedural aspects of the model were

refined during the 1980s (McCullough, 1980a, 1980b, 1984a, 1984b, 1984; 1991; McCullough & Carr, 1987). Incorporating the creative input and feedback of my clinical psychology graduate students throughout the 1990s (Drs. Arthur L. Kaye, J. Kim Penberthy, Sue Caldwell-Sledge, as well as Mr. W. Chris Roberts and Ms. Anmarie Hess), I developed a therapist manual, *Therapist Manual for Cognitive Behavioral Analysis System of Psychotherapy (CBASP)* (McCullough, 1995b). This manual was used by 70 certified CBASP psychotherapists in a national study of chronic depression (McCullough, Keller, et al., 1997; McCullough, Kornstein, et al., 1997). The recent history of CBASP will be discussed more fully in Chapter 10.

2. *Arrested maturational development is viewed as the etiological basis of chronic depression.* Chronic patients are not amenable to logical disputation, reasoning, or other critical-analytic cognitive techniques. Patients talk to their therapists in monologue style, and their thought processes are prelogical in nature. They are unable to interact empathically, and their behavior is not modified by the reactions or feedback they receive from spouses, friends, supervisors, or work colleagues. The chronic patient presents an interpersonally "closed" cognitive-emotional system. In short, chronically depressed adults function at a primitive mental level paralleling that of five- to seven-year-old children.

How did they get this way? For most early-onset patients (depression onset before 21 years of age), maltreatment in the family resulted in an arrest of the cognitive-emotive maturational process at the preoperational stage of development (Piaget, 1923/1926, 1954/1981; Inhelder & Piaget, 1955/1958; Cowan, 1978). The etiology of late-onset chronic depression (depression onset at or after 21 years) originates from a different direction but concludes in the same preoperational level as the early-onset patient. Late-onset patients have usually functioned in a normal cognitive-emotional vein prior to their first major depressive episode, usually during their mid-20s (McCullough, Klein, Shea, Miller, & Kaye, 1992). About 20% of these late-onset, first-episode patients will not recover from their major depression and will remain chronically depressed (Keller, Lavori, Lewis, et al., 1983). Structural deterioration of heretofore normal mental functioning usually follows on the heels of the unrelenting mood disorder. The refractory state of depression that the individual cannot overthrow results in the assumption of a worldview that is permeated by feelings of helplessness and hopelessness. The results of this phenomenological transformation are seen in a deterioration of normal functioning and a return to a preoperational level of mentalistic thinking. In both early- and late-onset conditions, it is structural cognitive-emotive problems, not functional ones such as negative attitudes or beliefs, that maintain and fuel the pathology of the chronic patient. Much more will be said about the etiology of chronic depression in Chapter 3.

3. *Depression and its modification are conceptualized in terms of a "person × environment" (P × E) perspective.* I assume that depression arises from the dynamic interplay of several factors operating in a person's interactions with his/her environment. Two interrelated domains are implicated in all depression experiences. In the intraorganismic domain, biological and psychological processes remain in constant and reciprocal interaction. The environment, representing the extraorganismic domain, regularly presents challenges to the person with which he/she either copes effectively or not. In a similar vein, Akiskal and colleagues (Akiskal & McKinney, 1973; Whybrow, Akiskal, & McKinney, 1985) hypothesize that depression stems from two sources: (1) faulty coping in the face of environmental challenges/stress, and (2) the deleterious effects of inadequate coping on the biological and psychological processes of the individual. Skinner (1953), not concerned with depressive etiology but with studying behavior modification variables, wrote that environmental consequences modify organismic behavior. Akiskal and Skinner each represent unique approaches to the "person × environment" relationship and have directly influenced my conceptions of depression and its treatment. Akiskal's biopsychosocial model led me to view depression as a "person × environment" disorder. Skinner's emphasis on the environment's role in behavior modification provided me with the rationale for behavior change in CBASP.

To summarize, chronic depression results from maladaptive social problem solving (D'Zurilla & Maydeu-Olivares, 1995) and the accompanying perceptual "blind spot" that prevents such individuals from recognizing a connection between *what they do* and *the effects of what they do* on others. If the perceptual connection between the person and his/her environment is never established or is broken, the environmental domain has no power to influence what the person does. This "person × environment" approach to depression and its treatment is expressed in two assumptions that underlie CBASP.

> *Assumption 1*: Chronic depressive disorder is best understood when it is viewed as the result of a person's long-term failure to cope adequately with life stressors.

Avoiding entrapment in a depressive disorder requires adequate *social coping ability* (Whybrow et al., 1985), which in turn is affected by several variables: (1) cognitive-emotional construction of the self as well as of others, which is derived, in large measure, from a person's developmental history; (2) the quality of the person's social skills repertoire; (3) his/her past history concerning interpersonal stress management; (4) his/her general health status when confronted with stress; and (5) the degree of social support available to the person.

Patients Are Responsible for Their Depression

Since I believe that chronic depression and coping failure are inextricably connected, I also endorse the view that *chronically depressed patients are ultimately responsible for their depression*. Many such patients try to affix the blame for their depression elsewhere by pointing to external causes. A currently popular excuse is, "I'm depressed because I have a chemical imbalance." The ultimate eschewal of personal responsibility is captured by one patient's words: "It's not my fault! I have nothing to do with the way I feel! If anything, I don't want to feel this way!" CBASP is grounded in an extreme view of personal responsibility, particularly with its notion that patients bear ultimate responsibility for the state of their lives.

The assumption of personal responsibility may appear difficult to support, however, when chronically depressed adults also have a developmental history of maltreatment. After all, how can adults be held responsible for coping failures when they grew up in families where abuse, hostility, and/or neglect predominated? One might easily conclude that these adults *never* had the opportunity to learn how to cope effectively or to live productive lives. So how can they be held responsible for their depression when they never had a chance to learn to live otherwise? The answer to this question is realized when psychotherapists help patients gain control over their lives in psychotherapy. Even though children do not select or choreograph their family milieus, wise clinicians assist individuals to realize that the only hope for improving the quality of their lives and terminating the depressive disorder is to assume total responsibility for the way they live in the present—regardless of the quality of their developmental history!

How does this assumption translate into CBASP strategy? Specifically, patients are taught that their behavior has interpersonal consequences, and they are shown how to recognize these consequences. Then it is up to them to decide whether they wish to continue to enact the same patterns or not. CBASP therapists create conditions in the session whereby patients must make a conscious choice: "Will I continue to live as I have, or will I choose to chart another course?"

Victor Frankl (1959), a renowned survivor of a German death camp, poignantly made a similar point when he described the existential moment when an individual assumes personal responsibility for his/her life: "So live as if you were living already for the second time and as if you had acted the first time as wrongly as you are about to act now!" (p. 173). This quote captures the treatment goals of CBASP. It first teaches patients to identify how they contribute to their own personal living dilemma; that is, the model clearly exposes the way individuals have been living. Once patients become aware of the type of life they have been creating, only then are they in a position to make a choice about living differently.

It is only from this perspective of believing that one has a viable choice about how to live one's life that I make the assumption that each chronic patient is personally responsible for his/her depression. In the absence of a choice, patients cannot be held responsible; they remain victimized by existence.

The second CBASP assumption follows from the first:

Assumption 2: Teaching patients to view their problems-in-living from a "person × environment" perspective results in behavior change, personal empowerment, and in the amelioration of emotional dysregulation.

Because there is no depression without stress and the failure to cope with it, the depression experience, as noted above, is best conceptualized as a "person × environment" phenomenon (Coyne, 1976; McCullough, 1984a, 1996b). The goal of CBASP is to focus the patient's attention on the consequences he/she elicits from the environment. Concentrating upon interpersonal situations and making explicit the patient's effects on others help the person recognize his/her "contingent" relationship with the environment. A general awareness that one's behavior has specific consequences in the world is termed perceived functionality in CBASP. The manner in which patients' behavioral consequences are made evident in the therapy sessions represents a unique aspect of the CBASP program. What I have termed the "consequation" strategies will be described in greater detail in Chapters 5, 6, 7, and 8.

4. Utilizing formal operations in social problem solving and interacting empathically with others indicate that one has mastered the CBASP pro-

gram. Both of these goals represent unique features of CBASP. Teaching preoperational patients formal operations problem-solving techniques (Cowan, 1978; Gordon, 1988) makes it possible for them to become perceptually aware of behavioral consequences. Thinking in formal operations ways also makes it possible for them to learn how to relate empathically with others. The ability to enact these skills is often accompanied by generalized treatment effects: Depressive symptoms decrease and the depressive disorder is resolved. Chapters 5, 6, 7, and 8 will discuss the techniques used to achieve these essential goals.

5. *CBASP therapists are encouraged to become personally involved with patients in a disciplined way in order to modify their behavior.* I know of no other therapy program recommending that clinicians become personally involved with their patients. Disciplined personal involvement, which involves a willingness on clinicians' part to disclose personal feelings, attitudes, and reactions to patients, facilitates the teaching of empathic behavior. Disciplined personal involvement is also necessary to modify the injurious history of maltreatment that many patients bring to therapy. In acquiring "significant-other" status with patients, therapists have a unique opportunity to teach them what it is like to interact with a decent and caring human being. Chapter 8 will describe in greater detail the uses of disciplined personal involvement in CBASP. In Chapter 13 I will show how personal involvement techniques can be used as intervention strategies to defuse patient crises and problems.

6. *Transference hypotheses are generated to target interpersonal "hot spots" that need special attention.* During the second session, a personal history of the patient's experiences with significant others is elicited by means of the Significant-Other History procedure (Chapter 5). Transference hypotheses are generated from the history information and used to target interpersonal problem areas or "hot spots" that may become problematic as clinicians and patients interact. The therapist then uses the transference hypotheses to challenge proactively the interpersonal trouble spots during the remainder of therapy. When therapists find themselves embroiled in these "hot spots," they can utilize their personal involvement with patients to initiate the Interpersonal Discrimination Exercise (IDE), which teaches the patient to distinguish between the negative reactions of significant others and the positive behavior of the therapist. The construction and use of the transference hypotheses and the modification of behavior via the IDE are discussed in Chapters 5 and 8.

7. *CBASP uses Situational Analysis (SA) to exacerbate the pathology of the patient during the session.* Talking about change rarely leads to the

modification of behavior. For this reason, CBASP exacerbates the pathological behavior of the patient during the therapy session by means of SA. SA first helps the patient focus on a particular problem situation and then elicits the original cognitions and emotions that occurred during that targeted event. Once the situation is pinpointed and the behavioral components are described, a situational outcome or consequence for the patient's behavior is identified. In this manner, the patient is assisted in examining the consequences of his/her behavior and in constructing alternative ways of thinking and behaving that would have led to a more desirable outcome. Frequently, emotional relief accompanies the construction of the solution strategies; this in turn reinforces and accelerates the entire change process. SA procedures will be addressed in detail in Chapters 6 and 7.

8. *CBASP utilizes negative reinforcement as an essential motivational strategy to modify patient behavior.* The most powerful motivator psychotherapists have at their disposal is to demonstrate the simple yet profound truism that *behavior change makes patients feel better.* Skinner (1953) defined a "negative reinforcer" as any aversive stimulus condition (e.g., in the present clinical context, distress or felt discomfort) that is superseded or terminated by some behavior. One of the major tasks of CBASP therapists is to look for those behaviors that lead to decreases in the patient's felt distress. When patients learn to behave more adaptively, emotional relief is often present. The therapist's job is to make certain that the behaviors that result in decreases in discomfort are made explicit to patients. In this way, negative reinforcement is used to motivate patients to modify their own behavior. An elaboration of the major ways CBASP administers negative reinforcement to patients is described in Chapter 5.

The Nature
of the Depression Experience

AKISKAL'S BIOPSYCHOSOCIAL VIEW
OF DEPRESSION

Psychotherapy models purporting to treat depression can be categorized as *intrapsychic* (e.g., Beck et al., 1979; Freud, 1916–1917/1960, 1933, 1917/ 1950, 1963), *interpersonal* (e.g., Klerman et al., 1984; Safran, 1990a, 1990b), *behavioral* (e.g., Ferster, 1973), or *biological* (Akiskal & McKinney, 1975) perspectives. Akiskal and McKinney (1975) note that there is a common thread running through these four categories, which is evident in the way they all define "depression." The common definition of depression includes a general sense of helplessness resulting from a self-perception of inadequacy whereby the person feels powerless to control his/her life (Akiskal & McKinney, 1975; Whybrow et al., 1985). The negative self-appraisals or cognitions are associated with reactions of social withdrawal. Akiskal and colleagues point out that the biological domain in which the interacting intrapsychic, interpersonal, and behavioral elements converge is located in the midbrain or diencephalon (Akiskal & McKinney, 1975; Whybrow et al., 1985). Whybrow et al. (1985) conclude: "Depression, then, is conceptualized as the feedback interactions of three sets of variables at chemical, experiential, and behavioral levels—with the diencephalon serving as the field of interaction" (p. 195).

Akiskal makes another point, briefly alluded to above, that is relevant to our understanding of the biopsychosocial nature of the depression experience. The multivariable interaction site in the diencephalon handles "two-way traffic"; that is, the diencephalon is the locus of a psychological-biological reciprocal interactive process that is always present in depression (Akiskal & McKinney, 1975).

> Bridges are supposed to handle two way traffic. Whereas in the psychiatric literature the focus has largely been on behavior alterations occurring secondary to changes in biogenic amines, there is another line of research that indicates the reverse may also be true. That is, one can selectively manipulate social variables and induce major changes in brain amines. (Akiskal & McKinney, 1975, p. 298)

Akiskal implies three things in his bridge metaphor. First, neither biological nor psychological factors can be considered primary; both must be viewed as reciprocally interacting fields of action. Second, not only do depression intensity, social withdrawal, and a sense of helplessness increase when there are changes in the biogenic amine system; they also increase during periods of psychosocial dysfunction. Third, the interactive psychological-biological linkage is evidenced by biogenic and other autonomic system alterations that follow psychosocial failure to resolve conditions of threat and stress (Barchas & Freedman, 1963; Bliss & Zwanziger, 1966; Lazarus, 1984; Lazarus & Alfert, 1964; Lazarus, Opton, Markellos, Nomikos, & Rankin, 1965; Schachter & Singer, 1962; Welch & Welch, 1968).

In short, depression is a biological-psychological-environmental disorder implicating state-dependent psychological and biological activity in the brain (Kiesler, 1999). Regrettably, most depression research conducted during the present century has not been based upon a biopsychosocial view of psychopathology; instead, it has stemmed from a dichotomized view in which depression has been viewed as *either* a biological illness *or* a maladaptive psychological problem. Today, the biopsychosocial model is being advocated more often in theoretical articles (Akiskal & McKinney, 1973; Blanchard, 1977; Engel, 1977; Gentry, 1984; Kiesler, 1999) and in research. Support for the multivariate model of depression can be found in contemporary research reports that show somatic measures of change respond just as robustly to CT (Beck et al., 1979) as they do to pharmacotherapy (Blackburn, Bishop, Glen, Whalley, & Christie, 1981; Hollon, 1990; Rush, Beck, Kovacs, & Hollon, 1977; Simons, Garfield, & Murphy, 1984; Wright & Thase, 1992). Wright and Thase (1992) note that "the overall results of these studies suggest that, when effective, both CT and pharmacotherapy appear to produce changes across response dimensions" (p. 452).

Why is Akiskal's integrative approach so important here? One reason is this: biopsychosocially oriented clinicians should no longer feel that they have to make a choice between biology *or* psychology when conceptualizing the psychopathology of chronically depressed patients or when selecting the most effective treatment. Because chronicity is usually associated with a poorer response to treatment than that seen in acute conditions (Keller & Hanks, 1994), it is probably safe to assume that the most effective therapy regimens for chronic patients, particularly in the more severe cases, will be those that combine both agents into one comprehensive treatment package (Garamoni, Reynolds, Thase, Frank, & Fasiczka, 1992; Keller et al., 1999; Miller, 1997; Sotsky et al., 1991; Wright & Thase, 1992). More will be said about combination treatment for the chronic depressive disorders in Chapter 10.

I turn now to a presentation of two illustrative cases of depression which allow me to differentiate between a pathological depressive reaction to stress and a normal depressive reaction.

THE CASES OF PHIL AND STEPHANIE

"Phil" is a 27-year-old mechanical engineer who told his therapist that he has felt sad since he was 13 years old. He was able to function well academically in elementary, middle, high school, and college, but he just never really felt happy. As best Phil could recall, when he first became depressed he had few friends and was not included in most of the social events in which his peers participated. During his senior year in college he broke up with his girlfriend, and this led to a deepening of his depressed mood that lasted for approximately five months. He did not consult a doctor about his depression. When queried about his mood after the deep depression subsided, Phil reported, "It was about like how I had felt before. I just didn't have any zest for living."

There had been no further deep depressions since the one episode six years earlier. At the time Phil sought therapy, Phil was working for a large engineering firm on the East Coast; he is married and has two small children. He entered treatment because his wife urged him to try and "get rid of your gloomy outlook." His diagnosis is double depression with one episode of major depression six years previously. He is currently functioning with a dysthymic disorder.

"Stephanie," a 36-year-old PhD chemist, divorced with one adolescent son, had recently been promoted to supervisor status in a chemical corporation. She was responsible for the work of nine fellow chemists who used laboratory animals to test the company's products for adverse effects. She reported that right after being promoted she felt like "a fish out of water" and had to take several days off from work because of a "down" mood. She was plagued with doubts about her ability to be a supervisor. Gradually, she realized that she could manage her new responsibilities effectively; she says that now she enjoys her work. When asked what happened to the down mood, Stephanie said, "It just went away." She also reported that she had never had an experience like this before, but that now she knows what depressed people must go through. She sought help from a psychologist right after the promotion and was seen for two sessions.

The depression experiences described in both examples are normal human reactions to common life stressors. More specifically, the initial depressive reactions of Phil and Stephanie are adaptive, biological-psychological responses to stress overload. For all of us, depression or feeling "down" is an emotional signal that stress has overextended our coping capacity. We have all experienced stress resulting from illness or disease, the death of a loved one, the ending of a relationship, a family crisis, or other situational events that have adversely affected us and extended our coping capacities beyond our limits. Additional components of depression experiences include feeling victimized and a tendency to withdraw from immediate responsibilities as well as social engagements; fatigue or a vague sense of tiredness; and thoughts of inadequacy or incompetence. The intensity of these natural symptoms of depression can range from very mild levels to life-threatening.

Both Phil and Stephanie had depressive experiences that signaled systemic overload. In addition, their ability to manage stress was sufficiently challenged to make them pull back and question their self-adequacy. Stephanie was able to recognize the circumstances exacerbating her depressive experience. All Phil could do was tell his therapist the approximate year when he started feeling down. The interpersonal-social confusion that this pubescent male had encountered at age 13 rendered the onset of his depression experience far less well defined than Stephanie's.

DEPRESSION AND THE NATURAL WISDOM
OF THE BODY

The withdrawal-rebuilding-coping-to-recovery cycle describes the phasic nature of the depressive experience (Akiskal & McKinney, 1983; Whybrow et al., 1985). The normal and pathological phasic cycles of the depression experiences of Stephanie and Phil are illustrated in Figure 2.1.

Whatever particular stressors lead to depression, the result is the same. The "natural wisdom of the body" (Cannon, 1929, 1932) dictates that rest and renewal must occur to allow time for recovery. Coping with stress affects the functioning of the central nervous system (e.g., Thase & Kupfer, 1996) and leads to numerous biogenic and antonomic nervous system alterations; the organ systems in the body may be affected dramatically (Alexander, 1950; Scheier & Carver, 1987; Selye, 1976; Shapiro, Lidagoster, & Glassman, 1997); functioning of brain structures may be altered (Bremmer & Narayan, 1998; Bremmer et al., 1995); and the adequacy or inadequacy of the individual's coping abilities may be exposed (Folkman & Lazarus, 1980, 1988; Whybrow et al., 1985). A period of withdrawal from the sources of stress results in rest and rejuvenation, and thus enables many individuals to recover from a transitory depression experience. After the respite has led to systemic renewal, the person is ready once more to "get back into the game" and try to resolve the problem.

The difference in the coping patterns in the two cases above can be found in the inadequacy of Phil's coping repertoire. Phil was never able to

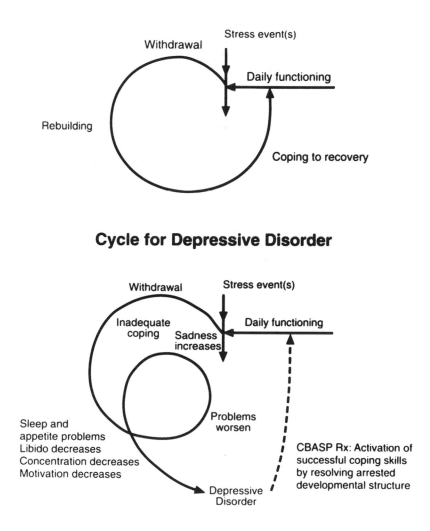

FIGURE 2.1. Normal and psychopathological cycles of the depressive experience.

"get back into the game" (in this case, the adolescent social game). His limited coping skills precluded rejuvenation and recovery from the depressive experience, resulting in entrapment in the withdrawal phase of depression, which eventually settled into a chronic depressive disorder. Stephanie, by contrast, realized that she could effectively manage her work challenges when she sized up the office situation and began to focus directly on solving her problems. Stephanie resolved the stress of the new job by enacting effective problem-focused coping strategies (Folkman & Lazarus, 1988), thereby avoiding entrapment in the withdrawal phase of depression. *Resolving stressful circumstances through successful coping (or at least concluding that the problem at hand can be managed effectively) is the sine qua non for avoiding extended entrapment in the withdrawal phase of the depressive experience—chronic depression.*

I turn in Chapter 3 to a fuller discussion of the psychopathology of chronically depressed patients, focusing on the etiology of the early- and late-onset forms of the chronic disorder.

CHAPTER THREE

Understanding the Psychopathology of Chronically Depressed Patients

I was like a piece of driftwood caught in the downflow of a flood. I was pushed here and there. Sometimes I got stuck behind other debris and stopped moving. Then the current caught me once more, and I began to be swept downstream again. My only hope was that I could keep my head above water and not drown. It has always been chaos.

—"ALLEN"

I was born riding in a horse-drawn cart. Ever since I was little, I was expected to ride in a jet plane. No one ever bought me a ticket or showed me how to get on the plane. It's been like this forever. All I know is riding in a cart.

—"SUSAN"

. . . symptomatic manifestations of various forms of psychopathology are determined, at least in large part, by different types of impairments of cognitive-affective structures of the representational world.

S. J. BLATT (1991, p. 450)

IMPORTANCE OF CORRECT DIAGNOSIS AND UNDERSTANDING THE PSYCHOPATHOLOGY OF CHRONIC PATIENTS

Accurate diagnosis of the chronic patient is now recognized as essential to successful treatment. This is made even more critical because of (1) the

increasing diagnostic complexity of the unipolar depression area (e.g.
Keller, Klein, et al., 1995; McCullough et al., 1996) and (2) the serious
developmental limitations of the chronic patient, which may cause a psychotherapist to overestimate the individual's immediate capacity for
change.

Diagnostic Complexity

The increasing diagnostic differentiation now required by the DSM-IV
provides the opportunity to compare the treatment responses of patients
with the chronic depressive disorders to those with the episodic disorders.
We are finding that the protracted course of a unipolar disorder functions
as a moderator variable (Baron & Kenny, 1986; Holmbeck, 1997) that
significantly influences response to treatment. For example, when the
medication responses of chronic patients are compared to those of episodic major depressives, chronic patients take longer to respond, show
higher nonresponse rates, and exhibit greater recurrence and relapse rates
(Keller, 1988, 1990). In short, chronically depressed individuals present
a more difficult medication challenge than do other unipolar groups
(Thase, 1992).

The same conclusions are emerging from psychotherapy studies conducted with chronically depressed subjects, wherein the general consensus
is that chronic patients are more difficult to treat and more often need
long-term treatment regimes than episodic major depressives (Thase,
1992; Thase et al., 1994, 1992). Failure to diagnose the chronic patient
correctly is likely to result in undertreatment and a poor treatment
response (Harrison & Stewart, 1993; Keller, 1990). Thase (1992) notes
that "it is likely that the majority of depressed individuals in the United
States continue to be either untreated or incorrectly diagnosed and/or
inadequately treated" (p. 32). More will be said about these treatment
issues in Chapter 4.

Developmental Limitations

It is my strong belief that chronically depressed patients have a primitive
representational worldview, and that most contemporary therapy programs do not address this worldview adequately (e.g., Beck et al., 1979;
Klerman et al., 1984; Safran, 1990a, 1990b). Without a discerning awareness of the developmental limitations of chronic patients, psychotherapists are likely to overestimate their change capabilities, at least at the

outset of treatment. This chapter clarifies the etiological origins and current pathological functioning of chronic patients.

In the next two sections, I will discuss how normal and abnormal psychological processes are related and then describe one aspect of mature interpersonal-social development. The material in these sections will serve as general background information to facilitate an understanding of the specific psychopathological mechanisms of the chronic depressions.

THE MUTUALLY INFORMING RELATIONSHIP OF NORMAL AND ABNORMAL BEHAVIOR

My views of the relationship between normalcy and disorder have been significantly influenced by the work of several researchers, most notably the writings of Wakefield (1992a, 1992b), Cicchetti (1993; Cicchetti, Ackerman, & Izard, 1995), and Weiss (1961, 1969). My conceptual reliance upon these individuals will become obvious in the comments below.

Jerome Wakefield's (1992b) general concept of disorder assumes that some mechanism, be it psychological or physical, is not performing "a natural function for which it is designed" (p. 374). In discussing the nature of disorder, particularly as it applies to mental disorder, Wakefield seeks to transcend the traditional debate over whether disorder concepts are biomedical issues or sociopolitical ones (Kendall, 1986). He concludes by saying that the disorder construct must include both biomedical *and* sociocultural domains. In order to accomplish this synthesis, Wakefield labels mental disorder "harmful dysfunction": ". . . a mental disorder is a harmful dysfunction in a mental mechanism or, equivalently, a harmful mental dysfunction" (1992b, p. 384). "Dysfunction" denotes a scientific fact of deviation (e.g., symptoms, observed aberrant behavior, emotional loss of control/dysregulation, etc.); it signifies that some mental structure or disposition is not performing its naturally designed function. Wakefield notes that the word "dysfunction" comes from the field of evolutionary biology and derives from the evolutionary concept of natural selection. The word "harmful" is value-based in sociocultural standards and describes the negative consequences resulting from mental dysfunction. Dysfunction causes or results in "harm or deprivation of benefit to the person as judged by the standards of the person's culture" (1992b, p. 384). Describing harmful dysfunction, he says: "On the other hand, facts alone are not enough; disorder requires harm, which involves values. Thus both values and facts are involved in the concept of disorder" (Wakefield,

1992b, p. 381). In conclusion, the concept of disorder implies that normal psychological development is intended to lead the individual to a state of "functional well-being" as defined by the social values and meanings of one's culture (Wakefield, 1992b). His view suggests that any type of psychopathology causes personal harm to the individual and, as such, is not the intended normative state for the human organism. From my perspective, chronic depression represents a state of harmful dysfunction and does not represent a normative condition for adults.

Wakefield's definitions of functional well-being and disorder contain two implications relevant to the task of conceptualizing the psychopathology of the chronically depressed adult: (1) both "disorder" and "functional well-being" must be conceptually linked, and an understanding of one domain (either normalcy or abnormality) should contribute to an understanding of the other domain; and (2) Wakefield's view that disorder results from an interruption in the intended function of some mental mechanism strongly suggests that *both* normal and abnormal behavior derive from similar origins or from the same developmental process.

Other researchers have proposed similar views (Cicchetti, 1993; Cicchetti et al., 1995; Weiss, 1961, 1969). For example, embryologist Paul Weiss states: "Pathology and developmental biology must be reintegrated so that our understanding of the 'abnormal' will become but an extension of our insight into the 'normal,' while . . . the study of the abnormal will contribute to the deepening of that very insight" (p. 50).

In similar fashion, Dante Cicchetti (1993; Cicchetti et al., 1995), a developmental psychopathologist, urges researchers to study atypical or psychopathological instances (or cases) to inform, expand, and challenge our current developmental theories of normal development. Cicchetti views instances of abnormal behavior as experiments, saying that "experiments of nature can make significant contributions to our understanding of normal ontogenesis" (1993, p. 477).

In conclusion, there is a strong precedent for assuming that psychopathology is an interruption of (or a deviation from) an intended process of functional well-being such that both normal and abnormal behavior originate from the same developmental process. Understanding chronically depressed patients requires a comprehension of how their abnormal patterns represent deviations from the intended functional norm and how their psychopathology enacts behavior from an earlier developmental stage.

I have approached the task of understanding the psychopathology of chronic patients by utilizing Jean Piaget's model of normal cognitive-emotional development (Piaget, 1923/1926, 1954/1981; Inhelder & Piaget, 1955/1958) and identifying where the intended process of functional well-being has been interrupted by harmful dysfunction.

THE TELEOLOGICAL GOAL
FOR INTERPERSONAL-SOCIAL DEVELOPMENT

Before describing Piaget's model of normal cognitive-emotive development, I first must describe my definition of the teleological goal of *interpersonal-social development*. My notion of the highest level of interpersonal-social maturity is based upon Piaget's (1923/1926) description of the nature of mature, socialized language exchanges that occur between adults. The mature adult, according to Piaget, uses language to understand and be understood while simultaneously placing "himself at the point of view of his hearer" (1923/1926, p. 9). "Indeed, the further a man has advanced in his own line of thought, the better able is he to see things from the point of view of others and to make himself understood by them" (1923/1926, p. 39). Piaget's description of the mature usage of language matches a current definition of "empathy." *Webster's New Universal Unabridged Dictionary* (McKechnie, 1979) defines "empathy" as "the projection of one's own personality into the personality of another in order to understand him better" (p. 594). Learning how to participate empathically with others is one of the major goals of CBASP.

Being able to interact empathically is learned in relationships where empathy is modeled and valued. The more one practices relating to others empathically, the better one gets at it. As noted above, empathy in an interpersonal encounter is best observed in the way an individual uses verbal and nonverbal language while interacting. Empathic behavior signifies that (1) the person is interested in making himself/herself understood, and (2) there is an equivalent motivation to understand the language of the other person. Two people interacting empathically engage in a reciprocal process of synchronous giving and receiving via verbal and nonverbal communication. The interpersonal roles enacted are those of understanding equals, sharing comrades, and fellow travelers.

From a structural, developmental perspective (Cowan, 1978; Piaget, 1923/1926), empathic encounter denotes the ability to use abstractive thought or, in Piaget's terms, to use formal operations thought (Cowan, 1978; Piaget, 1923/1926, 1954/1981; Inhelder & Piaget, 1955/1958). Persons who do not enact formal operations thinking in the social-interpersonal sphere, such as chronically depressed adults, cannot generate authentic empathic behavior.

Finally, the ability to generate empathic interpersonal behavior requires the skills of *perceived functionality* thinking (McCullough, 1984a, 1991, 1995a; McCullough & Carr, 1987)—the general awareness that one's behavior has specific consequences in the world. Perceived functionality thinking means that the person is sensitive to the effects his/her behavior has upon another, while concomitantly being aware of the other person's effects upon him/her.

Like other growth processes, the ability to generate empathic engagement is never fully actualized by anyone. The normal mature adult is always on a trajectory, progressively moving toward greater ability to encounter others in an empathic way. Because of the complex meshing of the cognitive-emotional and behavioral factors operative in empathic engagement, empathy represents the quintessential form of human interaction; therefore, in my view, it is the ultimate goal for interpersonal-social development.

Normal Development and Chronic Depression

JEAN PIAGET'S STRUCTURAL MODEL OF NORMAL DEVELOPMENT

Jean Piaget (1954/1981, 1923/1926; Inhelder & Piaget, 1955/1958) provides us with a structural and functional model of normal cognitive-emotional development that illuminates the interpersonal-social psychopathology of early- and late-onset chronically depressed patients. Noam (1988) succinctly articulates the basic reason I have turned to Piaget for help in describing the etiological predicament of the chronic patient: "Piaget's theory of intellectual development is as yet the only theory that has been able to describe the underlying logic, or so-called structural operations of a developmental sequence" (p. 97).

My summary of Piaget's conclusions is based on his book *Intelligence and Affectivity* (1954/1981). This text is Piaget's definitive statement of his views concerning the maturational development of both cognitive *and* emotional organization (schemas).

Piaget (1954/1981) was guided in his hypotheses concerning cognitive and emotional development by one overriding principle: *Cognition and affect are always in constant interaction; these two components are essentially indissociable and inseparable.* There is no cognition without emotion, nor do emotions occur disengaged from thoughts. The emotive content of children's attention is seen in the interest exhibited toward an object, while movement away from the object may denote emotional uninterest or fear avoidance. For Piaget, *emotions affect cognitive development by influencing what children seek out or avoid.*

The entire interpersonal cognitive and emotional universe of the child is centered on the early attachment to the mother (Cowan, 1978). The quality of this mother-child bond (Cicchetti & Barnett, 1991; Guidano & Liotti, 1983; Hammen, 1992; Hammen et al., 1995) affects all areas of functioning: the infant's interests (translating into energy for behavior) toward objects in the world (people and inanimate things), feelings of respect for parents (other-esteem), self-feelings of superiority or inferiority (self-esteem), generalized interpersonal feelings toward other people (other-esteem), and an ambient emotive tone permeating all cognitive constructions concerning the environment (i.e., the world is experienced as a safe place, a dangerous place, an empty place, etc.).

Emotions, according to Piaget (1954/1981), act as an "energizing force" driving cognitive behavior and development, and cognitive structure channels the way emotions are expressed. He likened affect to the gasoline that activates an automobile, while the engine (cognitive structure) provides the outlet for the energy (power, speed) as well as the direction of the car's motion. Understanding the indissoluble union of cognition and affect—the fact that they represent two sides of the same coin (Piaget, 1964/1967)—is central to an understanding of the etiology of chronic depression.

Piaget (1954/1981) observed that affect is progressively schematized (organized) over time, paralleling but distinct from the maturing cognitive differentiation and "decentration" process. Recently several investigators have expressed similar views that emotions are not epiphenomena of cognitions or language, but constitute a distinct developmental-neurological system (Cicchetti et al., 1995; Gardner, 1983; Izard, 1993). As such, normal emotional growth moves toward increasing regulation in synchrony with differentiating cognitive structure (Cicchetti et al., 1995). When derailment occurs during normal development, emotional dysregulation and asynchrony between cognitive and emotional processes characterize the individual's behavior (Cicchetti et al., 1995; Piaget,

1954/1981). One possible result of this derailment is seen in early-onset depression (depression beginning before age 21), which usually signals that one has experienced the beginning of an affective-cognitive disorder that will probably be long standing and nonremitting (McCullough et al., 1988, 1994a).

In normal development, increasing differentiation of the self from itself occurs through an essential and continual "decentration" process extending from birth throughout the life span (Cowan, 1978; Piaget, 1954/1981). "Decentration" designates the process through which one acquires increasing ability to disengage oneself from the experience of the immediate, present moment. The child moves beyond a "snapshot view of reality" (Cowan, 1978)—that is, beyond infantile thinking that constructs the world mainly through static and concrete images—by learning to organize knowledge into rules and categories that transcend the ongoing activity in the moment. The final step in the decentration process takes place when the growing child grasps and utilizes abstract concepts. This step, which signals the perceptual overthrow of the immediate dominance of the moment, is termed "formal operations thinking" (Piaget, 1954/1981; Inhelder & Piaget, 1955/1958).

Decentration proceeds gradually during the first two years and finally nudges the child dramatically into the interpersonal-social realm, where he/she views himself/herself *in relation to others*. Decentration of the self is overwhelmingly dependent upon a salubrious environment created by significant others who increasingly draw children outside themselves and into propitious interpersonal relationships (Cowan, 1978; Nannis, 1988; Noam, 1988; Piaget, 1954/1981). To these fortunate children, the world looks like a safe and inviting playground. To those unfortunate children whose early environments do not promote decentration, the world becomes a forbidding and dangerous place. In addition to the emergence of positive or negative feelings toward the caregivers, the decentration process is associated with feelings of superiority or inferiority toward the self regarding the mastery, or lack thereof, of the immediate environment (Piaget, 1954/1981).

The normal process continues throughout the preoperational stage that lasts approximately from 24 months to 6–7 years of age (Piaget, 1923/1926, 1954/1981) and, as noted above, is finally superseded by formal operations thinking. Moving beyond perceptual attachment to the immediate environment (the snapshot perspective) signals a structural shift involving greater cognitive-emotional differentiation.

This developmental shift has crucial implications for adaptive living.

The normally developing child (1) can now construct a world in which a particular emotional reaction (sadness or anger) is viewed as simply one response among a number of possible reactions, thereby avoiding the primitive conclusion that the way he/she feels now is the way he/she will always feel; (2) can categorize another individual as being one type among a number of different types, thereby avoiding the conclusion that everyone will be similar; and (3) can observe a present interpersonal event with a parent or family member as being just one experience in a continuous montage of interpersonal happenings, thereby avoiding the conclusion that all future interpersonal events will entail a replay of this one event. The three negative alternatives avoided in these examples represent preoperational snapshot views of reality and characterize the phenomenological worldview of most chronically depressed patients. Such patients are unable to construct a perceived future or to think about any potentiality except in terms of the past. Thus the emotions of the present moment (say, sadness), as well as memories of early developmental figures and specific hurtful interpersonal encounters, circumscribe what is or is not possible in the future. *The perception of time literally stops for the chronic patient, such that the past defines interpersonal possibilities in the present and future.*

TWO TYPES OF DERAILMENT
IN NORMAL DEVELOPMENT

In Cowan's preface to Piaget's (1954/1981) *Intelligence and Affectivity*, he summarizes one of the important implications of Piaget's theory: ". . . when the affective side of intelligence is considered along with the cognitive side, it becomes possible to develop new Piagetian approaches to the understanding of psychopathology—those instances when normal cognitive and affective development somehow goes awry" (p. xiii).

Piaget's theory of cognitive-affective development suggests two etiological sources of harmful dysfunction: one involving infants and the other involving adults. In the first instance, normal development is retarded; in the second, heightened emotionality leads to "paralogical" thinking (fallacious thought that is structurally determined) and general functional regression. As I've noted, the first type applies to early-onset patients, and the second describes the etiological patterns of late-onset patients.

In the first instance, Piaget hypothesized that stimulus impoverishment and deprivation (unfavorable environmental conditions) may disrupt and retard normal development. In describing the developmental retardation seen among Rene Spitz's (1946) marasmus children ("marasmus" is a condition of progressive unresponsiveness in infants that is due to physical and emotional deprivation), Piaget (1954/1981) provides a case illustration with strong similarities to the developmental histories I have encountered in many early-onset patients. Piaget concluded from this example that the structural and developmental arrest reported by Spitz can occur in any environment characterized by "stimulus deprivation." His assumption that the environment can interfere with normal maturational development is consistent with our observations of dysfunctional family environments and their effects upon children. The maltreatment milieu interferes with normal development and results in primitive cognitive-emotional representations in adults who become early-onset chronic depressives. Piaget wrote:

> Lacking necessary environmental stimulation, there is general developmental retardation. Unfavorable conditions impede functioning and lead to functional regressions, both cognitive and affective, but neither type of regression causes the other. (1954/1981, p. 42)

In the adult instance, normal functioning deteriorates when heightened emotionality (a major depressive episode) undermines the person's representational view of reality. Piaget's description of the impact of "impassioned reasoning" (heightened affectivity) on rational thought applies to the late-onset type: ". . . affectivity only makes rational thought deviate into all sorts of paralogisms" (1954/1981, p. 60). Cicchetti et al. (1995) are more explicit in commenting on the effect strong emotions have on general functioning:

> Emotions may become maladaptive in two situations . . . The second situation may involve emotional flooding, where an emotion overwhelms control structures and strategies. In Wakefield's terms (1992a,b), this situation represents "harmful dysfunction," in that an evolutionary control mechanism cannot perform its natural function. (p. 6)

Thus late-onset of an acute major depressive episode may result in a deterioration of adult functioning. When the disorder is sustained over time, normal adult thinking patterns are undermined and replaced by earlier, preoperational-like functioning.

PARALLELS BETWEEN CHRONICALLY DEPRESSED ADULTS AND NORMAL PREOPERATIONAL CHILDREN

Preoperational thought remains bound to perceptual experience.

—PIAGET (1954/1981, p. 55)

By observing children's use of language and problem-solving capabilities at various ages, Piaget conceptualized his theory of development. In a similar manner, the way chronically depressed adults talk and solve problems has influenced my views concerning the structural underpinnings of their psychopathology. To the observer, a person's use of language, emotional responses, and behavior can be used as an index of that person's covert representational worldview (Beeghly & Cicchetti, 1994; Cicchetti, 1991; Cowan, 1978; Guidano & Liotti, 1983; Lane & Schwartz, 1987; Hammen, 1992; Noam & Cicchetti, 1996).

I have found striking similarities between Piaget's (1923/1926) descriptions of the preoperational functioning of two- to seven-year-old children and the language patterns and behavior of chronically depressed patients. Other researchers have discussed parallels between preoperational thinking and psychopathology (e.g., Breslow & Cowan, 1984; Cowan, 1978; Gordon, 1988; Nannis, 1988; Noam, 1988), but I am aware of no one who has described the structural characteristics of chronically depressed adults, particularly in regard to the way they think and express their emotions.

Analogous features of the preoperational patterns of normal children and chronically depressed adults include the following: (1) Both groups use global and prelogical thinking; (2) their thought processes are not influenced by the reasoning and logic of others; (3) both groups are pervasively egocentric in their views of self and others; (4) verbal communication is largely conducted in monologue form; (5) authentic interpersonal empathy is beyond the capacity of both groups; and (6) both groups exhibit poor affective control under stress.

1. *Chronically depressed patients think in a prelogical and precausal manner.* That is, they move from a premise to a conclusion with no stops in between. Little value seems to be placed on proving the premise or even checking out hypotheses with others. As one patient told me, "The world is the way I see it just because I know what I believe is true." Patients also describe themselves and their problems in global terms (e.g., "No one will ever like me," "Nothing I do will ever work out," "My life is

a total failure"). The title of one of Ray Charles' biggest hits, "Born to Lose," aptly portrays the inexorable course of failure ordained by the preoperational worldview of the depressed individual.

2. *Chronic depressives are also generally unaffected by logical reasoning and the reality-based views of those around them.* The following excerpt from a therapy session illustrates how this male patient is unaffected by the logical cause-and-effect reasoning of his therapist. The prelogical, precausal thinking of this male patient makes it impossible for the individual to see how his behavior leads to his neighbor's reaction.

PATIENT: My next-door neighbor has been on my case lately.

THERAPIST: What's going on between you two?

PATIENT: Well, he's been calling me and telling me to turn my stereo down. I got some new speakers last week.

THERAPIST: Was he on your case before you bought the speakers?

PATIENT: No, not really. I think he's just a bastard.

THERAPIST: Do you see any connection between his complaints and your playing the stereo too loud?

PATIENT: Why are you taking his side? You're just like all the others—no one understands me.

The patient's prelogical, precausal thought patterns, as represented in this excerpt, make it impossible for him to see how his behavior leads to his neighbor's reaction. The neighbor is "a bastard" simply because he calls and requests that the stereo be turned down. There is no awareness of an *antecedent condition* (the loud stereo) *caused by* the patient and *evoking* the neighbor's reaction ("turn it down!"). The patient is not malingering or being stubborn in his final comment to the therapist. Instead, what we see at work here is an infantile-like mentality that is not affected by reality-based reasoning and logic.

3. *Chronically depressed patients are pervasively egocentric in their views of themselves and others.* From a preoperational vantage point, such a person's worldview is valid and logically unassailable solely because the individual believes it to be true. In behaving egocentrically, chronic patients, like normal preoperational children, cannot allow others into their phenomenological sphere. They talk as if they believe they are the center of the universe. But unlike normal children, the patient's preoperational thought arises from hurtful and injurious developmental

sources. Regardless, the outcome for both is the same. Others cannot gain entrance into individual's world and he/she remains focused on the self. The following excerpt illustrates the egocentric talk of a female patient when her therapist tries to direct the woman's attention to his positive perceptions of her. She is unable to shift her attention outside herself to consider a viewpoint other than her own.

PATIENT: No one will ever like me—I'm such a miserable person.

THERAPIST: How do you think I feel about you?

PATIENT: You're just a nice person; you're nice to everyone.

THERAPIST: You didn't answer my question.

PATIENT: If you're honest, there's no way you can like me.

THERAPIST: How do you know?

PATIENT: Because that's just the way it is. No one could like me. Nothing you say will make me believe otherwise.

4. When we compare the characteristics of preoperational children with those of chronic depressives, we see another similarity in the way both groups use language. *Conversing with therapists, chronic patients talk in monologues,* as if they were thinking aloud; therapists' responses have very little influence on the style or content of their speech. To refer again to Piaget, their verbal presentations are similar to the "noncooperative" talk that is so characteristic of preoperational children. To illustrate the point, look at this verbatim conversation of two normal five- to six-year-old children, Pie and Jacq, conversing in Piaget's laboratory (Piaget, 1923/1926, p. 59):

PIE: It was ripping yesterday [a flying demonstration].

JACQ: There was a blue one [an aeroplane] there was lots of them, and then they all got into a line.

PIE: I went in a motor yesterday. And d'you know what I saw when I was in the motor? A lot of carts that were going past. Please teacher can I have the india-rubber?

JACQ: I want to draw that [the aeroplanes]. It will be very pretty.

Both boys talk in monologues, with neither child's words particularly influencing the verbal content of the other's. What is missing here is what

Piaget calls verbal "cooperativeness," a characteristic of a later stage of development. Cooperative talk is observable when the words of one child obviously influence the verbal content and behavioral responses of another child.

5. Another aspect of this monologue style of speech that results in a similarity between preoperational children and chronic depressives is *the absence of authentic empathy with others*. The ability to achieve empathic engagement with another person does not exist in preoperational children or chronic patients. Empathy must not be confused with emotional sensitivity. Preoperational children as well as chronic individuals are highly sensitive to emotional impacts stemming from the behavior of others. What distinguishes a merely sensitive person from an empathic one is the sensitive person's inability to understand the emotions of another and to convey understanding in a congruent, interactive manner.

Following are two verbatim examples of noncooperative speech to show how chronically depressed patients are unable to generate empathic engagement with therapists in the early stages of treatment. The patient in the first example had a 20-year history of depression.

THERAPIST: You have really had a difficult week with your wife.

PATIENT: It's no different from any other week.

THERAPIST: I was really struck by how her comments to you on Thursday night must have hurt you.

PATIENT: I could have married someone else.

THERAPIST: It's hard for you to acknowledge my reactions to you—the way I feel seems to have very little effect on you.

PATIENT: My wife is not speaking to me any more.

The therapist might as well be looking at the wall and talking to herself. In the second example, the absence of empathy is almost brutal in its impact. This patient presented with a 17-year history of depression.

THERAPIST: I'm sorry that I'm running late for our appointment. My child was sick, and I had to take him to the doctor.

PATIENT: Nothing really matters . . . [voice drifting off]

THERAPIST: I was really frightened by the high fever my son has been running since last night.

PATIENT: You know, I've really had a miserable week.

These interactions make it seem possible that these two patients could have been exchanged with Piaget's children, Pie and Jacq, and still easily recreate Piaget's lab scenario! The adults talk just like the children; that is, they talk in parallel, using noncooperative speech, and are unable to generate empathic engagement. However, our imaginative analogy breaks down quickly because the patients are *not* children. Tragically, they are adults behaving like preoperational children.

6. The final similarity between preoperational children and chronic depressives is *emotional dysregulation—the lack of emotional control under stressful conditions*. We would not characterize the emotive vulnerability of normal preoperational children as being dysregulated. We would, how-ever, describe normal young children as possessing less emotive control and fewer aspects of affective organization (schemas) than they will develop as they mature. When adults think, feel, and behave like young children, emotional control is precluded; they are thrown automatically into perceived states of helplessness and hopelessness when challenged by the daily stress of living. The primitive emotional organization of chronic patients consigns them to a life of poor affective control and emotional dysregulation (Cicchetti et al., 1995).

Being unable to resolve daily problems and manage interpersonal encounters effectively results in repeated social failures and the conse-quent propensity to anticipate failure in every situation. The possibility of an out-of-control, dysphoric mood state awaits the person at the end of every road. A common emotional response for such patients was recorded in a therapy session with a chronically depressed male, who had finally obtained the raise for which he had worked. His emotional reaction is a consistent one for such patients in these kinds of situa-tions. We would expect pleasure to be his response, but this is certainly not the case.

PATIENT: I finally got the raise I wanted.

THERAPIST: Great! Do you feel that the raise is related to the hard work you put in at the plant?

PATIENT: Naw, my number just came up, I was just lucky.

THERAPIST: Is this the way raises are given at your workplace? I mean, do people get raises just because they are next in line—regardless of the quality of their work?

PATIENT: No. But ever since my supervisor told me about the raise, I have been as depressed as ever. I don't think I really deserved one.

DIFFERENCES BETWEEN NORMAL PREOPERATIONAL CHILDREN AND CHRONICALLY DEPRESSED ADULTS

Why don't preoperational thinking and the resultant "snapshot" view of reality predispose normal children to depression? The question is appropriate, particularly in light of the cognitive-emotional parallels I have drawn above. One difference between a normal preoperational child and a chronically depressed adult is that the normal child is developmentally in progress. The second distinction involves the home life of the normal child, which is not one of maltreatment. Development is progressing within a safe and nurturing interpersonal milieu. When a child is overwhelmed by the dangers of an abusive or neglectful home life, normal development is thwarted because the child's energies and behavior are directed toward basic survival, not growth (Drotar & Sturm, 1991; Money, 1992; Money, Annecillo, & Hutchinson, 1985). The outcome in this latter instance is a stunting of growth or a failure to thrive (Drotar & Sturm, 1991). Such children are damaged by ongoing stress, in that they never learn to cope adequately in a social world; hence, they are hypervulnerable to reacting to stress with an early-onset depressive experience. These early negative experiences remain prepotent when compared to ongoing more positive experiences in an adult patient's life. The chronic patient constructs current interpersonal experiences as if they were merely replays of the negative past. Future interpersonal experiences portend only more of the same kind of interpersonal negativity.

In working with chronically depressed patients, we are not just dealing with fallacious beliefs about the world or confronting habitually negative thoughts. The challenge of working with these patients is much more serious, *because the phenomenological problem we face at the outset of therapy is essentially a structural one. Psychotherapy must begin with an "adult child" and then help the adult to mature developmentally.*

NORMAL BIFURCATED COGNITIVE-EMOTIONAL DEVELOPMENT

One type of chronic patient I have treated warrants special mention. This patient functions normally, using abstract thought in the realm of inanimate objects; in the interpersonal-social arena, however, he/she thinks and emotes in a primitive way. Piaget (1954/1981) and others (Cicchetti et al., 1995; Gardner, 1983; Izard, 1993; Mayer & Salovey, 1993) have described what I term a "bifurcated" type of cognitive-emotional development in the normal child, which differentially affects the social (interpersonal) and nonsocial (inanimate) spheres of functioning. The derailment of this particular developmental task produces particular features of harmful dysfunction often observed among chronically depressed adults. Piaget (1954/1981) noted:

> Actually, there are not two kinds of schemes, cognitive and affective. There are, rather, schemes that have to do with people and schemes that have to do with objects. Both [schemes] are cognitive and affective at the same time. (p. 51)

I have observed that some chronic depressives function quite well in relation to nonsocial object areas. Whereas preoperational thinking dominates their interpersonal-social sphere, their abstract and symbolic processes are facilely engaged in professional work areas such as education, law, business, mathematics, and science. This observation suggests that the structural impairment I have hypothesized to exist in the interpersonal-social domain is not always accompanied by maturational impairment in nonsocial areas or in the manipulation of concepts. A number of other psychologists have drawn similar conclusions about social and nonsocial areas of development (Cicchetti et al., 1995; Gardner, 1983; Izard, 1993; Mayer & Salovey, 1993). In short, there seems to be substantial evidence that social and nonsocial mental organizations may represent a bifurcated developmental process that unfolds along different neurological tracks. This phenomenon is observed from time to time in therapy with chronic patients.

Let me illustrate. A 34-year-old man, depressed since early adolescence (a case of early-onset double depression), requested psychotherapy. The patient's academic and statistical wizardry (and formal thinking ability) in the nonsocial domain propelled him upwards in a large, national corporation. However, his interpersonal childishness and inability to cope with normal work-related interactions brought him to the brink of job termination. The interpersonal problems he had with both his supervisor and colleagues were the major reasons he sought treatment. His skills in formal operations thinking in mathematics were not impaired. This is not an infrequent occurrence. It is for this reason that I target the *interpersonal-social sphere of functioning* as the problematic area for treatment: It is an area of preoperational impairment for both early- and late-onset chronic depressives.

MALTREATMENT AND DERAILMENT OF THE MATURATIONAL PROCESS AMONG EARLY-ONSET CHRONIC DEPRESSIVES

The recalled memories of early-onset patients include injurious themes and motifs that pervaded their home life. When we observe these adults' current social expectations and behavior with family members, lovers, colleagues, friends, and finally with therapists, we find the same core theme: that *others will hurt them if given the opportunity*. This theme, characterizing both early and contemporary relationships, strongly suggests a developmental history of maltreatment (Cicchetti, 1993; Cicchetti & Barnett, 1991; Cramer, Manzano, Palacio, & Torrado, 1984; Dodge, 1990, 1993; Fox, Barrnett, Davies, & Bird, 1990; Hammen, 1992; Lizardi et al., 1995; Rubin, Coplan, Fox, & Calkins, 1995). It appears that early interpersonal maltreatment produces a structurally and functionally damaged adult who behaves like a wounded child.

Cicchetti and Barnett (1991) identify four categories of early childhood maltreatment that are frequently reported in the developmental histories of early-onset depressive patients: *emotional maltreatment* (active emotional abuse or passive neglect), *physical abuse, physical neglect*, and *sexual abuse*. Additional factors associated with early childhood conditions of chronic patients include homelessness and residence in a municipal shelter (Fox et al., 1990); a history of maternal depression leading to inconsistent parenting (Akiskal, 1983; Dodge, 1990; Hammen, 1992; Hammen, Burge, & Adrian, 1991; Lizardi et al., 1995); early parental separation, divorce, or abandonment (Hammen, 1992; Klein, Taylor, Dickstein, & Harding, 1988b; Klein, Taylor, Harding, & Dickstein, 1988); self-reported perceptions of a disturbed childhood home environment, poor relationships with both mothers and fathers, and/or lower levels of maternal and paternal care (Lizardi et al., 1995); and a high prevalence of psychopathology among parents of chronically depressed children (Klein et al., 1988b; Klein, Taylor, Harding, et al., 1988). It is also a well-known fact that "assortative mating" (Akiskal, 1983; Hammen, 1992; Merikangas, Prusoff, & Weissman, 1988; Rutter & Quinton, 1984)—the propensity of pathological individuals to seek out pathological mates—characterizes the marital patterns of chronically depressed individuals.

Such couples often produce chronically depressed offspring (Klein et al., 1988b; Klein, Taylor, Harding, et al., 1988).

Four Familial Themes among Early-Onset Chronic Patients

Most early-onset patients were not adequately parented or socialized; consequently, they have not thrived cognitive-emotionally or behaviorally. Patients frequently describe their childhood as being consumed by efforts to survive the physical and emotional "hell of the family." Four common themes of maltreatment consistently characterize the familial environments of chronic depressives:

1. The early family environment did not recognize or satisfactorily address a child's physical and/or emotional needs.
2. A child was subjected to a dangerous familial environment where significant others hurt him/her as well as hurt each other.
3. Physical and emotional pain leading to tension, anxiety, and fear/terror was a prevalent dynamic in a child's daily life.
4. A child was often thrust into an interpersonal role requiring him/her to meet the emotional needs of the caregiver(s).

The severity of one chronic patient's experiences during childhood is illustrated in the following excerpt, taken from the second session of therapy. The patient is an early onset, 27-year-old female with early-onset double depression, who had been depressed "all my life."

THERAPIST: Tell me about your early life history with your family.

PATIENT: I was the oldest child of four children. I had two sisters, and the youngest sibling was a boy. Both of my parents were alcoholic and they were always fighting—both physically and verbally. My earliest memory is sitting on my father's lap while he was rubbing my vagina. I must have been four or five years old at the time. He began having intercourse with me around six, and this went on until he left the family, when I was a sophomore in high school. I don't think my mother cared one way or the other. My mother would beat all of us kids when she was drunk, and that was frequent. She used to bring other men to the house and sleep with them. They would fool around with us girls when she was not paying attention. I grew up feeling like

I was a piece of meat. I still feel like I'm a piece of meat around men. I feel worthless. I've always felt that way about myself. No one could ever care about me with the life I've had. Both my sisters are depressed and alcoholic. Somehow, my brother has done all right for himself.

The following conversation, which took place between a 25-year-old male with early-onset double depression and his therapist, again depicts the common theme of early maltreatment.

THERAPIST: Tell me about the course of your depression and something about your history with significant persons in your life.

PATIENT: I've been feeling down for as long as I can remember. Maybe as early as the first or second grade—just knew that something was wrong with my life. My mother was alcoholic and was not home a lot of the time. When she was there, she used to beat all of us frequently—mostly over nothing! She was a very mean lady. She had multiple affairs with other men when she was drunk, and my father, when he found out about it, would smack her around a lot. My dad worked most of the time. He cooked the meals when he did come home and made us eat everything he cooked. He would punish us if we didn't eat it. He yelled a lot. Never played ball with me or took me places. I really don't think he cared for me. Seemed like I was just "trouble" for him. Now that I think of it, I don't think he was much of a dad. Our family wasn't much. I don't have much contact with either my brother or sister. We weren't close when we were kids. I never had any friends, and if I had had, I wouldn't have brought them around my house. I was sort of a loner. People used to tease me a lot when I was in high school. Sometimes I would get really depressed. I have been hospitalized twice because I wanted to kill myself. Never been able to hold a job. I bet you hear this kind of story a lot.

The ambience of disruption and stress surrounding the child's early development precludes normal growth and produces an individual who continues, over time, to function interpersonally like a child. In addition, the person continues to superimpose the destructive interpersonal-social world of early childhood on present relationships. Piaget's dictum that *preoperational thinking and functioning are dominated by the immediate perceptual experience* is seen when a patient recreates the past through current relationships. This occurs when people in the present world of the patient are perceived as individuals who will react to the patient in ways that parallel the old maltreatment themes. The excerpt below shows how one 30-year-old patient with chronic major depression expects the therapist to react to her the way her father did:

PATIENT: I read the *Patient Manual* last night, and I don't think I'm going to be able to complete all the work. I know I'm going to fail at this and disappoint you. I think this had better be my last session.

THERAPIST: Why are you so discouraged? This is only the third session we have met together, and I just gave you the *Manual* at the end of last session.

PATIENT: I never succeed at anything I try to do, and this therapy will not be any different.

THERAPIST: Where did you learn that you were beat before you started?

PATIENT: I can still hear my father telling me I would never amount to anything. He told me that over and over and over. When I failed, he would just gloat and tell me, "See, I told you so." So I finally just quit trying to do anything. I bet you have thought what a waste of time working with me will be. I can just hear you thinking that—it's better I quit therapy now than disappoint you later.

Here the therapist has a severe patient crisis on his hands in the beginning of the third session. Not only is the individual convinced she is destined to fail, but she is also convinced that her therapist expects her to fail. She perceptually constructs the clinician into the rejecting father who holds negative expectancies for her. Her early maltreatment by the father perpetuated a snapshot view of failure that has been reenacted with numerous persons over the years and that now threatens to terminate therapy. Her static view also precludes her perceiving that the therapist is *not* reacting to her in a manner similar to her father.

Clinicians are frequently told by their early-onset patients that they first became aware of their depression at about 15 years of age (McCullough & Kaye, 1993). The onset of puberty is invariably accompanied by stringent social demands that these individuals are unable to meet. A depressive experience is often the result. Without adequate treatment, preoperational arrest and the coping limitations it imposes commit the person to entrapment in the withdrawal phase of the depressive experience.

A Paucity of Research

Regrettably, no specific research is available to support the view that early maltreatment causes structural impairment in early-onset depressive patients. However, substantive descriptive evidence does exist, suggesting that structural deficits are indeed present among abused children and adolescents, many of whom are described as being depressed (Blatt, 1991; Breslow & Cowan, 1984; Cicchetti & Barnett, 1991; Cowan, 1978; Fox et al., 1990; Gordon, 1988; Noam, 1988; Rubin et al., 1995). What is sorely missing in the developmental literature are empirical data that would directly link early maltreatment to the phenomenological problems that characterize chronically depressed adults.

In one of the few studies investigating the relationship between early childhood functioning (at three years of age) and abnormal adult functioning (Caspi, Moffitt, Newman, & Silva, 1996), the authors concluded: "Some forms of adult (21 yrs.) psychopathologic abnormality are meaningfully linked, albeit weakly, to behavioral differences observed among children in the third year of life" (p. 1033). At age 21, approximately 30% of those rated as being "inhibited" (shy, fearful, easily upset) as three-year-old children were given DSM-III-R diagnoses of unipolar depression (major depression, dysthymia, or double depression), and 5% reported one or more suicide attempts. Among the children rated as "undercontrolled" (impulsive, restless, distractible), 46% had received at least one DSM-III-R diagnosis at age 21, and 9% of this group reported a history of suicide attempt(s). The authors did not explore the family environment of the three-year-olds, nor did they describe the phenomenological world of the pathological adults. What they did find was a significant relation between problematical childhood social patterns and adult psychopathology! This study was descriptive only and did not investigate causal mechanisms. In the absence of empirical data, two etiological hypotheses are offered that summarize the inferences I have made from my observations of the in-session behavior of early-onset adult patients:

Hypothesis 1: Early-onset patients enter adulthood with the interpersonal-social "mindset" of children, as a result of environmental maltreatment that was severely stressful and personally damaging.

Hypothesis 2: Early-onset patients behave in ways that indicate structural impairment, and they are maximally ill-equipped to cope effectively with the daily stressors of living.

Adults who are structurally impaired are at extreme risk of becoming chronically mired in the withdrawal phase of the depressive experience. These individuals are programmed to fail miserably in mature social spheres, be they the family milieu, marriage, the workplace, the social milieu, or the psychotherapy setting. Such persons are simply not functionally equipped to behave as an adult around other adults.

LATE-ONSET DEGENERATION
OF COGNITIVE-EMOTIONAL FUNCTIONING

Many late-onset patients describe a set of events that are thematically similar—in essence if not in content—to the following description given by a 43-year-old male, depressed for seven years, during the initial therapy session.

THERAPIST: Will you tell me how long you have been depressed and when you began having problems with depression? Then describe your experiences with persons who played a significant role in your life.

PATIENT: I have been depressed since I was 36 years old. I was released from a company seven years ago, and shortly after that they hospitalized me for depression. You know, downsizing and all that. I have not worked since that time—can't get up the courage to get out there and find a job. My wife has been carrying the economic load for us. Been tough all around. You want to hear about my family, I guess. Well, I was raised in a regular family. My father worked, and mother raised four of us kids. Can't remember anything really bad that happened. They loved us and tried to teach us the right things. We never had a lot of money, but got along all right. I am closer to my older brother than anyone else in the family now. Talk to him almost every week. He has been really supportive of me. I really think I got screwed when my boss told me that I was being terminated. Was literally thrown out on the street. I worked as a clerk for 10 years for that company—ever since I was in my early 30s. I don't have any real skills that would get me a good job—I've just given up.

THERAPIST: Have you ever been depressed before?

PATIENT: Not really. Oh, I had my ups and downs, but nothing like this. People always told me I was a "pretty okay guy to be around."

Piaget (1954/1981) proposed that acute periods of excessive emotionality may lead to a deterioration of normal cognitive-emotive structure and functioning. His description neatly fits the late-onset experience of many of these adult patients. If one looks closely at the early memories recalled by late-onset patients, they usually report a milder and less ruthless developmental history than their early-onset counterparts. Late-onset patients often remember growing up around one or more loving adults, as well as having other facilitative relationships. These patients rarely present with antecedent dysthymia as part of their clinical history. They frequently tell clinicians that their first major depressive episode occurred at about 25 years of age (McCullough & Kaye, 1993), and more often than not, they are able to pinpoint a stressful event that precipitated the depression (McCullough et al., 1992; McCullough, Roberts, et al., 1994). Current research has also shown that most late-onset cases are part of the 20% of adult patients who are treated for their first major depressive episode and don't fully recover. The episodic disorder then takes on a chronic course (Keller & Hanks, 1994; Keller, Lavori, Rice, et al., 1986).

Late-onset chronically depressed individuals are now faced with an unprecedented and unabating emotional condition. I hypothesize that for these patients, the relentless assault of dysphoria (an unremitting major depressive episode) leads to a deterioration of cognitive-emotional functioning and thus to a return to preoperational functioning. As stated by Cicchetti et al. (1995), "abundant evidence shows that the emotions system has a causal influence on cognitive interpretations and processes, independent of the influence of cognitive appraisals on emotions" (p. 5). The view that emotions affect cognitive functioning has been elaborated more fully by Izard (1993), who notes that emotions are activated by multiple neural, sensorimotor, and affective processes in addition to cognitive mechanisms. Wakefield (1992a, 1992b) would label the structural deterioration in late-onset patients as an instance of "harmful dysfunction." He would argue that in such cases, the chronic disorder is exacerbated because the internal regulatory mechanisms affecting emotionality and behavior no longer perform their intended functions.

As briefly noted earlier, Cicchetti et al. (1995) described two instances in which the emotion-induced degenerative process occurs. One is highly relevant to the etiology of late-onset chronic depression. This is the instance in which normal regulatory mechanisms are simply washed away by an emotional reaction that "floods" or overwhelms them.

Three brief excerpts from sessions with late-onset patients serve to illustrate how emotional dysregulation pervades the lives of such individuals.

PATIENT 1: I end up feeling depressed regardless of what I do. If I try to be outgoing at a party, I feel depressed. If I hang back and don't talk to anyone, I feel depressed. It really doesn't matter what I do—I always end up feeling depressed.

PATIENT 2: I was going to the store with my wife the other night, and she was really on my case. She let me have it. I don't know what I had done to get her this upset. All I know is that the more she talked, the more guilty I felt. Sounds stupid, doesn't it—I mean, feeling guilty and not even knowing what I had done wrong.

PATIENT 3: The evening started out well. The banquet had been given in my honor. People were really complimentary with their remarks, and I was feeling right proud of myself. Boy, that didn't last long. Here comes the depression, and it wiped me out the rest of the night. I withdrew at my own party.

What processes are operating in the late-onset patient that erode and undermine normal functioning? To continue along the lines suggested by Piaget (1954/1981) and Cicchetti et al. (1995), the unyielding emotional state of depression leaves the late-onset adult concluding not only that the world he/she lives in is unworkable (hopelessness), but that its problems are unresolvable (helplessness). The "immediate" distress of the uncontrollable dysphoric condition (the major depression) becomes all-consuming and leads to erosion of the patient's normal structural view of the world.

Entrapment in the withdrawal phase of depression is actualized when late-onset patients conclude that there will be no successful coping alternatives available to them to resolve the depressive dilemma in the future. Late-onset chronic depressives lose the future perspective that they once had (but that their early-onset comrades never had) and with the loss they end up concluding, "The way things are now is the way they will always be." As the deterioration process unfolds, such individuals become progressively enmeshed in a sense of overwhelming distress. The patient's cognitive-emotional perceptions are now chained to the chaos of the present dysphoria, and the heretofore normally functioning person is transformed into an adult child. The present perceptions of hopelessness and helplessness become their snapshot view of reality. It is not surprising to hear these patients say, "Who I am now is all I will ever be," "There is no hope of ever being different," "The way I see things now is the way they will always be," and so forth. This downward spiral of the depressive disorder cycle has been illustrated earlier in Chapter 2 (see Figure 2.1). These individuals find it increasingly impossible to consider seriously any alternatives or views that might mitigate their current mood problem (e g , "It feels bad to be fired, but I have the skills to obtain other employ‐ ment," "My children still count on me to come through for them," "My wife still loves me in spite of this crisis," etc.). Instead, the once adequate representational worldview has imploded under strong affective bombard‐ ment and turned the patient inward and away from others. The pernicious late-onset process has left the adult patient helpless, hopeless, and with no sense of the future.

SIMILAR TREATMENT GOALS
FOR EARLY- AND LATE-ONSET PATIENTS

The good news is that because both early- and late-onset chronic patients function at a preoperational level, they can be treated in the same man‐ ner. CBASP therapists attempt to overthrow the preoperational entrap‐ ment by interacting with patients in a direct manner that requires them to engage, systematically and repeatedly, in formal operational thinking and behavioral patterns.

In the next chapter, I will discuss the historical development of the chronic depression nomenclature in *DSM-IV* and review some of the research literature involving chronically depressed subjects.

CHAPTER FOUR

Course Patterns, Comorbidity, and Psychological Characteristics

> Dysthymia is a low-grade chronic depressive disorder that has a
> pernicious long-term course often complicated by bouts of
> superimposed major depression. ... it is difficult to treat and is
> often treatment resistant.
>
> —M. B. KELLER (1990, p. 15)

FIVE COURSE PATTERNS
OF CHRONIC DEPRESSION

Chronic depression is defined as a unipolar mood disorder lasting two or more years and with less than a two-month period during which the individual reports no symptoms. This disorder, in its several patterns of manifestation, will affect approximately 50–75 million individuals now living in the United States (Bland, 1997; Kessler et al., 1994).

The chronic disorders can be categorized in terms of five course patterns:

1. *Dysthymic disorder.* This is a mild to moderate disorder of two or more years duration, usually beginning during adolescence.
2. *Double depression.* This consists of a single major depressive epi-

sode or recurrent major depression without interepisode recovery, superimposed on dysthymic disorder.

3. *Recurrent major depression lasting for two years or more without full recovery between episodes.* In *DSM-IV*, this profile is given a longitudinal course specifier for major depression; it is called "major depression, recurrent, without full interepisode recovery, with no Dysthymic Disorder."

4. *Chronic major depression.* Full criteria for a major depressive episode are met continuously for two or more years in this pattern.

5. *Double depression/chronic major depression.* A fifth course pattern (McCullough et al., in press) was identified in a recent national study (Keller et al., 1998) among a cohort of patients who met criteria for both double depression and chronic major depression at screening.

I will briefly describe the five course patterns below; I also provide figures illustrating the clinical course for each pattern.

Dysthymic Disorder

Dysthymia is a relatively recent addition to the *DSM*. Until 1980, with the publication of the *DSM-III*, chronic depression was frequently classified as a personality or characterological disorder. The *DSM-I* (APA, 1952) and *DSM-II* (APA, 1968) classified a long standing "affective" depressive condition as "cyclothymic personality disorder, depressive type." It is also interesting to note that only since the publication of the *DSM-III* in 1980 have the chronic mood disorders been considered "treatable." This is because of the fact that during the *DSM-I* and *DSM-II* era (1952–1979) the general belief was that personality disorders would not respond to pharmacotherapy (Akiskal, 1995).

In the *DSM-III*, dysthymia was characterized as a mild to moderate type of chronic depression, present more days than not, and lasting for two or more years; it was categorized as an axis I "affective disorder" (Akiskal, 1983; Kocsis & Frances, 1987; McCullough et al., 1996). The symptom checklist for the disorder underwent significant revision in the *DSM-III-R*, but the mild to moderate features as well as the two-year duration criterion remained unchanged (Kocsis, 1993).

The recently completed *DSM-IV* Mood Disorders Field Trial (Keller, Klein, et al., 1995), studying dysthymia and major depression, reported that the most frequently observed symptoms of 190 dysthymic subjects involved cognitive, functional, and social features. Vegetative symptoms, including sleeping and eating problems, were less frequently reported. Despite this empirical evidence, the APA's *DSM-IV* Task Force Committee voted to retain the *DSM-III-R*'s two vegetative symptoms of an eating disturbance (poor appetite or overeating) and a sleeping disturbance (insomnia or hypersomnia) as part of the dysthymia symptom checklist.

Most dysthymics report an insidious onset of the disorder in mid-adolescence (mean age = 15 years). (McCullough & Kaye, 1993; McCullough et al., 1992); if onset is reported as occurring before age 21, the correct diagnosis is early-onset dysthymia. Late-onset dysthymia, a rarer form of the disorder (Klein et al., 1999), begins after 20 years of age. Two course patterns have been observed: Dysthymia may occur in its pure state without syndromal involvement (i.e., major depression), or it may precede one or more episodes of major depression. Only 11% of 526 *DSM-IV* Field Trial subjects were diagnosed with the "pure" disorder, whereas 35% of those diagnosed with a current episode of major depression at screening reported an antecedent course of dysthymia. Data now provide the statistical verification that pure dysthymia is relatively uncommon: 90% of dysthymia patients have a major depressive episode sooner or later (Keller, 1988; Thase, 1992). Over time, the usual pattern among patients with double depression (those with both major depression *and* antecedent dysthymia) is to experience remission of the syndromal episode, either with or without treatment, and a return to the antecedent dysthymic baseline (Keller & Shapiro, 1982; Keller, Lavori, Endicott, et al., 1983).

Considerable information comparing early- and late-onset dysthymics (Klein, Taylor, Dickstein, & Harding, 1988a; Klein et al., 1999; McCullough et al., 1990) has been reported. Compared to late-onset patients, early-onset patients seek out treatment more often and report significantly higher rates of lifetime major depressive disorders, as well as more anxiety symptoms (Klein et al., 1988a). In addition, first-degree relatives of early-onset patients have a greater prevalence of major depression; more importantly, these patients experience a higher rate of comorbid Axis I and II disorders (Klein et al., 1988a, 1999). Both groups demonstrate an external locus of control orientation as measured by Rotter's Internal-External Locus of Control Scale (I-E: Lefcourt, 1976; Rotter, 1966; Reid & Ware, 1974) and both evince similar coping styles (self-blame, wishful thinking, and seeking social support) when confronted with stressful events (McCullough et al., 1990). The course pattern of pure dysthymia is shown in Figure 4.1.

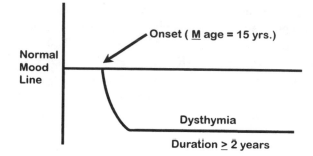

FIGURE 4.1. Clinical course profile for dysthymic disorder.

Double Depression

Double depression is diagnosed when one or more episodes of major depression occur after the onset of dysthymic disorder. The dysthymia condition must be present for two years prior to the onset of the first major depressive episode. Two course profiles for double depression, illustrating both a single major depressive episode and recurrent episodes, are illustrated in Figure 4.2.

Chronic Major Depression Patterns

The *DSM-III* was revised in 1987, and for the first time, chronic major depression became a formal diagnostic category (McCullough et al., 1996). The *DSM-III-R* nomenclature for the chronic disorder suggested two course patterns. The first type of chronic major depression (the third course pattern in the list at the start of the chapter) described a patient whose "index episode" of major depression included a history of recurrent episodes with incomplete/partial recovery periods occurring between episodes. Determining the duration of an index episode meant calculating the time between the onset of an uninterrupted episode of major depression and the date of the screening interview. In the *DSM-III-R* the index episode was considered "continuous," even though the original episode was characterized by one or more instances of partial remission (McCullough et al., 1996). If the patient reported a remission of symptoms for a period lasting two or more months during the previous two years, chronic major depression could not be diagnosed.

The *DSM-IV* changed the labeling process for this course. The current diagnosis is now "major depression, recurrent, without full inter-episode recovery, with no Dysthymic Disorder" (APA, 1994, p. 388). The two-year criterion for this disorder is no longer specified in the *DSM-IV*. In labeling the third course pattern as a chronic disorder, I am assuming that the index episode has persisted for a minimum of two years. Patients whose index episode of depression remains at a full syndromal level for a minimum of two years are simply diagnosed as having chronic major depression (the fourth pattern listed earlier). These two course patterns are diagrammed in Figure 4.3.

Double Depression/Chronic Major Depression

Recent data (McCullough et al., in press) from a national treatment study (Keller et al., 1998) in which sertraline (an SSRI) or imipramine (a TCA) was administered to 635 chronically depressed patients indicated a fifth course pattern for chronic depression. Twenty percent of the patients met criteria for antecedent dysthymic disorder and also for a superimposed

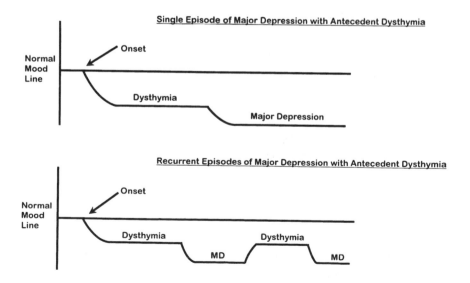

FIGURE 4.2. Clinical course profiles for a single episode of major depression with antecedent dysthymia and recurrent episodes of major depression with antecedent dysthymia.

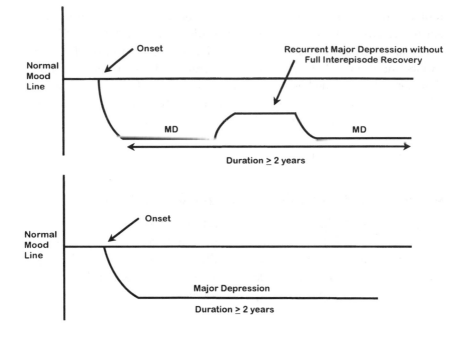

FIGURE 4.3. Clinical course profiles for recurrent major depression without full interepisode recovery and chronic major depression.

index episode of chronic major depression. The course pattern for this fifth group is diagrammed in Figure 4.4.

Differential Diagnosis among the Chronic Disorders

Our current knowledge concerning the longitudinal course patterns has surpassed our knowledge of the contribution differential diagnosis makes to treatment outcome (McCullough et al., 1996). The current differential diagnostic requirements for the chronic disorders in the *DSM-IV* raise an important issue: Do these categories represent different disorders, or are they simply variations of the same disorder?

The only diagnostically based study comparing differences between the types of chronic depression described in DSM-III-R was reported recently (McCullough et al., in press). Diagnostic differences among those with double depression ($n = 216$), chronic major depression ($n = 294$), and double depression/chronic major depression ($n = 125$) were assessed across a wide range of measurement indices (e.g., sociodemographic variables, clinical course, symptomatology, psychosocial factors, general health functioning, Axis I and II comorbidity, depressive personality traits, family history of Axis I disorders, and acute phase response to treatment variables). *Similarities among the three diagnostic groups far outweighed the differences.* Another finding was that double depression/chronic major depression appeared to be a more severe condition in regard to the following variables: lower Global Assessment of Functioning scores (GAF: Axis V in the *DSM-III-R*), greater work impairment, a higher prevalence of depressive personality, and a greater likelihood of having sought psychotherapy in the past. In addition, the group with double depression/chronic major depression reported a significantly earlier age of onset for dysthymia than the group with double depression. Overall, however, the data suggest that *the three conditions are variations of the same disorder.* Before definite conclusions can be drawn about the differences among the chronic disorders, more comparative work needs to be done.

Ascertaining the value of differential diagnosis is important because of dysthymia's demonstrated moderator variable effects on the treatment response of patients with acute major depression (Keller, 1990; Keller, Lavori, Rice, et al., 1986; Keller & Shapiro, 1982; Keller et al., 1982b; Keller, Lavori, Endicott, et al., 1983). By the term "moderator variable" (Baron & Kenny, 1986; Holmbeck, 1997; Whisman, 1993), I mean that antecedent dysthymia has been found to interact with treatment of the syndromal disorder and to influence outcome (Keller & Hanks, 1994). Future research is needed to determine whether the second through the

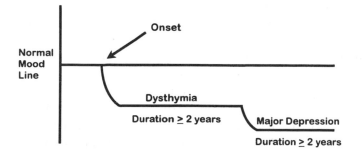

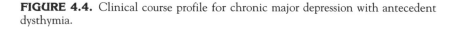

FIGURE 4.4. Clinical course profile for chronic major depression with antecedent dysthymia.

fifth chronic patterns listed earlier influence the (1) quality of the response to treatment, (2) time to response, (3) time to relapse and recurrence, and (4) overall relapse and recurrence rates.

Clearly, much work remains to be done before we will be able to show if the present differential diagnostic procedures now required by the *DSM-IV* are of value beyond the important function of discriminating the acute disorders from the chronic ones and determining whether or not dysthymia precedes an acute episode of major depression (McCullough et al., in press). I turn now to a discussion of the importance of identifying Axis I and II comorbidity when treating the chronic depressions.

DIAGNOSING COMORBIDITY

Dysthymia Cormorbid with Major Depression

Since the early 1980s, research has consistently found that when dysthymia and major depression are comorbid, failure to treat both disorders with aggressive, long-term regimens of pharmacotherapy and psychotherapy constitutes undertreatment; it not only results in a continuation of the dysthymic condition, but exacerbates the likelihood of recurring major depressive episodes (Harrison & Stewart, 1993; Keller & Hanks, 1994; Keller, Lavori, Lewis, et al., 1983; Simons & Thase, 1990; Thase, 1992; Weissman & Akiskal, 1984). Keller, Lavori, Endicott, et al. (1983), summarizing these findings, stated that "patients with double depression should receive intensive treatment after recovery from the episode of major depressive disorder, because it appears that they are predisposed to rapid relapse by the continued existence of the chronic preexisting depression [dysthymia]" (pp. 693–694).

These same authors also reported that 61% of major depression patients with antecedent dysthymia relapsed into a syndromal episode within one year. In addition, Keller and Shapiro (1982) warned that it is much easier to achieve remission of the major disorder than it is to achieve remission of the chronic, minor dysthymic condition. In the Keller, Lavori, Endicott, et al. (1983) study, in which patients with double depression were treated pharmacologically, 97% recovered from the major episode while only 39% recovered concomitantly from both major depression and dysthymia.

As noted above, dysthymia acts as a moderator variable when it is comorbid with major depression (Keller, 1990; Keller et al., 1982b; Keller, Lavori, Rice, et al., 1986). Dysthymia's moderating influence is also seen in the fact that patients with double depression recover more rapidly from the major episode than do patients with no history of dysthymia, but their time to relapse is shorter than it is among the latter group (Keller & Shapiro, 1982; Keller, Lavori, Endicott, et al., 1983). Antecedent dys-thymia clearly places both the treated and untreated individuals with major depression at high risk for repetitive episodes of major depression (Akiskal, 1983; Keller & Shapiro, 1982; Klein et al., 1998; Thase, 1992).

It is imperative that clinicians evaluate the presence or absence of the variables of *chronicity* and *antecedent dysthymia* in all patients they treat for major depression. When the antecedent mild to moderate disor-der is diagnosed in the history, the clinician should be alerted to the seri-ousness of the case, as well as sensitized to the prognostic dangers that often accompany misdiagnosis and undertreatment (Harrison & Stewart, 1993; Keller, Harrison, et al., 1995). Before treatment is terminated, the clinician should reassess the patient to determine whether or not the dysthymia has remitted. If the mild disorder is still present, treatment must continue.

Comorbid Axis II Personality Disorders

Another important diagnostic concern is determining whether or not an Axis II personality disorder is present (Markowitz, 1995; Markowitz, Moran, Kocsis, & Frances, 1992; McCullough, 1996a, 1996b). In a recent literature review (McCullough, 1996a), I reported that comorbid person-ality disorders are present in approximately 50% of chronically depressed outpatients. Most of the personality disorders are in the Cluster B (dra-matic, emotional, erratic) or Cluster C (anxious, fearful) categories. Riso et al. (1996) noted that many dysthymic patients present with Cluster B personality disorders and that individuals with borderline and antisocial personality disorders frequently exhibit higher rates of comorbid dys-thymia.

When a comorbid Axis II disorder is diagnosed in a chronically depressed patient, the treatment task becomes even more arduous, and successful outcomes are even more difficult to achieve (Akiskal, 1983; Alnaes & Torgensen, 1991; Farmer & Nelson-Gray, 1990; Keller, 1990). With the foreknowledge that a personality disorder may be part of the presenting problem, clinicians can proceed armed with an awareness of the interpersonal-behavioral issues that are likely to arise. Addressing the interpersonal-behavioral aspects of treatment will be discussed fully in Chapter 8.

The next section describes the psychological features of a group of chronic depressives who volunteered to be studied under nontreatment conditions. The primary aim of the research was to deepen our understanding of the refractory nature of these disorders by examining the personality trait, cognitive features, interpersonal features, and social coping styles of chronically depressed individuals who had agreed to forgo treatment for an extended period.

PSYCHOLOGICAL CHARACTERISTICS OF UNTREATED CHRONICALLY DEPRESSED ADULTS

In a series of longitudinal studies, my colleagues and I (McCullough et al., 1988, 1990, 1994a, 1994b) described the psychological features of 58 untreated chronically depressed adults. Also identified were the spontaneous remission rates for the disorders in the absence of treatment. Another concern was to determine whether the symptom and psychological patterns of subjects remained stable over time, as would be expected, given the label of "chronic disorders." Untreated subjects diagnosed as having either pure dysthymia or double depression were prospectively followed for 9–12 months and were rediagnosed and assessed psychologically over time.

Summarizing the data, we found unchanging symptom profiles and stable levels of depression intensity for most subjects. We also observed that some subjects (about 13%) showed spontaneous remission during the first year of the study. Seven of nine remitters were available for diagnostic interviews two and a half to four years after the studies ended; of these seven, two were diagnosed as having relapsed. We concluded that the prognosis for spontaneous recovery rate among untreated subjects appears to be poor and that, when remission does occur, relapse occurs in approximately 29% of the cases.

Our untreated chronic depression subjects typically scored high in neuroticism (poor emotional control) and low in extraversion (denoting introversion and poor sociability patterns) on the Eysenck Personality Inventory (Eysenck & Eysenck, 1968). High neuroticism and low extraversion scores are consistent with the conclusions discussed earlier in Chapter 3: Chronic patients begin treatment in a state of emotional dysregulation (high neuroticism), and poor sociability patterns are prominent and are associated with trait introversion.

Our subjects also complained of feeling helpless, and they verbalized the belief that they had little or no control over what happened to them. A common complaint was this: "I cannot control my depression, and I have no control over my life." We examined the subjects' perceptual orientation via Rotter's I-E Scale (Reid & Ware, 1974; Rotter, 1966, 1978) and substantiated the source of the feelings of helplessness as well as the eschewal of personal responsibility for the depression. Subjects obtained external locus of control scores on this scale and these scores remained stable over a one-year period. A person with an external locus of control perceives the major causal influences in life as residing outside his/her sphere of influence; thus fate, luck, chance, or sociopolitical forces were endorsed as major causal variables in the worldviews of these subjects.

In a series of replicated single-case studies (Sidman, 1960) in which the CBASP approach was used to treat 10 chronically depressed adults (McCullough, 1991), the mean externality score on the I-E Scale for the group at screening was 14.5 (SD = 2.9). The group scores fell into the internality range by the end of treatment, when the group mean reached 5.9 (SD = 3.1). These shifts toward internality suggest that perceptions of control can be modified when patients are taught how to manage their environment more effectively. The movement from an external toward an internal locus of control is one of the essential goals of CBASP. Patients are taught systematically to relinquish the fiction that they exert little or no influence or control over what happens to them. Movement toward internality on Rotter's I-E Scale is one indication that a shift is occurring in the perceived locus of control.

Statements about feeling hopeless are another type of complaint often heard during therapy. In our studies, these feelings of hopelessness were reflected in subjects' high scores on the stability and globality subscales of the Attributional Style Questionnaire (Peterson et al., 1982). Not only do chronic patients see no end to their depression (stability), but they also view the depression as affecting most areas of daily living (globality). Again, these stability and globality scores remained constant over a one-year period.

I have already mentioned that chronically depressed adults bring inadequate social coping repertoires to psychotherapy. Administering the Ways of Coping Questionnaire (Folkman & Lazarus, 1980) to our untreated subjects, we found that the coping subscales most subjects endorsed mirrored our in-session observations of patients in psychotherapy. These chronically depressed adults relied on wishful thinking and blaming themselves as major strategies for coping with stress.

Subjects also displayed very poor problem-focused coping skills—another characteristic shared by beginning psychotherapy patients. Therapists typically find that chronic patients are unable to focus on any *one* problem situation; rather, they describe their problems in global, not problem-focused, terms. To illustrate the point, we asked our untreated subjects to pinpoint "two major life stressors" and rate their severity. One year later, we queried them about the severity of the two designated stressors and the degree to which they had been resolved. Most subjects reported no change in severity of the stressors, not to mention the lack of any resolution. These findings are consonant with complaints of helplessness and hopelessness made by chronic patients who invariably describe themselves in impotent and despairing terms. Once again, the subjects evinced stable scores in their poor coping patterns over time.

Interpersonal functioning also does not appear to change over time. Investigating the interpersonal styles of subjects with pure dysthymia or double depression (McCullough et al., 1988, 1994a, 1994b), at screening and one year later, we found that interpersonal functioning did not change. Following the diagnostic interviews, clinical raters used the Impact Message Inventory (IMI: Kiesler & Schmidt, 1993), an instrument measuring a range of interpersonal styles, and rated the subjects as submissive, interpersonally detached, nervous, and/or anxious during the interviews. The ratings placed subjects on the "submissive" or "hostile-submissive" octants of the IMI Interpersonal Circle (Kiesler, 1996; Kiesler & Schmidt, 1993), which is discussed fully in Chapter 8.

These interpersonal styles program individuals to live out a "victim lifestyle" when interacting with others. Characteristically, submissive interpersonal styles naturally "pull" or "push" others into a dominant role, thereby placing the individual (realistically) in a one-down position. In the therapy context, this means that the clinician is sitting with a person who consistently waits to be told what to do and how to do it. What is the clinician's response likely to be? After a while, most therapists become impatient and find it tempting to take over and begin telling patients what to do. In the course of supervising therapists who treat chronic patients, I have learned to be alert for dominant behavior on the part of practitioners because such behavior only reinforces the submissive stance of these patients.

Coyne (1976) also described a destructively submissive interpersonal style of behavior in depressed patients. He argued that this submissive behavior is subtly reinforced even by well-meaning individuals who wish to see them behave more autonomously. All too often friends react to the submissive behavior by directly intervening and telling the depressed person what he/she should and should not do. I find myself repeatedly reminding CBASP clinicians that the submissive patterns of chronic patients are maintained every time they assume a dominant interpersonal role.

Consistent with the data regarding the stability of diagnosis and psychosocial functioning over time among untreated chronically depressed subjects, a recent study by Klein et al. (1998) followed 86 outpatients with early-onset dysthymia in a 30-month naturalistic study. A baseline evaluation was conducted soon after admission to the clinic. The stability of their diagnosis and the prevalence of symptoms were assessed at 30 months. Diagnostic status was fairly stable (only 39% recovered during the course of the 30-months follow-up period), and many of the early-onset patients still exhibited mild to moderate depressive symptoms. The chronic course of dysthymia was once again confirmed.

NEED FOR AN INTEGRATIVE THERAPEUTIC PROGRAM

The plain truth is that we have had much better success in describing the chronic depressive disorders than we have had in treating them (McCullough et al., 1996). Furthermore, most of the post-treatment data available today come predominantly from pharamacological research. Very little information is available from psychotherapy research because few clinical trials have been undertaken with chronic patients (Markowitz, 1994; McCullough, 1991).

To date, no integrative psychotherapy program has been developed to address the multidimensional problems (cognitive-emotional, behavioral, interpersonal) of chronically depressed patients. It is not surprising, therefore, that traditional domain-specific techniques (e.g., IPT for interpersonal problems; CT for cognitive and behavioral problems) have not been particularly effective (Hoberman, Lewinsohn, & Tilson, 1988; Sotsky et al., 1991; Thase et al., 1994). Robert Howland (1996), in his review of several treatment approaches with dysthymics, emphasizes the need for a more integrative model that addresses the myriad functional deficiences of patients:

... as noted, dysthymia can be distinguished from major depression in several important ways, which can pose a problem for therapists accustomed to dealing with the acute time-limited nature of major depression. As such, it is useful to consider an integrative psychotherapy model that draws on specific characteristics of different theoretical orientations that can be applied to the unique problems seen in chronically depressed clients. (p. 235)

If clinicians seek to treat chronic patients successfully, they first need to be aware of the multiple levels of problems they are likely to encounter:

- A history of developmental trauma and repeated interpersonal failure
- Primitive cognitive functioning evidenced by a pre-causal view of the world
- A tacit expectation that the major causal influences in life always remain beyond the patient's personal control
- Coping skill repertoires that are deficient and that prevent these persons from being able to focus specifically on any one particular problem
- Distressing emotional dysregulation that interferes with social, familial, and occupational functioning
- A profound sense of hopelessness and helplessness, inhibiting any optimism that treatment will change anything
- Interpersonal–social behavior that is ineffective at best and blatantly offensive at worst
- A submissive style of interacting that makes it difficult for clinicians to avoid assuming a dominant role
- Interpersonal distrust arising out of real-world experiences

Given that as many as 95% of persons with emotional and mental problems in the United States are treated by primary-care doctors and general practitioners (Wilkinson, 1989), many patients have previous treatment histories characterized by the following factors and experiences:

- Patients enter psychotherapy with a previous history of misdiagnosis.
- Those who have previously received an antidepressant drug are more than likely to have been prescribed less than an adequate therapeutic dose and to have spent insufficient time on the drug.
- Those who report having undergone some form of psychotherapy

will probably admit that they obtained very little benefit for their efforts.
- Rarely will patients report receiving a combination form of treatment that included an adequate dose of both psychotherapy and medication.

In light of these common factors, it is not surprising that the outcome track record for psychotherapy and pharmacotherapy has been only fair to moderate with this class of patients.

The CBASP model is offered as an integrative and comprehensive plan to modify the multiple problem areas that afflict chronically depressed patients. The offensive therapeutic game plan to be described in Part II has been carefully constructed to address every defensive maneuver of these patients I have encountered.

PART TWO

CBASP METHOD AND PROCEDURES

CHAPTER FIVE

Strategies to Enhance Motivation for Change

Teaching is arranging contingencies so people learn.
—B. F. SKINNER (1968, p. 5)

THE IMPORTANCE OF MOTIVATION

Motivating chronically depressed adults to change their behavior is one of the most difficult tasks psychotherapists face. These patients' pervasive sense of helplessness and hopelessness, combined with their detached interpersonal style, presents a formidable barrier. The motivational predicament is captured by the words of one patient: "It doesn't matter what I do; I will stay depressed." This sentence describes the central motivational predicament of the patient. The truth of the matter is that chronically depressed individuals have usually tried everything they can find to stop being depressed, but nothing has worked. Naturally, they give up trying sooner or later. If the lack of motivation to change is to be modified, something must be added to the patient's perspective. The addition entails *awakening patients to the fact that their behavior has consequences.* Once patients begin to associate their behavior with consequences, two things happen: Behavior change occurs, and motivation to change increases.

B. F. Skinner was correct in his contention that consequences influence behavior. What Skinner did not discuss was the circumstance in

69

which persons do not perceive a connection between what they do and subsequent effects. Before consequences can have a formative influence on behavior, individuals must make a connection between their behavior and the subsequent consequences. At the beginning of treatment, contingency thinking—"If this . . . then that"—is beyond the capability of chronic patients. As long as chronic patients are able to maintain the *preoperational fiction* that how they behave doesn't matter, they will remain helpless victims, hopelessly mired in the negative spiral of their depressive disorder. It is the task of therapy to undercut the preoperational fiction by demonstrating to patients that everything they do produces effects in the environment.

PERCEIVING ENVIRONMENTAL CONSEQUENCES

The importance of teaching patients to recognize behavioral consequences can be gleaned from the following attempt at dialogue between a beginning patient, "Cora," and her therapist. The patient is obviously unaware that her behavior has any effect on the environment.

CORA: The company photographer went around at the meeting and was taking pictures of all the people in my department. He never once asked to take my picture.

THERAPIST: What did you do?

CORA: He took pictures of Fred and Judy. She always gets her picture in the company magazine. I'm always overlooked—no one ever thinks about including me.

THERAPIST: Did you say anything to anyone about wanting your picture taken? Did you talk to the photographer?

CORA: People are really inconsiderate. They never think of what I might want or need!

THERAPIST: Cora, did you say anything to anyone about what you wanted?

CORA: People just ought to be more considerate. Why should you have to ask people to be nice? Anyway, I'm being childish about this. It's really not that important anyway.

Before consequences can be used to change behavior, individuals must view themselves and their relationship to the environment in a *perceived functional manner* (Bandura, 1977b; Baron, Kaufman, & Stauber, 1969; Kaufman, Baron, & Kopp, 1966; McCullough, 1984a). Perceived functionality in CBASP must be differentiated from Bandura's (1977a, 1982, 1986) "outcome expectancy" construct, wherein attention is focused on the role of personal efficacy in determining the choice made between continuing to work at some task and disengaging from the task. Perceived functionality also differs from "dispositional optimism," a term used by Scheier and Carver (1987, 1992) to describe behavior arising out of a person's subjective probability expectancy that some outcome in the environment will or will not occur. Perceived functionality, as it is used in CBASP, simply denotes one's perception of a contingency relationship between behavior and its consequences. Chronically depressed adults live without a well-developed perception of this contingency relationship. Perceived functionality is referred to in CBASP as "If this . . . then that" thinking.

Patients like Cora don't understand their functional connection to the world. The next example presents a striking contrast to Cora's preoperational worldview by showing what happens when a late-in-therapy patient, "Shirley," not only perceives her impact on the environment but also uses it effectively.

SHIRLEY: The company exec officer asked several persons in our office if they would be interested in taking an advanced computer training course using the company's software. I don't really have the computer skills that some of my work colleagues do, but I wanted to check with the exec and see if he felt I might be eligible. So I went into his office that afternoon and asked him if I qualified for the course. He said that I would not qualify for the course, but if I would be interested in moving into such work in the future, there were some specific things I could do to prepare myself. He said I could take a home study preparatory course that would make me eligible. I told him I would take his suggestion and begin the course right away.

THERAPIST: Well, this outcome was obviously not what you wanted, right?

SHIRLEY: No, it wasn't. But at least I found out what I have to do to put myself in a position so that when he offers the course again, I'll be ready.

Cora did not act directly on her environment, whereas Shirley did. Why? The answer lies in their descriptions of their respective situations. Cora saw no connection between her silence and not getting her picture taken, stating instead that people just ought to be more considerate; Shirley, on the other hand, understood the connection between taking action now and making herself eligible for a position later. She verbalized that taking the advanced training course would increase the probability of her being selected later. Shirley was thinking in an "If this . . . then that" manner, whereas Cora was thinking preoperationally.

Cora frequently discussed her interpersonal problems with the therapist and often said, as in the example above, that others *should* behave differently toward her and be more considerate. Two problems are embedded in her complaints: (1) Cora's perception of her relationship with others remains on a precausal level (i.e., "Others ought to behave the way I want them to, simply because *I* want them to"), and (2) she doesn't have the assertive skills to obtain what she wants. Cora's therapist mistakenly overlooked her preoperational orientation and pointed out her behavioral omission in a logical, causal analysis of the situation:

THERAPIST: Cora, the photographer may not have known you wanted your picture taken, or he might have just accidentally overlooked you.

The therapist forgot that she was dealing with a preoperational individual, and she fell into a trap that therapists encounter. Cora's next response was predictable. She reiterated her preoperational worldview:

CORA: Well, people just ought to know how to be nice. You shouldn't have to remind people to be considerate. Anyway, I shouldn't be worried about such a silly thing. It's not important anyway.

Is there a way to change preoperational behavior other than by just telling patients logically what they must do? The following section illustrates one way it can be done.

PATIENT MISERY AND THE NEGATIVE REINFORCEMENT PARADIGM

The basis for changing the behavior of chronic patients resides solidly in their state of misery. Their general psychological distress (Derogatis, 1983;

McCullough et al., 1988, 1994a), their despair over ever feeling normal "like other people," their distrust of others, and their history of negative interpersonal encounters constitute a powerful reservoir of misery that can be used to administer negative reinforcement (Skinner, 1953) and thereby to provoke change in their behavior.

How is this accomplished in the session? Any behavior that leads to relief from chronic distress can be strengthened if therapists remain vigilant and help patients recognize which behavior led to the reduction in their discomfort level. For example, "Carol," a reticent and timid patient, asserted herself to a colleague for the first time and discovered that the verbal abuse or rejection she expected did not occur. Instead, the other person listened to her and thoughtfully considered what she had said. This led to a profound sense of relief and joy as the expected interpersonal catastrophe did not occur. At first Carol did not perceive the connection between her assertion, the colleague's reaction, and the decrease in discomfort that resulted. When she analyzed the situation during the next therapy session, she easily recalled the felt relief but saw no link between her assertive behavior and her felt relief:

"I felt such relief that my colleague did not rake me over the coals for what I said. God, what a wonderful feeling!"

On these occasions, it is the job of the clinician to make sure that the "If this . . . then that" association is made explicit to the person. In Carol's case, the therapist helped her recreate what had led to her feelings of relief; in this way, the moment of negative reinforcement is palpably reexperienced. Carol learned that relief from her discomfort was under *her* control, contingent upon her willingness to assert herself. Skinner (1953) assumed that the association between behavior and the contiguous termination of the aversive state would be made automatically by the organism. A contemporary example of his negative reinforcement paradigm is the sequence of (1) feeling the discomfort of a headache, (2) taking two aspirin, and (3) feeling relief from the headache. The next time a headache occurs, the person reaches for the aspirin bottle. The contiguous association between the behavior (taking aspirin) and termination of the aversive state (the headache) is strengthened over time. As noted above, these basic associations are not readily apparent to chronically depressed, preoperational adults. In a case like Carol's, the assertiveness and the subsequent felt relief must be made explicit to the individual; otherwise, the "If this . . . then that" relationship between behavior and consequence is likely to be over-looked.

I call these in-therapy instances "relief moments": Observable decreases in discomfort levels that result from some internal or external behavior of the patient. Such potential negative reinforcement events signal that the individual has emitted some type of salubrious behavior. If the patient cannot readily identify the contingencies that led to the felt relief, then the therapist must stop and examine what produced the cessation of distress. Helping the patient target the antecedent behavior that preceded the relief moment is the place to start. The following example illustrates how a relief moment can be used with another patient, "Leah," to actualize the delivery of negative reinforcement in the session.

LEAH: I never thought I could tell my husband I didn't like the way he was treating me—he's always been so rude to me. He has always treated me like dirt.

THERAPIST: Well, you just said you told him how badly he was treating you. What was his reaction?

LEAH: He said he never realized what he was doing to me. I felt more encouraged, and I laid it all out to him—how I had avoided him because of his rude behavior. He just listened and looked sad. It all turned out so unbelievably! He and I talked for the first time. It is the first time I have felt hopeful about the marriage in years (*observable relief with a corresponding increase in energy and general excitement*).

THERAPIST: You're almost coming out of your seat with relief and excitement right now. Every time you've talked about your marriage with me, you've cried and talked like you're miserable. Now you're hopeful and energetic. Why the change? (*The therapist knows why but plays a naive role—it is crucial that the patient sees the "If this . . . then that" connection.*)

LEAH: Because I told him how I felt—it made a difference, a real difference in how I'm feeling. I've gone from despair to feeling hope. It's the first time I have felt this way since I've been coming to see you.

THERAPIST: You say you are feeling the relief and hope right now?

LEAH: Yes.

THERAPIST: Let's go back and review the steps that led to these feelings. Briefly, take me through the steps.

LEAH: I told him how I felt, he listened, and we talked for the first time! My despair went away and I started feeling hopeful right then.

THERAPIST: Tell me what brought on the hope feelings.

LEAH: Telling him how I felt and what I wanted.

THERAPIST: Did putting your cards on the table with your husband lead you to start feeling hopeful?

LEAH: I never thought of it that way before. Letting him know what I felt and wanted led to my feeling hopeful.

THERAPIST: Are you telling me that it really matters how you behave— that it can make a difference in how you feel about your marriage and how your husband responds to you?

LEAH: That's exactly what I am saying!

THERAPIST: I've got to ask you one more question—it's so important that you know the answer. You did something new and different in this situation. Is your behavior change what decreased your despair about the marriage and led to your feelings of hope?

LEAH: Yes!

Targeting the antecedent behavior that led to a decrease in misery reinforces the new, more adaptive behavior. The next time this patient is feeling miserable about her marriage, she will have this new tool in her "tool belt" of life experience to use to decrease her discomfort.

Leah's example contains both positive *and* negative reinforcement events. The husband proffered the positive reinforcement by listening to his wife's feedback. Negative reinforcement was also present with the acknowledged decrease in Leah's discomfort. I focus here on the negative reinforcement event because of the overwhelming impact that distress and depressed mood have upon these patients. Among chronically depressed adults, the importance of the negative reinforcement event always overshadows whatever positive reinforcers are present. Why? Because without a decrease in the intensity of the patient's distress and depression, the patient remains stuck in the withdrawal phase of the depressive experience, with its concomitant feelings of hopelessness and despair. The CBASP program prompts the patient to enact more adaptive behavior in the environment. If the behavior does not lead to a termination of the distress, it will not ultimately matter whether the environmental response is a positive reinforcer. *This has been the patient's problem all along!* That is, nothing the individual has done has been able to overthrow the depression. *Until the depressive cycle is broken, any positive reinforcement present in the situation will have no forma-tive influence on the individual.*

The above scenario illustrates one way in which the "relief moment" can be used to actualize the delivery of negative reinforcement in the ses-sion and to increase motivation to change. This strategy can be adminis-tered many times during treatment if therapists remain observant and look for the relief moments when they occur. In addition, relief moments can also be achieved by deliberately intensifying the patient's discomfort through examination of aversive interpersonal events or through a focus on negative aspects of the patient's dyadic relationship with the clinician. Relief moments occur in sessions as patients are assisted in resolving the problem in the present by enacting more adaptive behavior. The adminis-tration of negative reinforcement in these instances will be described in the remainder of the chapter.

When relief moments are managed optimally, the results can be dra-matic. The contrasts between normal mood and chronic dysphoria, between hope and interminable despair, and between interpersonal em-powerment and isolating helplessness can serve as significant learning experiences when patients are taught to recognize *what produced the shift* from negative to positive affect. I have worked with some patients who, when they experienced hope for what felt like the first time in their lives, broke into a radiant smile that was like a ray of sunshine streaking through the clouds on an otherwise gloomy afternoon. The change pro-cess in other patients may be more gradual and less dramatic—though no less gratifying. Regardless of the pace, low motivation levels are difficult to maintain as individuals learn that they have the power to decrease their suffering through enactment of more adaptable behavior.

Recognizing causal sequences between interpersonal behavior and consequences requires formal operations thinking. Before patients can catch the full impact of what has led to a cessation of their distress, they must first think logically and causally in an "If this . . . then that" man-ner. I turn now to a discussion of how formal operations training is under-taken in the CBASP program.

TEACHING FORMAL OPERATIONS THINKING TO MODIFY THE PREOPERATIONAL DILEMMA

The CBASP program requires preoperational patients to solve their depression problems by engaging in formal operational problem-solving exercises. The basic principle underlying these exercises is that of "mismatching demands" (Cowan, 1978; Gordon, 1988; Nannis, 1988). The principle can be stated as follows: If didactic exercises are presented at a level matching the person's current level of functioning (i.e., the preoperational level), change will not occur. However, if the didactic exercises are "optimally mismatched"—that is, are offered on levels exceeding the patient's current level of functioning—cognitive operations will be sufficiently challenged and maturational-cognitive shifts will follow (Cowan, 1978). Teaching preoperational patients to solve interpersonal problems on a formal operations level results in a structural reorganization of thinking and moves individuals to a more mature plane of cognitive functioning.

Two formal thinking exercises are used; both require patients to engage in *perceived functional thinking* and to describe their interpersonal encounters from an *empathic perspective*. By the time patients master the two tasks, they are using formal operations processes in their thinking, emoting, talking, and behaving. The exercises also help patients identify what they need to do in order to avoid their customary felt discomfort in specific situations.

The first exercise consists of exacerbating and then resolving a patient's psychopathology in the therapy session by means of a response-consequence technique called *Situational Analysis* (SA). The second response-consequence task, called the *Interpersonal Discrimination Exercise* (IDE), contrasts the behavior of the therapist with that of significant others. Since the patient has typically endured a fair amount of maltreatment, it is not difficult to compare and contrast the facilitative behavior of the clinician with experiences from the old history. Before I discuss and illustrate the two exercises, a caveat to clinicians concerning administration is essential: *Do not take over the responsibility of effecting change in a patient's behavior; let the in-session strategies do the work for you!*

AVOIDING TAKEOVER PITFALLS

One of the most seductive temptations practitioners face in working with chronically depressed patients is the temptation to "take over" and do the work for them. Another way to say the same thing is to say that psychotherapists often assume responsibility for changing patient behavior. The outcome of this tactic is *always* predictable: Patients are protected from confronting the consequences of their own behavior. As a result, they don't learn, and they certainly are not motivated to change.

Examples of these takeover strategies are seen (1) when clinicians tell patients what they ought and ought not to do to resolve their problems; (2) when clinicians make interpretations to explain behavior, or when they dispute dysfunctional cognitions or beliefs by using logic; (3) when clinicians preach, cajole, encourage, shame, or make outright demands on patients to behave differently; and, finally, (4) when clinicians arbitrarily try to make patients feel better by acting as well-intentioned fortunetellers who assure them, "Things will get better," "I know the future holds good things for you," and so on. Each of these strategies is intended to facilitate change, and though they may work with some populations, they fail utterly with chronic depressives. It is my opinion that one reason traditional CT seems to have limited success with chronically depressed patients (Thase, 1992; Thase et al., 1992, 1994) is the fact that, in CT, therapists typically assume an active takeover role with patients, inadvertently relieving them of the responsibility for change and thus protecting them from facing the consequences of their behavior.

Frankly, it is understandable why therapists resort to takeover strategies with chronically depressed patients. Such tactics are most likely to be attempted under three sets of circumstances. First, at the outset of treatment, many patients present such an extreme picture of dejection, distress, despair, and helplessness that most caring psychotherapists want to intervene and lessen the discomfort as quickly as possible. It can seem natural to assure these patients that things will improve or that they will soon feel better. Second, during SA, therapists may try to ease the patient's burden with too much assistance (much more will be said about this takeover tactic in Chapters 6 and 7). Third, during later sessions, a lack of improvement may push a therapist into feelings of frustration that can sometimes lead to takeover maneuvers.

When I watch a videotape of a session and see this takeover error enacted by a newly trained psychotherapist, it appears to me as if the therapist were saying to himself/herself, "All right, dammit, if you're not going to change, then I'll change you myself. This is what you have to do!" My advice to the therapist is always the same: "Avoid taking responsibility for doing the work that only the patient can do!"

Once patients are able to discriminate clearly between the consequences of maladaptive behavior and the consequences of more adaptive strategies, clinicians have done their job and have avoided the temptation to take responsibility for change. Now the patient has arrived at a crucial choice point. If the patient decides to continue to behave maladaptively, then he/she does so with the awareness of the consequences. The task for the psychotherapist on such occasions is simply to remind patients that if they tire of producing these unsavory outcomes, then they know what to do. I turn now to a brief description of SA, a central exercise in formal operations training, employed to modify behavior.

SITUATIONAL ANALYSIS: EXACERBATION AND RESOLUTION OF PSYCHOPATHOLOGY

There are two major phases in SA: the "elicitation phase" and the "remediation phase." During the elicitation phase, SA is used as an interpersonal, cognitive behavioral diagnostic tool for both clinicians and patients. As patients proceed through the elicitation steps, describing their specific contributions to particular aspects of a social encounter, various forms of interpersonal, cognitive, and behavioral pathology are revealed. During the remediation phase, pathological behaviors are targeted for change and then revised until the patient's new behavior brings the situation to a desirable conclusion. What follows is a glimpse into the methodology and administration of SA. Chapters 6 and 7 will elaborate extensively the steps described below. To show how the two phases of the exercise, elicitation, and remediation are administered, let's look at a situational event that "Paul," a late-onset patient, brought to his therapy session.

> "Well, the event started five days ago on Monday when my boss ['Fred'] asked me to compile a list of outstanding real estate contracts in his district so that he could include the information in his report to the City Council on Thursday. He said that presenting this information was important to him. I didn't have a chance to tell him that I have been so busy that I didn't have time to do the research on the contracts—I never pulled the information together. When I got to work about 9:00 A.M.—let's see, today is Friday—my boss called me into the office and yelled at me. He told me I was irresponsible, and that I had embarrassed him at the City Council meeting last night. He said he had had to give the report without the real estate data. I told him I was sorry—he was too mad to hear me. I don't think he appreciates the work I do for him. The situation ended when I left his office feeling like I had been a bad boy."

The consequences for Paul's behavior are obvious. He didn't complete the real estate research, and his boss chastised him for the failure. However, the conclusion Paul draws about his boss's reaction (the consequences) is completely off the topic:

"I don't think he appreciates the work I do for him."

Because Paul is not aware of the specific and relevant consequence that was linked to his behavior, it is unlikely that he will modify his behavior in the future to avoid similar mistakes.

If you look closely at Paul's description of the event, two problems crop up as a result of how he processed his boss's request that he compile the outstanding real estate contracts. First, Paul missed the point of Fred's informative evaluation of this task as important; Paul did not register the request as being a "must do" type of job. Second, he failed to connect his boss's anger to his failure to do the work. Cognitive and behavioral deficits were thus evidenced in Paul's experience of the event as it unfolded, as well as later in his reflection on it. What was also obvious to the therapist during the elicitation phase was Paul's general distress over the fact that Fred didn't appreciate his work.

Answers to six therapist prompts comprise the core of the SA during the elicitation phase. The prompts are as follows:

1. Describe what happened in the situation.
2. Describe your *interpretation(s)* of what happened.
3. Describe what you *did* in the situation.
4. Describe how the event came out for you, that is, what was the *actual outcome?*
5. Describe how you would have wanted the event to come out for you. That is, what is your *desired outcome?*
6. Did you get what you wanted here? (Why?/Why not?)

As the therapist began the SA, Paul's cognitive interpretations and behavioral strategies were specified. Then the therapist asked Paul, "How did the event come out for you?" We call this step pinpointing the "actual outcome" (AO). Attention is focused on the patient's perception of the outcome. Even though Paul missed being able to see *why* his boss had chastised him, his answer to the AO question was not corrected: "Fred yelled at me, and I left the office." (he then went on to say, "Fred doesn't appreciate what I do for him.")

Next, Paul was asked, "How would you have liked the situation to have come out?" This step is called pinpointing the "desired outcome" (DO) and is part of every SA exercise. Paul's answer was interesting: "I wanted the boss to thank me for the work I did for him." Does this sound incredible? It is not at all unusual for patients to desire outcomes that are precluded by their own behavior. We can see immediately that what Paul wants from the boss is not achievable, given his failure to do the assigned work. The problem is that Paul doesn't see it this way. All he sees and feels is that he is an unappreciated employee. When a patient like Paul is asked, "Did you get what you wanted here?", distress frequently becomes obvious because of the failure to obtain the desired outcome. Ideally, the second phase of SA—remediation—will lead to a reduction of the discomfort, along with the concomitant opportunity to administer negative reinforcement for more adaptive behavior.

How can Paul's therapist make the behavioral consequences explicit to him without engaging in the takeover strategy of just *telling him* why Fred became upset? The therapist wants Paul to catch the full gale winds of the consequences he has produced; that is, the therapist wants to increase his felt discomfort. This is done this by asking him, "*Why* didn't you get what you wanted here?" Paul has to explain to the therapist why he failed to produce the DO. His response to this question is, "Fred just doesn't appreciate the work I do for him."

The SA thus exacerbated Paul's situational dilemma, and it made explicit his pathological cognitive and behavioral maneuvers. At this point, the therapist is aware of the pathological components of Paul's behavior. Paul will become aware of his problematical behavior in the next phase of SA. The second phase of every SA, remediation, begins with a review of the problematical event and an assessment of the attainability of the desired outcome. The goal for this phase in Paul's case is to reduce his distress by having him "fix" his own behavior so that he can achieve the DO. The therapist reviewed the situation with Paul, examining the adequacy of his cognitive interpretations and behaviors, in order to show Paul how they resulted in his failure to obtain the DO.

The remediation phase is directed by the clinician who helps Paul examine his situational behavior. Paul is prompted to evaluate his behavior in a stepwise fashion, following the therapist's prompt questions:

1. How did each interpretation contribute to your obtaining the desired outcome?

2. How did your behavior help you obtain the desired outcome?
3. What did you learn in going through this SA?
4. How does what you have learned in this situation apply to other similar situations?

As the therapist takes Paul though the remediation steps of the exercise, Paul will finally recognize the impossibility of achieving his DO, given the fact that he had failed to do the work. Paul was thereby guided to revise his interpretations of Fred's request. With assistance, he finally recognized that the request had a top-priority status and that he would have had to put aside his other work and complete the research on time in order to garner his boss's gratitude (the DO).

A relief moment often accompanies the insight that what a patient has perceived as an "impossible" interpersonal situation is actually resolvable. What behaviors are then reinforced? The specific cognitions and behaviors that resolve the problematical event and help patients achieve their DOs.

When the exercise was completed, the therapist asked Paul what he had learned. Paul summarized the "solution components" that were needed to obtain the DO. In this manner, SA helps patients resolve problematical interpersonal events and reduces general distress by demonstrating to them that they can solve their own problems through making certain changes in the way they think and behave. The last step of remediation was completed when Paul was able to generalize what he had learned in this situation to other similar events he recalled.

Dealing with Negative Affect

SA often exacerbates the negative affect that was present during the targeted situation. When the event is analyzed, whatever emotions that were present during the event often resurface: confusion, frustration, anger, fear, rejection, guilt, and shame. CBASP therapists learn to highlight the negative affect during SA, so that when solutions are identified, patients can then compare and contrast the original situation *without a solution* to the revised situation *with a solution*. When relief moments occur during SA, therapists assist patients in identifying the specific cognitive and behavioral processes that precipitated the relief. In this manner, negative reinforcement is administered for the adaptive patterns, with the result being that motivation to change is increased.

SA Must Be an Existential Encounter for Patients

What needs to be avoided in SA is a discussion of stressful events in which a therapist and patient just "talk about" the interpersonal situation. Patients cease to be existential participants at such times and simply become observers. When individuals talk about their problems, the goal of experiencing consequences is thwarted, motivation to change remains low, and the change process is aborted. The SA exercise can engender high drama when it is administered in a sensitive and disciplined manner. Another case example can best illustrate the existential nature of the SA exercise.

"Jane," a 24-year-old executive secretary for a computer firm, described a situation involving her boss. We will proceed stepwise through the SA to illustrate again how SA is administered and experienced. Jane was an early-onset patient with double depression.

Prompt: Describe what happened in the situation.
Step 1. *Jane's situational description.*

"Last Wednesday afternoon I was approached by my boss ['Bill'] and asked to stay after 5:00 P.M. to help him finish some work. He told me it would take about three hours. I had an important date with my boyfriend ['John'] that night. We were supposed to go to a play at the Kennedy Center in Washington. My boss asked me in a nice way, and I agreed to stay late. And so I worked late and missed going to the play."

Prompt: What did the event mean to you?
Step 2. *Elicitation of Jane's cognitive interpretations.*

Jane was asked to formulate each interpretation in one sentence that described what the event meant to her. After several attempts to do this, she was able to reduce her lengthy explanation to three sentences that became the interpretations for the analysis:

1. "I can't say 'no' to Bill."
2. "John and I won't be able to go to the play."
3. "Bill was in a jam and needed my help."

The clinician wanted to focus next on how Jane behaved with Bill. For example, he wanted Jane to tell him how she had stood and gestured while they talked. Then he asked her to tell him exactly what she had said and to describe the manner in which she had said it. Jane's verbal style turned out to be passive and whiny.

Prompt: What did you do in the situation?
Step 3. *Elicitation of Jane's behavioral strategies.*

> "I sorta whined, looked down at my feet and told him that I really didn't want to—that I had something else to do. Bill was insistent, and I whined again and said, 'Oh, all right.' I never really looked him in the face during the conversation. I was too scared to."

Prompt: How did the event come out for you?
Step 4. *Elicitation of the actual outcome (AO) in behavioral language.*

> "I worked late and missed the play."

Prompt: How would you have liked the event to come out?
Step 5. *Elicitation of the desired outcome (DO) in behavioral language.*

> "I wanted to tell Bill 'no' and go to the play."

Prompt: Did you get what you wanted here?
Step 6a. *Highlighting the consequences (to increase discomfort) by inquiring whether the patient achieved what she wanted in this situation.*

> "No! I missed the play! I failed again, and now John is mad at me for messing up our plans (starting to cry). I keep failing to get what I want. I've always done this. I can't keep from doing it."

Prompt: Why do you think you didn't get what you wanted here?
Step 6b. *Highlighting the consequences again by assessing the degree to which the patient is aware of why she failed to achieve the DO.*

> "Because I never can say no to anyone who wants something from me. In high school, I slept with any guy who asked me, because I never could get up the courage to say 'no.' I hate myself. I am weak and no good."

Jane is on the "hot seat"; she has described an aversive event that suggests a personal failing. Now the clinician will use her discomfort in the present moment as the focal point for constructing a remedial cognitive and behavioral solution that reduces the distress—telling Bill "no" and attending the play. If Jane's affect changes in a positive direction when she realizes that she can say "no" to Bill, the therapist will highlight the relief moment and assist her in identifying what led to this decrease in discomfort.

Jane reports a lifetime history of interpersonal misery stemming from repetitive enactment of behavior similar to what she described in this SA. Jane's inability to take seriously what she wants and act assertively to obtain it has always placed her in a "one-down" position when faced with interpersonal demands. Jane's situation with her boss is representative of a long standing and pathological coping pattern, which was highlighted and exacerbated in the SA. Ideally, the exercise will have three effects upon Jane: (1) She will perceive that her behavior produced the "undesirable" AO; (2) she will see that assertive behavior would make her DO attainable; and (3) her obvious relief in seeing how to avoid these distressing outcomes in the future will result in her learning how this failure to assert herself leads to feelings of personal distress. The therapist used the observed decrease in Jane's discomfort level during the remediation phase to administer negative reinforcement. Jane was able to pinpoint the strategies that mitigated her aversive feelings during the session.

Generalizing learning outside of the therapy context is the next step in SA. If Jane grows tired of being manipulated by others (and we know that she already is), the generalization step helps her see how to apply what she has learned to other interpersonal situations. SA makes this point explicit to Jane: *"If you don't say 'no' when you want to, you will continue to feel miserable."*

PROACTIVELY ADDRESSING INTERPERSONAL TRANSFERENCE ISSUES

The second strategy for illuminating consequences, teaching formal operations thinking, and increasing motivation to change involves using the therapist-patient relationship in salubrious ways via the Interpersonal Discrimination Exercise (IDE) described below. The IDE brings into sharp focus the interpersonal consequences of the patient's behavior by making explicit the therapist's personal reactions to a particular segment of their interaction.

Negative reinforcement can also be administered by putting patients on the "hot seat" and examining their transference issues. Most chronically depressed adults enter the therapeutic relationship in severe distress. They may fear being rejected by the clinician; they may fear they will be abused in ways that are similar to previous experiences of abuse; or they may be concerned that if they come to rely upon or trust the therapist, abandonment will follow (again, in ways that mirror earlier experiences with significant others). This means that a clinician who treats a chronically depressed adult enters into a problematic and usually unpleasant relationship. Yet the negative interpersonal features and expectancies of the patient's worldview are precisely what can be used to change his/her behavior. When the patient learns that rejection is not forthcoming when he/she expects it, that abuse does not happen, that punishment is not inevitable for mistakes made either within or outside the session, and that the therapist doesn't withdraw in times of emotional need, distress is lessened and motivation to change is increased—*but only if the therapist makes explicit what has just occurred!* Otherwise, the negative reinforcement opportunity will be lost upon a preoperational patient and he/she will overlook or discount what has just taken place. An example will illustrate this point:

THERAPIST: You look like you just felt relief. What happened?

PATIENT: I have never disclosed to anyone what I just told you. I do feel relieved telling you this stuff.

THERAPIST: What does it mean to you that you can say these things to me?

PATIENT: Well, I'm paying you to listen to me, aren't I?

This response will take the wind out of the sails of any well-meaning clinician, for it demonstrates unequivocally that the patient is missing important aspects of the relationship. However, if the therapist uses the occasion effectively, the relief moment can provide a wonderful opportunity to highlight the fact that the expected interpersonal rejection or censure has not occurred. The therapist calls attention to the fact that his/her personal reactions toward the patient play a significant role in alleviating the patient's distress. These learning experiences with the therapist help the patient replace negative interpersonal expectations with feelings of trust; novel experiences of interpersonal closeness that stem from sharing one's thoughts or feelings typically follow, as does a newfound freedom to act assertively.

The therapist can precipitate these change events by employing the IDE—that is, by comparing and contrasting his/her own in-session behavior with that of significant others in the patient's history. Changes in affect often become obvious in the IDE, usually signifying that the person has begun to discriminate the positive behavior of the therapist from the negative patterns of others.

ELICITING A SIGNIFICANT-OTHER LIST

The second psychotherapy session is a highly structured one designed to elicit information concerning significant individuals who played a decisive and influential role in the patient's life. Asking a preoperational patient to provide historical-causal information about how significant others influenced him/her entails the abstract reasoning of formal operations thinking. This exercise is the first "mismatching exercise" (Cowan, 1978; Gordon, 1988) the CBASP patient encounters in treatment. At the beginning of the second session, the therapist says something like this:

> "I want you to think back over your life and identify those individuals or persons whom you feel have had the most influence on the direction your life has taken. We call such people 'significant others.' All of us have friends and acquaintances. The significant others I am asking you to designate are more than just friends and acquaintances. They are persons who have had a major influence on you—have left their stamp on you, so to speak—and whose influences have literally shaped the course your life has taken. The influences may be either positive or negative, good or bad, helpful or hurtful. Now name the individuals for me, and I will write them down. Then we will go back through our list, and I will ask you certain questions about each person."

Each person on the list will be discussed in the order in which he/she is mentioned. For example, the therapist may preface the discussion of the first person on the list by asking the following:

> "Tell me how your mother has affected the course of your life. I mean, how did growing up around her influence the direction of your life, or influence you to be the kind of person you are?"

One patient hesitantly formulated the following sentence:

"My mother never liked anything I ever did [antecedent causal phrase], and I have never had any confidence in myself or anything I do—I'm always questioning myself [consequence phrase]."

Most patients need continued encouragement and prompting to formulate "consequence phrases"—that is, conclusions concerning specific effects others had upon them. However, these conclusions are what constitute the essential material from which the transference hypotheses are derived. A therapist will frequently have to interrupt a patient's description and ask for a consequence phrase. For example, the therapist may need to inquire, "Now, what effect has your mother's behavior had upon the way you live?", "How has your life been influenced by your mother?", "What kind of person are you today because of your mother's influence?", or the like.

Asking patients to make explicit causal connections between the behavior of significant others and its effects on them produces interesting reactions. Some are frankly surprised by the behavior patterns that come into focus as they relate their interpersonal histories. For example, abuse by one or more significant others may be recalled, with the person exclaiming in shock that he/she never realized these individuals had had such a destructive effect upon him/her. Patients are often amazed, angry, frightened, or saddened by the consistency of their avoidance and withdrawal behaviors with significant others, as well as by the direction their lives have taken as a result of these early significant relationships.

When preoperational patients are asked to think causally in this highly structured exercise, it requires them to engage in problem solving at a higher level in the developmental chain (which is why Cowan calls it a "mismatching" exercise). In all likelihood, this will be the first time patients have identified historical precursors of their present behavior.

PITFALLS IN ELICITING
THE SIGNIFICANT-OTHER HISTORY

Two types of therapist behaviors must be avoided in eliciting the Significant-Other history.

- Therapists should avoid verbalizing causal implications (i.e., drawing consequence conclusions) for patients after they have discussed significant others.
- Therapists should avoid allowing patients to describe and free-associate about life events with significant others without requiring them to draw causal inferences between the behavior of significant others and their own behavior.

The first error occurs when clinicians, in doing the work for patients, move too quickly to supply the antecedent-consequent connections for them. Patients must be allowed to struggle with answering this probe: "How did this person [parent, sibling, spouse, friend] influence the course of your life?" Therapists ought to begin to see connections between the antecedents and consequent patterns of behavior as they move through the Significant-Other list. However, they must simultaneously inhibit the impulse to do the causal work for the patient. The goal of treatment here is to guide patients to begin forming causal inferences between themselves and their significant others.

The second error made during the Significant-Other history occurs when therapists allow patients to ramble on in a stream-of-consciousness manner, describing "what happened" when they lived around particular persons. Here are two examples:

JACK: My father never played catch with me, never went anywhere with me, never helped me when I needed it. He drank a lot, he was on the road most of the time, he never talked much when he was home, and he surely got mad when things didn't go his way.

PAUL: My aunt used to sew when she visited my family. She and my mother argued a lot, and she hated my older brother and criticized him a lot. She used to wear funny-colored clothes, and she smoked like a fiend. Another thing—god, did she talk loud. When she left the house, I noticed such a change in the noise level.

As noted above, such open-ended descriptions often occur during the Significant-Other history and the clinician's essential job is to keep the patient focused on the task at hand: probing for the antecedent-consequent connections. It can be done by saying something like this:

THERAPIST: All right, you have described what it was like having your aunt visit the family. Now, try to answer this question: How did being around your aunt affect your life, influence the course of your life, even today?

PAUL: I don't like being around women. She was just like my mother. Loud, inconsiderate of others, and downright mean. Being around a woman means that I'm probably in for a lot of unpleasant criticism.

This is what the therapist is looking for: causal associations for the "If this ... then that" format of the transference hypothesis (in this case, "If I am around a woman, then I will be criticized"). Most patients can begin to make preliminary causal associations if therapists continue to probe for the specific connections.

CONSTRUCTING THE INTERPERSONAL TRANSFERENCE HYPOTHESES

Following the second session, the patient's causal theory conclusions are utilized to generate specific hypotheses about how the patient might transfer his/her expectations of, and habitual response patterns to, significant others to the therapy relationship. In formulating these hypotheses, the practitioner should consider the four transference domains of interaction that are targeted in the CBASP program:

- Moments in which *interpersonal intimacy* are felt/verbalized by either the patient or the therapist
- Situations in which the patient expresses *particular emotional needs* to the clinician, either directly or indirectly
- Situations in which a patient *fails at something* or *makes an obvious mistake* during the session
- Situations in which *negative affect* (e.g., fear, frustration, anger, etc.) is obviously felt or expressed, either directly or indirectly, by the patient toward the therapist

These domains of interaction have been selected in part because of the maltreatment themes chronic patients typically report (Chapter 3). Getting close to parents and/or siblings, experiencing emotional needs with caregivers, failing or making mistakes around a significant other, and having negative feelings toward caregivers are frequently cited as problematical or conflictual areas by patients. *Intimacy* issues typically accompany a long history of rejection or abuse; issues around *making mistakes* or *failure* often result from chronic patterns of criticism or ostracism by significant others; issues around *emotional needs* may be associated with earlier patterns of withdrawal by one or both parents, or even ridicule or punishment of the patient; reluctance or fear associated with *expressing negative affect* usually reflects early learning that to do so leads to rejection. When a patient experiences these situations in which they are most vulnerable in the session with the therapist, such moments indicate natural "hot spots" that can be turned into profound experiences of change. The therapist must be sure to construct the transference hypotheses before the third session, in order to respond appropriately when a hot spot flares.

Case Example: Transference Hypothesis Construction

C. H. is a 49-year-old woman, divorced, who had been depressed "for as long as I can remember." She was an early-onset patient with double depression. C. H.'s Significant-Other list consisted of her mother, father, older sister, older brother, maternal grandmother, maternal grandfather, and W. (ex-husband). In the verbatim material that follows, the statements labeled "Causal Theory Conclusions" denote C. H.'s responses to the question "What was it like growing up around this person?" or "How did the individual influence the direction your life has taken?"

> *Mother*: "She drank a lot, she lied, and always made me feel I was wrong. I always felt she was lying when she said she didn't drink. I had to take care of her; she never gave back to me emotionally. It was take, take, take. She made me tell her I loved her. I really didn't. I never could be honest with her about my true feelings. I always had to lie to her. Whenever I tried to be honest with her, she would get angry with me and tell me I was wrong and stupid.

> *Causal Theory Conclusions Regarding Mother*: "When I am around people now, they never know how I really feel. I keep having to make things all right with others. Somehow I feel pressure to take care of them—I don't know how to let others know what I need, what I want. She taught me to serve others at my own expense."

Father: "He was an alcoholic all my life. He was mean, had a bad temper, called my mom awful names, and beat her sometimes. When I was a little girl, I felt he loved me—I was his 'little princess.' When I was 10, he fell in an ice-skating incident and was hurt badly. Everyone said that his fall was my fault. I never understood why they blamed me. I backed away from him because I didn't want to cause him any more trouble. Once when I came home from college, he kissed me on the lips and embraced me for a long time. I felt very uncomfortable around him after that. I still don't understand what he was doing. I don't remember any sexual abuse from him, but I'm not sure. All I know is I don't want to be around him."

Causal Theory Conclusions Regarding Father: "I always feel that men want something from me—something sexual. At the same time, I feel I have to serve them, take care of them. I also think that if I have my own opinion about something, they will 'pooh-pooh' it and tell me I'm stupid."

Older Sister: "Very powerful person to me. She was good in everything she did. I always came up short when I compared myself to her. I made good grades in college, but she was a summa cum laude. I did one thing she could never do! I had children [*laughs derisively*]."

Causal Theory Conclusions Regarding Older Sister: "I always come out on the short-end of the stick when I compete with women. I always feel like it's really no contest. I'm a loser when it comes to women."

Older Brother: "He always teased me. When I was little, he would protect me in the family and stand on my side. He and I loved each other. Now he and I don't have much to do with each other."

Causal Theory Conclusions Regarding Older Brother: "Nothing that's any good lasts. I think this is a general attitude I have now about any decent people I meet."

Maternal Grandmother: "She was a kindly lady. She loved me, I think. She would hug me. And she taught me how to crochet.

Granny made me feel special, but I didn't see her all that much. She died."

Causal Theory Conclusions Regarding Maternal Grandmother: "Again, good things with people don't last. It's been the story of my life—I seem to lose all the good stuff I care about."

Maternal Grandfather: "He was an arrogant, self-centered, and controlling man. I was afraid of him. I was always afraid that he and my father would get into a real fight. They never did."

Causal Theory Conclusions Regarding Maternal Grandfather: "Just another man that I stayed away from. I learned early that I needed to keep my distance from all men."

W. (Ex-Husband): "I was married for 21 years. Had one son. W. was an alcoholic and was never emotionally open with me. He convinced me that I could never do anything right. He always questioned any decision I made. The way I fought back was to refuse to have sex. Finally, we just quit altogether. Things went from bad to worse; he drank more and more, and finally I left him and took my son. We got a divorce the following year."

Causal Theory Conclusions Regarding W.: "I was always his mother—he remained an angry little boy. He still is. I think my opinions and ideas are stupid. I feel I can't do anything right. I have always been very afraid that something is very wrong with me—I mean, really wrong. There must be a part missing or loose in me that can't be fixed. I just can't trust myself on anything."

Next, the major causal themes applying to the transference domains of intimacy, emotional need, failure/making mistakes, and negative affect were extracted. As C. H.'s clinician, I made the final decisions (using the causal theory conclusions) regarding hypothesis construction, based on my clinical judgment. Using a hypothesis construction grid (see Table 5.1), I summarized C. H.'s causal themes in relation to each person on her Significant-Other list. Following the grid summary, I then constructed two interpersonal transference hypotheses that represented potential "hot spots" between C. H. and myself. I offer no specific procedure for selecting one interpersonal domain over another, other than using your clinical

TABLE 5.1 Hypothesis Construction Grid for Causal Theory Conclusions

Significant other	Intimacy	Failure	Emotive need	Expression of negative affect
Mother	Hide my feelings; play servant role	—	Lie about needs	Does no good
Father	Play servant role	—	Disregard my feelings	Does no good
Older sister	—	No contest- always lose	—	Does no good
Older brother	Nothing good lasts	—	—	—
Grandmother	Nothing good lasts	—	—	—
Grandfather	Keep my distance from males	—	—	—
W. (ex-husband)	Play servant role; get hurt repeat- edly	—	Disregard my feelings	Does no good

judgment to decide which areas appear to be the most salient and problematical. However, I always recommend parsimony: It is better to select one or two domains and cover them thoroughly in the IDE than to select all four and have time for only cursory treatment. In the case of C. H., I selected the *intimacy* and *emotional need* domains for hypothesis construction. I was aware that getting close to me would evoke caretaking and sexual issues for C. H., since I was a male. Expressing negative affect or telling others what she wanted had also been hurtful to C. H. in the past. I felt that I would be able to address both of these potential "hot spots" in a thorough manner if I limited my focus to them.

The first "If this . . . then that" transference hypothesis involved any intimacy or closeness the patient might verbally or nonverbally disclose. Note the personal manner in which the hypothesis is formulated; in the way it is stated, it injects me into a personal encounter with the patient.

"*If* I get close to Dr. McCullough, *then* he will want something from me (i.e., I'll have to serve him and take care of him, and I'll end up getting hurt)."

This hypothesis was based on C. H.'s comments concerning her mother, father, and ex-husband, in answer to my question evoking causal connections. The mother had been an immature individual who demanded love from C. H. while prohibiting honest disclosure. The mother's alcoholism also thrust the child into a parent role and conveyed the message that the mother's issues, not her own, were of ultimate importance. Despite the early positive relationship C. H. had had with her father, she had also learned that she needed to placate him to avoid precipitating his anger. In short, as with her mother, her early life was spent focusing upon her father's needs and not her own. In addition, ever since her college days she had withdrawn emotionally from her father, due to an interaction with confusing sexual overtones that she never "understood." She reenacted the servant role in her marriage when she "mothered" her alcoholic husband. Her fear of males was well learned and substantiated by numerous memories of occasions on which she was unable to establish effective boundaries with men. Since I was a male, it was not hard to imagine the servant or caretaker role she might be likely to act out with me.

The second hypothesis was based on the causal theory conclusions involving her mother, father, grandfather (of whom she was overtly afraid), and ex-husband.

> "*If* I am really honest with Dr. McCullough and let him know how I feel or what I honestly think about something, *then* he will 'pooh-pooh' what I say (i.e., make me feel that I am stupid, wrong, overreacting, or a bad person)."

C. H. had learned that expressing her feelings honestly to others led to pain and ridicule. She could not remember any constructive outcomes following honest disclosures. C. H. concluded that these undermining experiences had resulted in her inability to trust her own feelings and thoughts. Her lifelong experience of being told that she was stupid, wrong, or overreacting made her reticient to reveal her feelings to others (she described the ridicule she received from others as being "pooh-poohed"). C. H. and I had numerous opportunities to visit these two interpersonal transference "hot spots" over the next 14 sessions, some of which will be described in Chapter 8. Whenever we did, the IDE was employed, and my behavior as her clinician was discriminated from that of significant others. Over time, C. H. learned that since the negative consequences would not occur in these situations, she could relax and assert herself in ways that were new and exciting.

Case Example: Treating a Transference "Hot Spot"

In another case, "Orwell," a 30-year-old early-onset patient presented a Significant-Other history in which he described being ridiculed by both his mother and father for making even the slightest mistake. He answered the causal theory questions of the clinician by describing how his parents' reactions had affected the course of his life. Over the years, the ridiculing had left him feeling incompetent, and this feeling generalized to include intense feelings of dread whenever he had failed and then thought about how others would react. Orwell viewed himself as having to be "perfect" in all things to avoid rejection, pain, and ridicule. He also admitted that he imposed the same perfectionistic standards upon others. The domain of failure or making mistakes was a salient transference issue implicated in the Significant-Other history. Following the second session, the therapist constructed a transference hypothesis:

> "*If* I make a mistake, mismanage something, or fail around my therapist, *then* she will ridicule me and make me feel stupid and incompetent."

Orwell then related the following situational description in which he had irreparably ruined a relationship with a close friend. The SA automatically took the therapist and patient into a "hot" transference area:

> *Situational Description during the 10th Week:* "I was talking to my best friend [Jerry] several weeks ago. He had come over to my apartment to drink beer and watch a ballgame. He told me about a conversation he had had with a colleague of mine whom he ran into in the grocery store. He knew I was really interested in this person and was going to ask her out on a date. The lady asked Jerry if I was in psychotherapy. He told her I was and that he was really glad I was seeing someone about my depression. I became furious with him for breaking confidence with me like this. I told him I no longer wanted him for a friend, that I would not be able to trust him any more. He tried to tell me that she knew we were best friends and that lying to her would be foolish—she would find out anyway when we went out. I just got angrier and finally told him to leave. He told me we had been too close to let this stuff mess us up. I said that I didn't care—didn't want him for a friend any more. He

tried to apologize again for what he had done. I asked him to leave once more. He left. I haven't seen or talked to Jerry in two weeks. I think I really screwed up a great friendship and have made a real mistake. This has happened several times in the past when I have gotten mad at Jerry. I bet we won't be able to repair this one. God, have I have really screwed up this time!"

Following the completion of SA, the therapist, aware of the transference hypothesis given above, administers the IDE and addresses the patient's negative interpersonal expectancy for making mistakes. The therapist asked the following question: "How would your mother have reacted to you if you had told her about how your reaction to Jerry messed up the friendship?" Orwell proceeded to recall numerous hurtful and painful memories of past times in which he had mishandled situations and his mother had found out about it. (If the therapist had judged it necessary to increase the patient's distress further, she could also have inquired about what the father's likely reaction would have been.) The aversive state of discomfort was clearly present and the stage is set for the IDE, which will decrease the discomfort and reinforce more adaptive interpersonal behavior with the therapist. After letting the patient ponder the hurtful memories and painful affect for a few moments, the therapist asked Orwell to focus upon and describe the reactions he had noticed from his therapist as they had analyzed this difficult failure situation.

At first, Orwell had trouble identifying any of the therapist's reactions. This is usually the case; chronically depressed patients tend to overlook the obvious behavioral differences between destructive significant others and the positive reactions of therapists. The therapist then reviewed her reactions to Orwell's behavior toward Jerry and again asked him to compare her reactions to those he would have received from his mother.

Orwell realized that, indeed, there had been no ridicule, nor had the therapist made him feel stupid or incompetent. What did Orwell learn in this exercise? Probably the most important thing is the knowledge that not everyone will respond to his failures as his parents did. More specifically, he learns that the therapist cares about him and will not ridicule his mistakes.

During and after the IDE, the practitioner watches for any mitigation of distress that has accompanied the recall of painful experiences with significant others. In Orwell's case, there was a decrease or cessation in negative affect, and the clinician took the opportunity to call attention to the change, to summarize what had happened, and to ask a question:

THERAPIST: The interpersonal consequences you received when you made mistakes around your parents were feelings of being stupid and incompetent. The feelings you experienced with me involved acceptance instead of ridicule—understanding and assistance to focus on the solution to the problem instead of being made to feel stupid and incompetent! Now, what are the implications here for you and me?

ORWELL: I feel better having told you about my mistake. You didn't punish or ridicule me. Your reaction was different from my parents.

What behavior was negatively reinforced in Orwell by the termination of the distress? Owning up to his mistakes by learning that it's "okay" to make mistakes. This was not the last time such a transference situation came up between Orwell and the therapist. Orwell gradually learned to believe that the practitioner would not react to him the way his parents had, and he became increasingly bolder in disclosing his failure. Over the process of treatment, Orwell learned to discriminate between the actual positive reactions of the therapist and the expected negative responses based on his childhood experiences with his parents. Transfer of learning was achieved as he also began to admit to friends when he had been wrong or made a mistake.

To reiterate, *if therapists do not call patients' attention to the obvious differences between their reactions and those of significant others, patients will overlook the positive reactions every time.* The IDE provides fruitful opportunities for highlighting consequences, modifying interpersonal behavior, and increasing motivation to change.

Methodological Issues and Rationale

TRANSFERENCE HYPOTHESES AS TACIT KNOWLEDGE

I assume that the "If this ... then that" interpersonal hypotheses deduced from the Significant-Other history represent *tacit knowledge* (Polanyi, 1966, 1968) on the part of most patients. Polanyi defines "tacit knowledge" as that about which we cannot speak or don't know on a conscious level. "Explicit knowledge" denotes knowledge about which we do know on a conscious level. When it comes to the transference hypotheses, preoperational patients are *not* aware of the connections between their behavior and the consequences they experience, but they usually do have a general knowledge of their developmental histories that they can describe in rather global terms.

As an example, let's look first at an intimacy transference hypothesis constructed by a female psychotherapist regarding a male patient, "Aaron":

> "If I get close to Dr. Smith, then she will reject me; she cannot possibly care for me."

This hypothesis is not based upon any one specific event that Aaron recalled, nor could he point to a single individual and say that this person caused him to view the world in this manner. Such cause-effect perspectives represent tacit knowledge, which the transference hypothesis makes explicit. To put it another way, this transference hypothesis was a causal theory construction that the therapist *adds to* Aaron's developmental history.

Let's examine Aaron's description of his relationship with his parents. This represents the transference domain of rejection during intimate encounters.

> "I went to my mother to ask for help. I asked her what I needed to do to solve a problem at school. She laughed at me and told me I was stupid. Another time, I tried to tell her how scared I was to try out for the football team. She looked at me like I was crazy and told me that I was a sissy and that I would never be a man. Finally I just quit talking to her. She was always mean. My father was no better. He never cut me any slack. He was always riding me about something I had done wrong. We were never close—still aren't."

The obvious theme in Aaron's developmental description was that intimate encounters with his mother and father typically led to verbal abuse and rejection. The female therapist took the historical information and constructed the intimacy hypothesis given above.

In contrast to the therapist's transference construction is a precausal statement that Aaron made about himself during the first session: "No one likes me, nor could anyone ever like me." Not surprisingly, his autobiographical statement contains no antecedent causal event(s) connected to the generalized interpersonal expectancy—only the global proclamation. The transference hypothesis, on the other hand, is constructed with particular interactants in mind (therapist and patient) and with a categorically specific event (patient-therapist intimacy) targeted. The tacit knowledge component for the patient, in both the precausal sentence and in the transference hypothesis, is the following: "Intimate behavior leads to interpersonal rejection." Because of his preoperational global thinking, Aaron is unaware of the fact that his early strivings for guidance and support had resulted in rejection. All that remained in his mind concerning the original association between asking for help (intimacy) and rejection was the generalized expectancy "no one cares, or can care, for me." The sources of his worldview lie buried somewhere in his remote past, out of range of explicit awareness.

As tragic as his preoperational belief itself are the interpersonal consequences that result. The belief is not assailable in logical terms, and the result is that *everyone* receives a "rejector" label, regardless of any positive responses they make toward Aaron. The "no one likes me" perception applies equally to the psychotherapist and to Aaron's spouse, colleagues, friends, previous mentors, elementary and high school teachers, adolescent peers, and childhood friends. The patient has inadvertently "checkmated" all positive responses from the environment with a prepotent worldview forecasting universal rejection. What can be done to loosen this fossilized perception so that another, less rejecting perception of others may develop?

In a case like Aaron's, when the tacit "If this . . . then that" worldview is made explicit during the IDE, the individual learns to discriminate facilitative behavioral consequences from destructive ones. This new perspective undercuts the preoperational snapshot view of reality where everyone is perceived as being the rejector.

There are notable exceptions to the assumption that patients are not explicitly aware of the transference issues. One exception involves female patients who come to therapy with a history of sexual abuse or rape and who work with male therapists. In such a case, it is not at all unusual to find that the patient is quite aware of the transference issues concerning interpersonal intimacy and emotional vulnerability. This is the case because of the salience of the previous abusive event(s), coupled with the extreme negative reactions of the individual to the event(s) (Nisbett & Wilson, 1977). Many of these patients are admittedly afraid of seeing male therapists, or even of being alone in the room with them, and they can readily tell the therapists why. Nevertheless, the IDE can still be effectively used with these female patients. When the expected catastrophe repeatedly fails to occur in the session (the therapist does not "hit on" such a patient), *and* the clinician highlights the absence of the expected catastrophe during moments of interpersonal closeness, the negative expectations associated with being close to the therapist are mitigated.

A RATIONALE FOR CAUSAL THEORIZING

Asking patients to introspect and draw causal theory conclusions regarding the effects significant others have had upon them raises an important question: Are these causal constructions accurate (valid)? Cognitive psychology has dealt extensively with this issue, and the conclusions about the accuracy of the introspections range from "no" to "yes, but with a biased kind of accuracy." In a pessimistic paper discussing the capacity of research subjects to introspect, Nisbett and Wilson (1977) have concluded that people have little or no direct introspective access to their higher-order cognitive processes. What the authors mean is that the mental processes involved in decision making, in people's conclusions about why they do things, and in the reasons people give for why they prefer one thing over another are not consciously available to them. In short, the mental processes driving much of human behavior represent, according to Nisbett and Wilson, tacit and not explicit knowledge. The authors state that it is the *results of thinking* that people are consciously aware of (i.e., attributions concerning why we behave as we do, value judgments that we make, decisions we make, preference choices, etc.), not the thinking process itself.

Other researchers are not so pessimistic about the accuracy of people's introspective capabilities (e.g., Ericsson & Simon, 1980; Guidano, 1987; Guidano & Liotti, 1983; Miller, 1981; Solso, 1995; White, 1980). They argue that while introspection is by no means a window that opens directly to tacit processes, it can provide, under focused attentional conditions, essential information that can be used to increase awareness of oneself and others, as well as to determine causal relationships involving personal attitudes and behavior. Even Nisbett and Wilson (1977) note that what individuals report when they are asked to identify *why* they behaved as they did (i.e., to report on their cognitive processes) are "a priori, implicit causal theories, or judgments about the extent to which a particular stimulus is a plausible cause of a given response" (p. 231). They state that causal theorizing may be fairly accurate under two conditions: (1) when the relevant stimuli are *salient*, and (2) when the stimuli represent a *plausible cause* for the produced response. The Significant-Other history procedure is basically a focused attentional exercise. The patient's attention is focused on recalled interpersonal experiences with a significant other (relevant stimuli that are made salient), and then he/she is asked to assess and scrutinize what plausible effects this person has had upon him/her. The causal connection is completed when the patient gradually recognizes and verbalizes a plausible theory that links the long-ago behavior of the significant other with some aspect of his/her own behavior.

A patient and therapist can never get "back there" to recapture the actual person(s) and/or event(s) that shaped any aspect of the individual's behavior. The next best thing, however, is for the clinician to ask the patient to go back there under conditions of focused attention and then to provide the material for plausible causal hypotheses that the therapist can then use to modify the patient's behavior.

FREUDIAN VERSUS CBASP
TRANSFERENCE PERSPECTIVES

I must stop here and address an important question that readers are probably asking: Why is a transference construct introduced in a cognitive behavioral program of therapy, and how does it differ from psychoanalytic usage?

My approach to addressing transference problems differs significantly from Freudian psychoanalysis (Freud, 1916–1917/1960, 1933) while still sharing similarities—at least, in regard to how both models emphasize using the patient-therapist relationship as a vehicle for change. Freud's (1916–1917/1960, 1933) elucidation of the patient's transference reaction to the clinician via interpretation was employed to stimulate awareness that the patient's behavior with the clinician parallels earlier patterns with primary caregivers. He postulated that a patient's current behavior is largely motivated by tacit affective cathexes existing between the individual and one or both parents. An analyst *passively* allows transference to actualize itself in the therapist-patient relationship. Then the analyst administers interpretations to highlight certain aspects of the patient's interpersonal behavior toward the clinician. The goal of interpretation is to sever the cathected link with the caregiver(s), so that increased psychic energy will be available to the patient in the here-and-now.

Unlike Freud, CBASP defines "transference" as a representational worldview that is acted out with the clinician and others (Guidano & Liotti, 1983); we do not discuss transference cathexis. CBASP also addresses transference issues *proactively*, not passively. Furthermore, the IDE does not utilize interpretation to modify behavior; instead, patients are required to make explicit *discriminations* between the behaviors of significant others and those of the clinician. They do this by specifying the consequences they experienced while living around significant others and then by noting the interpersonal consequences they experience in working with the clinician. The IDE overthrows the preoperational worldview of patients by helping them compare old relationships to their relationship with the therapist, so that they learn to perceive that a new interpersonal reality exists between themselves and the clinician. One similarity between the psychoanalytic approach to transference and that of CBASP is the fact that patients' negative worldviews are thereby exposed as nonapplicable in the relationship with the therapist. The ideal outcome for both therapy systems is to demonstrate the obsoleteness and destructiveness of these negative interpersonal expectations and to replace them with new interpersonal perspectives.

Source for the CBASP Approach to Transference

The view of transference in CBASP is derived largely from the work of Guidano and Liotti (1983), who have taken the position that the present worldview and behavior of pathological individuals are valid reflections of what it was like for them to experience maltreatment during childhood. Guidano and Liotti have relied heavily on the work of Piaget and thus are keenly aware of the influences maltreatment imposes upon one's view of self in relation to others. They characterize the behavior of depressed patients in terms of debilitating "interpersonal life themes" that are lived out daily with others and that serve as autobiographical "windows" through which clinicians can view their primitive worldview. There is an assumed representational linkage between the *current preoperational worldview* of the patient and the *way things actually were* for the individual during the early years. Guidano and Liotti also propose a technique that can be used to elicit interpersonal life themes material. The technique involves asking patients to focus on various problem events they have experienced over the years (preschool years, childhood, adolescence, young adulthood, middle and late adulthood). Next they ask patients to describe their "methods of solution" in handling the difficulties (e.g., fighting, crying, ignoring the problem, resignation, withdrawing from others, despairing, etc.). In this way, interpersonal themes emerge that can subsequently be used as predictors of how patients will behave when problems crop up with the practitioner.

I have incorporated this technique in an indirect way in the Significant-

Other history, when patients are asked to describe their relationships with significant others (most of whom probably will have had a negative impact upon the individual) and then to describe the formative influences of these persons. Clinicians can discern definite interpersonal themes in the individual's descriptions of early relationships. The transference sentences represent hypotheses about how the destructive interpersonal themes are likely to be played out with the practitioner during treatment. Because the CBASP transference formulations are essentially "hypotheses," they can be revised whenever necessary. In closing, I restate the central point: *When the IDE is used in an effective manner to expose and resolve the transference problems, a patient's motivation to change will increase, and the individual will learn greater interpersonal adaptability.*

In the next two chapters, I will return to a discussion of SA. The rationale for SA will be presented, and the SA administration procedures will be fully described.

CHAPTER SIX

Elicitation Phase
of Situational Analysis

A psychotherapy process therefore subsumes a set of stages
which are defined both by therapist operations and by patient
performance shifts. In brief, it depicts a theory of therapy in
operational terms.

—S. CASHDAN (1973, p. 4)

... therapy process is structured so that the patient is guided
through a series of sequential steps, each of which contains its
own operationalized therapist rules and patient performance
goals.

—J. P. MCCULLOUGH (1984b, p. 387)

... a Piagetian perspective suggests that changing an
individual's way of thinking is facilitated by optimal mismatch
between the individual's existing level of cognitive functioning
and the cognitive structures required for solving a particular
interpersonal problem... the enhancement of formal
operational abilities may be directly addressed within the
therapeutic context.

—D. E. GORDON (1988, p. 68)

SITUATIONAL ANALYSIS

Having the tangible means to demonstrate to patients that there is order
in their lives, when all they have been able to discern are disorder and
chaos, is an operational definition of hope. Imparting hope to those who
have lost theirs constitutes one of the motifs of SA. Using SA demonstrates how patients play a determinant role in their relationships and
makes explicit the fact that they have been controlling interpersonal

events all along—they have just been doing it wrong. As noted in Chapter 5, the SA method is also designed to exacerbate a patient's psychopathology in the therapy session so that the probability of behavioral change is increased.

SA revises the preoperational orientation of chronically depressed patients by requiring them to function at a more advanced level of formal operations thinking (Cowan, 1978; Gordon, 1988; Inhelder & Piaget, 1955/1958). The revision of preoperational thinking is undertaken from several directions: (1) by focusing patients' global thinking patterns (e.g., "People will always end up rejecting me," "Nothing will ever work out for me," "Things will never improve in my life") upon specific spatiotemporal events; (2) by highlighting moments of interpersonal causality, as well as demonstrating to patients their functional connection to their environment; (3) by confronting patients with the destructive social consequences of their interpersonal submissive style; (4) by maneuvering patients into collaborative dialogue with their clinicians instead of allowing them to talk in their habitually detached monologue fashion; and (5) by undermining the outlook of hopelessness through showing them that they feel better when they behave adaptively.

THE COPING SURVEY QUESTIONNAIRE

The Coping Survey Questionnaire (CSQ) used in the SA exercise is shown in Table 6.1. All patients are given a supply of CSQs at the end of their second session, at which time they also receive the *Patient Manual for Cognitive Behavioral Analysis System of Psychotherapy* (CBASP) (Kasnetz et al., 1995). The CSQ presents a skeletal outline of the exercise. A patient is asked to complete at least one CSQ prior to each session. The completed form will then be utilized by the therapist and patient in a step-by-step analysis.

I will follow the format of the CSQ throughout the chapter in describing each step of the SA procedure. Included will be a discussion of the rationale for each step. I will then specify the "therapist rules for administration" and describe the verbal prompts clinicians use to initiate each individual step. Finally, "patient performance goals" for the steps will be delineated and discussed. When readers finish the chapter, they should have a general understanding of how the elicitation phase is administered.

All therapists who begin their CBASP training begin their SA instruction by working from the structured therapist form of the CSQ;

TABLE 6.1. Coping Survey Questionnaire

Patient: _____   Therapist: _____

Date of Situational Event: _____   Date of Therapy Sesion: _____

INSTRUCTIONS: Select one interpersonal problematical event that has happened to you during the past week and describe it using the format below. Please try to fill out all parts of the questionnaire. Your therapist will assist you in Situational Analysis during your next therapy session.

Situational Area: Spouse/Partner _____ Children _____ Extended Family _____
Work/School _____ Social _____

Step 1. Describe what happened.

Step 2. Describe your interpretation of what happened (how did you "read" the situation?).

　　1.

　　2.

　　3.

Step 3. Describe what you did during the situation (what you said/how you said it).

Step 4. Describe how the event came out for you (actual outcome).

Step 5. Describe how you wanted the event to come out for you (desired outcome).

Step 6. Was the desired outcome achieved? YES ____ NO ____

Therapist Prompts for Administering Situational Analysis (PASA; see Appendix A). Referring to the PASA while proceeding through the next two chapters will be helpful.

STEP 1: SITUATIONAL DESCRIPTION

The task in Step 1 is to teach a patient to focus on one specific "slice of time" during which he/she interacted with another individual. Patients typically ask how dealing with one stressful situation at a time is going to help them resolve their overall depressive state. The following excerpt demonstrates the importance of the clinician's response.

THERAPIST: I want you to think of one particular event where you had trouble saying what you wanted to your lover.

PATIENT: What good will that do? I need to talk about all the troubles I've been having. I just can't sit on all this stuff. It's just too much to sit on!

THERAPIST: I know you've got a lot to talk about. I want to hear it all, and I will. But not at one time. We can deal with only one problem at a time, so I must ask you to be specific and talk about one example where you have had the difficulty you mentioned. Tell me about the last time it happened to you. [This anchors the patient's problem in time and space.]

PATIENT: How is this going to help me get over my depression?

THERAPIST: There is only one way to find out. Describe for me the last time you didn't tell Billy what you wanted. One problem at a time is all we can tackle during this session.

PATIENT: Okay, but I still don't see how this will help.

Such a conversation is typical during the early sessions. Patients initially don't believe that by focusing upon one event at a time, clinicians can help them resolve their interpersonal problems and, ultimately, their depressive disorder.

The need to keep chronically depressed patients focused is not understood by those psychotherapists who allow patients to talk about "things in general." Verbal permissiveness and lack of focus do not result in behavioral change. Therapists who enable patients in this manner often ask general, open-ended questions, such as "How are you feeling?", "I wonder why you are feeling this way?", "Do you think behaving this way might help?", "What difficulties have you had this past week?", "How long have you been having trouble with your spouse?", and "Why don't you get along with your colleagues?" Change is precluded in these instances because *as long as patients talk about their problems, they avoid having to confront the consequences of their behavior.*

The crucial point is that something must be *added* to the way patients talk about any problem. That "something" is focusing attention on one "slice of time." Focusing specifically on discrete time periods then makes it possible for patients to identify the consequences of their actions. Therefore, in Step 1, the goal is to enlist the patient's cooperation and to focus on only one event at a time.

Another reason to narrow a patient's focus to a specific "slice of time" is that such an interaction typically serves as a microcosmic sample representing the *core interpersonal difficulties* of the patient. In several longitudinal studies, we (McCullough et al., 1988, 1994a) have demonstrated that interpersonal patterns among untreated chronically depressed patients remain stable over time. It is generally accepted that psychopathology and interpersonal rigidity are closely associated (Conway, 1987; Kiesler, 1996; Mischel, 1973; Wachtel, 1973). Wachtel (1977) has noted that the rigidity "is brought about in the present, both by the patient's own behavior and by the behavior he evokes in others" (p. 43). Wachtel labels this interactive pattern a "cyclical re-creation of interpersonal events." This view of interpersonal rigidity epitomizes the lifestyle of the chronic patient, for whom "time has stopped." Therefore, by focusing on one problematic event at a time, therapists capture and address a universe of similar interpersonal and perceptual problems.

Making certain that an event has a *beginning point* in time is important in Step 1. Circumscribing an event in time requires that the beginning point of the situation be clearly demarcated. This will be a difficult undertaking for persons who usually talk globally. Even more difficult is teaching patients to designate an *endpoint* or "exit point" for the event. Once a situational event is tightly framed within temporal boundaries ("It began here. . . and ended there"), the therapist can help the person analyze the cognitive and behavioral responses that led to some outcome (i.e., the endpoint or actual outcome). *The slice of time delineated in Step 1 literally becomes the living culture examined under the analytic microscope that defines the chronically depressed patient's pathological state of functioning.*

Defining the endpoint of the event is as crucial as defining the beginning point. Not anchoring the endpoint would be analogous to conducting an operant experiment without building in contingencies. When the endpoint is not established, patients tend to describe their situations in never-ending stream-of-consciousness monologues. Therapists must cut into this verbal stream and help patients identify the end of a situation. Finally, the endpoint must be described in objective or behavioral terms. This requires that the patient step back and objectify what has taken place between himself/herself and another person.

Practitioners should also discourage "editorializing" or guessing about the motives of others during this situational description step. They should stress that patients should provide just the interactive facts. Consider this example:

THERAPIST: Tell me what happened.

PATIENT: Well, I spoke to her in the hall but began to think to myself, "Why am I doing this now? She will certainly not want to discuss the issue in the middle of our coffee break." I really started feeling anxious, and. . .

THERAPIST: Just stick with what happened: what you did and what she did in response, then what you did next, and so on. We'll come back and fill in all the other aspects of the interaction in a moment. Learn to describe your situation objectively in this step without any editorializing. Just describe the action between you and the other person as it unfolded. Then tell me objectively what happened when the encounter ended.

Therapist Rules for Administering Step 1

1. During the early sessions, the therapist provides the patient with a rationale for the task, as in this example:

"Thinking about your life in terms of specific events will help you learn to manage your life more effectively. No one can solve problems while thinking about 'problems in general.' Solving a problem means learning to concentrate upon one difficulty at a time, working it through until you decide upon a solution strategy, and then implementing action. Not surprisingly, many patients discover that the solutions that work in one situation are applicable to other problem areas."

2. The therapist teaches the patient to describe one interpersonal event that has a beginning point and an endpoint, as well as an internally coherent story in between.
3. The therapist teaches the patient that an event selected for SA may be either problematical or successful.
4. The clinician teaches the patient to describe the event from an "observer" perspective; that is, to describe the behaviors observed during the unfolding situation by using action words: "I did this,

he did that, then I did this. . . and the situation ended when he said that."

5. The therapist actively discourages editorializing during the situational description (i.e., describing "how I felt," "how I thought the other person felt," "what I thought the other person was thinking," etc.).

6. The clinician is encouraged to use a chalkboard, an eraserboard, or a piece of paper and write out the major events in the situation on a "time-line," in order to engage the visual mode in addition to the auditory in describing the event.

While the patient is going through Step 1, the therapist can create a time-line (in view of the patient). On this line, working from left to right, the major interactive exchanges between the person and another are noted (Figure 6.1). The beginning point and endpoint of the time-line should be clearly labeled to show what behaviors initiated the encounter and those that terminated it. Visual procedures often enhance the patient's understanding of the flow of the situation. The individual can easily see that the entire situation is made up of a series of small events that leads to some final denouement. The following description by a patient is illustrated by the time-line shown in Figure 6.1.

"My 34-year-old daughter called up the other night and told me she had had a car wreck and had spent all of her month's salary on repairs. She said she could not pay the rent for April and asked if I would send her a check. I told her that I wished she would get a better job than the waitressing one she had. I stammered around and finally said I would write her a check. I asked for the name of her landlord—didn't want to make the check out to her. Then she said that she could not pay her income tax either. She asked me if I would loan her some money to pay it. I said nothing for a long time. Then, and with a big sigh, I said, 'Okay.' We hung up the phone, and I told my wife that my daughter is a loser."

7. At the end of Step 1, the therapist summarizes the patient's story, making certain he/she has correctly understood the temporal narrative.

The patient should be encouraged to correct the therapist if the summary alters, omits, or misses important aspects of the story.

SITUATIONAL TIME-LINE

Step 1: SA description by father (patient).

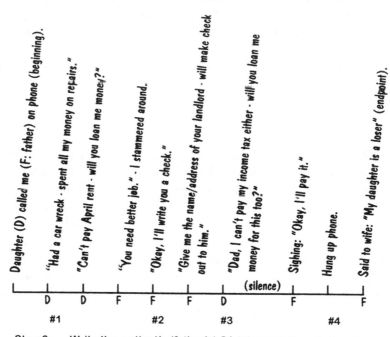

Step 2: Write the patient's (father's) SA interpretations "where" they occurred on the time-line.

#1. "God, I'm going to get screwed again."
#2. "I can never say 'no.' "
#3. "My daughter is a loser."
#4. "Nothing ever goes my way."

FIGURE 6.1. Graphic illustration of a situational time-line, showing how SA description can be written out (Step 1) and noting "where" the patient's interpretations occurred (Step 2).

8. The therapist teaches the patient to perform Step 1 independent of the therapist's guidance/prompts.

The therapist functions as a sensitive teachers throughout the SA exercise by directing the patient's narrative and helping him/her stay on task. Over the course of treatment, the individual should gradually be able to complete the step with little or no assistance from the clinician. Asking the patient to "tell me what happened in this situation" and then sitting back and letting the patient talk in generalities will be counterproductive. Situational descriptions that last longer than three or four minutes are indications that the therapist is not keeping the patient on task. By the end of the sixth or seventh session, the person should be able to complete Step 1 without coaching.

Step 1 has been accomplished successfully when the patient's story gives the therapist the experience of watching a silent movie. What are described are the behaviors and counterbehaviors observable in the story. Patients differ in regard to the quantity of their verbal descriptions. Some are overly parsimonious, while others are extremely verbose and descriptive. The clinician must strive for balance between the two extremes. Parsimonious patients may overlook relevant interpersonal information with their constricted description; verbose individuals may also miss salient points in their excessive detail. The first type must be taught to attend to relevant details, which often necessitates active intervention and shaping by the clinician. The second type will require frequent reminders that only a sequential description of the interactive events that led to the outcome is needed.

Patient Performance Goal for Step 1

1. The patient learns to describe a situational event in an objective and succinct manner.

This goal means (1) staying focused on only one situation, (2) delineating a clear beginning point and endpoint, and (3) avoiding the temptation to editorialize. Teaching the patient to focus on only one event at a time helps modify the global thinking of the preoperational adult. Being able to particularize a problem in time and space sets the focus so that the patient is optimally prepared to examine his/her cognitive and behavioral responses, which led to the actual outcome.

STEP 2: SITUATIONAL INTERPRETATIONS

The patient is now asked to think about the situational description, to *interpret the event*, and to answer the question "What did the event mean to you?" by constructing three or four concise sentences. Here is an example from the first SA exercise undertaken in the third session for one patient:

THERAPIST: What did the event mean to you?

PATIENT: [Interpretation 1] It means that no one really likes me. [The therapist already knows this is an irrelevant interpretation, but he lets it stand during the elicitation phase.]

THERAPIST: Think about the event you have just described—it had a beginning, some in-between events, and then an ending. Looking back now at your description, interpretations should indicate to you *what* was happening between you and Shirley. Interpretations should act like situational "rudders," guiding you from the beginning to the end by indicating what the other person is doing, what you are doing, and what direction the encounter is taking. Try again, and let's see what the event meant to you. [The therapist is providing a rationale to the patient for Step 2.]

PATIENT: [Interpretation 2] It means that Shirley has conflicting plans and cannot go out with me Saturday night.

THERAPIST: Did the event mean anything else to you?

PATIENT: [Interpretation 3] I was really disappointed that she already had plans.

THERAPIST: Now you are getting the hang of it. Your first interpretation was that "no one really likes me." In the situational description, you said that she told you she had already made plans, and then you indicated how disappointed that made you feel. You told her how disappointed you were. You also said that she asked you to call her earlier in the week next time. Look at the last comment she made to you about calling her earlier. What does that comment mean to you?

PATIENT: [Interpretation 4] I've got to call Shirley on Monday or Tuesday in order to make a date with her.

THERAPIST: Now you're constructing accurate and relevant interpretations in the situation. You have four interpretations that we can work with.

Teaching a patient to "read" accurately the ongoing flow involved in interpersonal encounters plants the person's perceptual "feet" solidly in the moment. I call Step 2 "determining the *what* of the situation." Only the cognitive constructions that describe actual ongoing events in the interaction are useful. The others must be revised. Later in SA, the therapist focuses upon each of the patient's cognitive interpretations and examines its potential to produce the desired outcome. This point will become clearer when we reach Step 5 and discuss the construction of the desired outcome.

Therapist Rules for Administering Step 2

1. During the early sessions, the therapist provides an explanation of the function interpretations serve in SA.

As illustrated in the excerpt above, therapists must explain to patients that their interpretations or "reads" function like the steering wheel on a car; that is, their interpretations steer their responses and behaviors in an event and thus are directly related to the situational outcome. When used correctly, interpretations enable participants to remain grounded and focused on the moment-to-moment exchanges taking place. In addition, interpretations denote *what* is occurring between a patient and another person. I am not suggesting here that interpretations should provide the answer to *why* someone is behaving toward the patient in a certain way; rather, interpretations tell the patient *what* another person is doing while interacting with him/her.

2. The therapist teaches the patient to compose a single, simple declarative sentence to express each interpretation.

Patients frequently find it difficult to reduce an interpretation to one sentence. It is easier to explain what the situation means and then elaborate upon other aspects of the event. It is the clinician's job here to help the patient "collapse" all the stream-of-consciousness material into one sentence. Encouraging the patient by prompting, "The situation means what. . . ?" has been found helpful. Practice and active feedback are the keys to mastery of Step 2.

3. The clinician should let the patient do the work. That is, he/she should interact collaboratively, but make the patient construct the final sentence.

The strong temptation in working with chronically depressed adults is always to do the work for them. My advice to therapists in this case is simple: "*DON'T!*" Doing a patient's work in Step 2 means that after a therapist has asked the question "What does the situation mean to you?", and the patient has provided several descriptive sentences, the therapist then summarizes or paraphrases the material into one sentence. Again, my advice is "*DON'T!*" Most of these patients are limited cognitively and will need repeated practice at this task. Patience on the part of the practitioner is therefore necessary. The inverse way of stating this rule is this: *Anything the clinician does for the patient, the patient will not learn to do for himself/herself!*

4. The therapist restates each interpretation for the patient, using the patient's own language and not paraphrasing.
5. The therapist must insure that he/she understands *every* word of the patient's sentence before asking for the next read.

This fifth rule is an elaboration of the fourth one. New therapists often give patients the benefit of the doubt when it comes to understanding idiosyncratic words. This is not recommended. The meaning of every word in a sentence must be understood by the therapist before moving on. An example will illustrate the point.

PATIENT: I was an "avenging angel" in the way I reacted to Mike.

THERAPIST: What does "avenging angel" mean to you? Help me understand this phrase in your interpretation.

PATIENT: It means I was acting like an angry protector of all children who are abused. Mike was making light of abused children and their problems.

THERAPIST: So you were behaving like you wanted to take care of them in the face of Mike's remarks. Is this what you meant when you used the phrase, "avenging angel"?

PATIENT: Yes.

THERAPIST: Okay, I got it. Did the situation mean anything else to you?

6. When the interpretation list is complete, the clinician briefly summarizes it for the patient, *using the patient's own language.*
7. The therapist teaches the patient to make interpretations that are both *accurate* and *relevant.*

The topic broached in the seventh rule is addressed more fully in the next chapter, where the remediation procedure for inaccurate and irrelevant interpretations is described. However, a description of the criteria for accurate and relevant interpretations is included here to complete the elucidation of what constitutes adaptive interpretations. Patient interpretations obtained during the elicitation phase, regardless of their inaccuracy or irrelevancy, are allowed to stand as long as they meet the requirements spelled out in the first six rules in this step. Active revision of maladaptive interpretations is undertaken during the second phase of SA, described in Chapter 7.

Accurate and relevant interpretations reflect correctly what is happening between the patient and the other person (accuracy) and are derived from, and anchored to, specific ongoing exchanges occurring in the situation (relevancy). Interpretations that are accurate are always relevant; however, interpretations may be relevant but not accurate. Some reads may be anchored within the context of the event (relevancy), yet may not interpret correctly (accuracy) what is happening. An example is a type of interpretation I label "mind reading"—a read that will *always* be inaccurate. Mind reading means that patients are guessing what other people think or feel or what their motives are when they have not asked specifically for, or been given, this particular information. An example of mind reading is given below to illustrate the point.

PATIENT: Molly really rejected me last night while we were on a date. She said that my shirt color really didn't match my tie.

THERAPIST: Did you check out your interpretation with Molly that she was personally rejecting you?

PATIENT: No. But I know she did because she said my colors did not match.

Adverbs such as "maybe," "never," "always," "again," "perhaps," "probably," and the like, when used in interpretation sentences, usually transform interpretations into conjectures about some future state or condition. Such adverbs lead to the construction of irrelevant reads because the interpretations will be disconnected from the immediate event. Table 6.2 provides examples of adaptive and maladaptive interpretations.

In summary, adaptive interpretations ground the person spatially and temporally in the event, describe what is actually happening, and specify

TABLE 6.2 Examples of Adaptive and Maladaptive Interpretations

Adaptive Interpretations	Maladaptive Interpretaions
"I asked him why I had not been selected, and he said that someone else should lead the group." [Accurate and relevant: Assumption checked out.]	"I always feel angry when I'm rejected." [Irrelevant: Read not grounded in the situation, and adverb makes it a conjecture.]
"I really felt angry the moment she told me she wouldn't go with me any more." [Accurate and relevant: Time-anchored introspection.]	"I know that he was thinking that I shouldn't be leading the discussion group." [Inaccurate: A *Mind-read assumption* not checked out.]
"My husband likes to spite me, and he admitted doing it this time." [Accurate and relevant: Time-anchored.]	"Here my husband goes again, rejecting what I say just to spite me." [Inaccurate: *Mind-reading* the motive, even though the rejection component may be a valid observation.]
"My boss knows I didn't have the skills to complete the assignment, and he told me so." [Accurate and relevant: Time-anchored.]	"I can never complete an assignment the boss gives me." [Irrelevant: Interpretation is conjecture.]
"We [both the spouse and patient] are handling this problem now without fighting." [Accurate and relevant: Time-anchored.]	"I'll never get married." [Irrelevant: Interpretation not time-anchored and is conjecture.]
"I've got to tell my husband that we must discuss this matter without arguing." [Accurate and relevant: *Action interpretation*, which is usually a precursor for assertive behavior. Action reads mobilize specific behavioral action.]	"I wish my husband and I could discuss something without fighting." [Irrelevant: Read not time-anchored, as patient is not focusing on disagreement at hand.]
"She really cares for me." [Accurate and relevant: Follows endearing actions by other person, and read is time-anchored.]	"I probably can't convince him to stay." [Irrelevant: Read not time-anchored in the situation.]
"I'm confused by what he said." [Accurate and relevant: Time-anchored introspection.]	"Perhaps this will work out for us someday." [Irrelevant: Read not time-anchored and is conjecture.]
"I'm not good enough to make this team." [Accurate and relevant: Time-anchored after not making the cut.]	"Maybe I should not have gotten mad at her when she said it." [Irrelevant: The adverb disengages the read from the situation at hand.]
"I don't like my wife being overweight the way she is now." [Accurate and relevant: Time-anchored.]	"Perhaps my husband should respect me at times like this, but he doesn't." [Irrelevant: The adverb disengages the read from the event and makes the interpretation a conjecture.]
"I'm not happy with how I look." [Accurate and relevant: Time-anchored introspection.]	"I wish I could make myself love her." [Inaccurate and irrelevant: Interpretation is not time-anchored—it is wishful thinking.]
"I don't want to be laid up in bed right now." [Accurate and relevant: Time-anchored introspection.]	"I wish I was a better baseball player." [Irrelevant: Read not time-anchored, wishful thinking.]
"My doctor told me at that time that I'll never walk again." [Accurate and relevant: Time-anchored.]	"Life is unfair. I should not be a cripple and confined to a wheel chair." [Irrelevant: Read not time-anchored.]
"I've got to speak up now or the motion will fail." [Accurate and relevant: *Action interpretation*, leading to assertive behavior.]	"Maybe I'll never walk again." [Irrelevant: Read not time-anchored, and is a conjecture.]
	"Nobody will ever love me." [Irrelevant: Read not time-anchored and adverb makes it a conjecture.]

what the person must do or wants to do in the situation. Adaptive interpretations also result in behavior that directly addresses the interpersonal task at hand. In short, accurate and relevant interpretations enable the individual to remain "fully present" in the moment.

Very few chronically depressed patients construct accurate and relevant interpretations during early SA exercises. Their snapshot preoperational view of problems and their perceptual disengagement from the environment preclude them from focusing upon discrete events. For most patients, Step 2 will be a difficult and revolutionary learning experience made possible by sensitive and persistent feedback from the therapist.

> 8. The therapist limits the number of interpretations to three or four.

Neophyte CBASP clinicians tend to elicit five, six, or more interpretation sentences by asking patients, "Does the situation mean anything *else* to you?" The result is the production of too many interpretations to manage in any one SA. More than three or four reads increase the risk of having too much information on the table. Information overload inhibits learning in SA. A practitioner does not have to resolve everything in one SA. I always tell CBASP trainees to "Keep it simple! Don't make SA too difficult for your patient!"

> 9. If a visual time-line procedure has been used during Step 1, the therapist makes notations on the time-line indicating when each interpretation was made.

This visual aid may enhance the patient's understanding of how interpretations are embedded in the ongoing flow of the situation. Figure 6.1 includes interpretation notations showing "where" each read occurred during the flow of the situation.

> 10. The clinician uses the interpretations to assess cognitive pathology and to determine how the individual attempts to solve interpersonal problems.

As discussed earlier in Chapter 3, the goal of interpersonal development is to be able to establish empathic encounters with others and use language as a vehicle to understand and be understood. Integral to this interpersonal developmental goal is the notion that empathic ability necessarily involves a perceived connection to one's environment. The patient's reads will indicate the degree to which the individual falls short of the goal.

Not being able to construct accurate and relevant interpretations makes it impossible for a patient to achieve an empathic relationship with another person. Maladaptive reads disengage the patient from others and lead to behavior that does not specifically address the situation at hand.

Pathological Patterns Arising during Step 2

Two pathological patterns may occur during Step 2 that present unique problems for therapists. First, some patients are unable to produce interpretations that can be used in SA; this means that their reads will be vague and disorganized. In such cases, extreme emotional distress is often present. It is not unusual for these individuals to wonder out loud what good will come from anything they do, as in this example:

THERAPIST: Sally, you have described a difficult interaction you had with your husband in which he reacted to your suggestion about moving furniture in the living room by telling you that your idea was stupid. You agreed with him that it was stupid. Let's take the next step in SA: I want you to think about what this situation means to you. Give me one sentence that reflects what it means.

PATIENT: (crying) I don't know what it means. Nothing ever works out for me [Interpretation 1].

THERAPIST: Did the situation mean anything else to you?

PATIENT: I'm not sure, I'm just stupid [Interpretation 2].

THERAPIST: Did the situation mean anything else?

PATIENT: I'm just not sure. I'm going to fail in this therapy because of my stupidity [Interpretation 3].

THERAPIST: Let's go back over the event and see if we can break it down into small parts. For example, you presented your idea about moving the furniture; then Fred reacted negatively to your suggestion; finally, you agreed with his opinion about your idea. Let's take the first part. What did it mean to you when you first presented your idea to Fred? Just focus on that part of the story.

Sally's misery over the event precluded her from constructing interpretations that could be assessed. She was so upset that she kept saying she wasn't sure what to make of the situation. The clinician then had to divide the situation into several phases and have Sally focus on one phase at a time. Much subsequent work had to be done to enable Sally to maintain her focus on the situation at hand and construct interpretations that could be used in the SA.

In the second pathological pattern, some patients construct interpretations with a destructive interpersonal motif, in which others are viewed as justly deserving of punishment or abuse. These individuals often produce interpretations that are vengeful and hateful.

THERAPIST: [. . . Summarizing the situational description. . . .] Your situational description involved a conversation you had with a store employee. He had made a sales error that cost the store $50. You talked with him about the mistake. You told him that this was his third mistake on the floor, he lost you money, and you were angry about it. The conversation ended when you said you would take the $50 from his weekly salary. Looking back on the situation, what does it mean to you?

PATIENT: It means that he's a stupid jerk who lost me money [Interpretation 1].

THERAPIST: Did the event mean anything else?

PATIENT: Yeah, one can't hire good workers any more [Interpretation 2].

THERAPIST: Anything else?

PATIENT: My employees don't like me and don't seem to care how their sloppiness loses me money [Interpretation 3]. I ought to fire them all.

In addition to the patient's anger, this excerpt provides clear evidence of preoperational thought. Part of the mismatching logic of SA is realized during the remediation phase, when patients are asked to provide a formal operations answer to this question: "How did each interpretation contribute to your obtaining your desired outcome?" In the above scenario, the owner wanted the employee to demonstrate greater caution with money exchanges at the cash register. His reads did not contribute to DO achievement; instead, they were directed toward punishment and rejection of the employee and the staff. All of the interpretations had to be revised.

The store owner's interpretations expressed a generalized reaction of anger that did not address the specific sales error. What was missing in the interpretations was a recognition of the need to teach the worker how to behave differently at the register; an *action read* was needed. The eight categories of maladaptive interpretations shown in Table 6.3 can be readily discerned during early SA exercises.

Patient Performance Goal for Step 2

1. The patient learns to construct accurate and relevant interpretations without assistance from the clinician.

The performance goal for this step is to enable the patient to construct relevant and accurate interpretations, and then to be able to self-correct any errors made along the way.

TABLE 6.3 General Categories of Maladaptive Interpretations

1. *Global* interpretations of conflict situations which preclude direct assessment of the specific problem (e.g., "I'll never suceeed in life") [irrelevant].

2. *Avoidant* interpretations, which remove the patient from the problem at hand and maintain a temporal focus in the past or future, or which entrap the person in a web of cynicism (e.g., "I should have taken the other job when I had the opportunity") [irrelevant].

3. *Self-blame* interpretations, which reflexively affix blame to the self and fail to take into account the foibles and limitations of oneself and others (e.g., "It's always my fault; I screw up any relationship I'm in") [irrelevant].

4. *Mind-reading* interpretations, which assign unconfirmed motives, thoughts, and feelings to others (e.g., "I know she thought I was trying to get out of work") [inaccurate].

5. *Self-negation* interpretations, that overlook the person's abilities and goals (e.g., "I know I'm stupid when I make such suggestions") [inaccurate].

6. *Perfectionistic* interpretations, holding the patient and those with whom he/she interacts to an unattainable standard and preventing the individual from dealing directly with the situation at hand (e.g., "My husband never does it right when it comes to housecleaning") [irrelevant].

7. *Conjecture* interpretations, prophesying one's status at home, at work, or interpersonally in the near or extended future (e.g., "I'll never be able to get close to anyone") [irrelevant].

8. *Wishful thinking-avoidant* interpretations, representing a retreat into fantasy and avoidance of the problem at hand (e.g., "I wish this had never happened to me") [irrelevant].

STEP 3: SITUATIONAL BEHAVIOR

The Step 3 task is to elicit a verbal description of behaviors the patient enacted in the situation. The therapist prompts the patient by saying simply, "Describe what you did in the situation."

General information about the individual's behavioral style will already be evident by observing how he/she behaved while completing the first two SA steps. For example, practitioners will know if patients give up easily in difficult situations, cry or weep when things go wrong, refuse to be assertive with others, become upset or frustrated when dealing with stress, react with anger or become impatient when describing the situation, protest that they ought not to behave so stupidly, have difficulty concentrating on the task, comply with the instructions of SA but do so reluctantly, ignore requests to stay on task and instead launch into new topics, or wonder out loud how the exercise can possibly help them. These general behaviors, though not necessarily connected to the situation being analyzed, are more often than not similar to the patterns the individual will describe in the SA.

Depending upon the therapist's hypothesis regarding the patient's interpersonal problems, additional information should be requested as needed to amplify behavior in these areas. For example, while going through the first two steps in SA, one patient had already made several references to the fact that he always fails at everything he does. His SA involved an exchange in which his boss assigned him a job but then, after talking with him, decided to give the assignment to someone else. From the patient's preceding behavior in the first two steps, the therapist knew it was highly likely that the patient's "sighs of failure" might have played an essential role in the boss's reassignment decision. In completing Step 3, the therapist had the patient carefully reconstruct both his verbal (what he said) *and* nonverbal (how he said it) behavior with the boss, once the job request had been made.

This step functions as an *assessment device* for the therapist (to target behavioral areas needing work) as well as a *means to an end* of demonstrating to the patient how his/her behavior contributed to the situational outcome.

Therapist Rules for Administering Step 3

1. During the early sessions, the clinician provides a rationale for the step.

Patients need to learn to think of their behavior as being one step in a process that leads directly to a situational outcome. Focusing on how a patient behaves in light of his/her newly identified interpretations provides the individual with essential information showing *why* the situation turned out the way it did.

2. The therapist teaches the patient to self-monitor his/her behavior while interacting with others.

Patients learn quickly in SA to start paying attention to how they behave. Over time, they also become cognizant of destructive patterns that lead to undesirable consequences. Hasty and impulsive reactions toward others are frequently encountered behaviors that preclude attainment of the desired outcome. Learning to *stop, look,* and *listen* before responding, particularly in important situations, is a valuable skill many patients pinpoint during latter sessions when they discuss which behavioral strategies have been most helpful.

3. The clinician uses the behavioral information obtained to formulate a behavioral skills training program.

The behavioral information obtained during Step 3 is used to formulate a treatment strategy to improve interpersonal functioning. CBASP behavioral training programs focus on developing (1) assertiveness skills, by training patients to communicate clearly with others in succinct declarative sentences; (2) job interviewing skills and social skills, by using role-playing techniques; (3) self-disclosure skills, by helping patients learn to share their emotional needs with others; and (4) listening skills, by teaching patients to track the emotional content of a conversation. The third and fourth types of skills involve the generation of empathic behavior, which is a central behavioral goal of the CBASP program. (It should be noted here that the implementation of a remedial behavioral program should only be undertaken after the SA exercise is completed.)

4. The clinician should let the patient do the work. That is, the clinician should participate and work collaboratively, but should not do the work for the individual.

Again, this point is important. Patients' generally submissive style always pulls for dominant takeover behavior on the part of therapists. The rule I have stated earlier is applicable here: *Whatever therapists do for patients, patients will not learn to do for themselves.*

Patient Performance Goal for Step 3

1. The patient learns to focus on relevant aspects of his/her interpersonal behavior that help to achieve the DO.

Since behavior and consequences are always linked in the SA exercise, patients are repeatedly given practice at identifying which responses led to a particular situational outcome. In addition, they are also required to evaluate whether or not a particular behavior resulted in a desirable or undesirable outcome. Over time, patients become adept at discriminating which of their behaviors lead to positive ends and which do not.

STEP 4: SITUATIONAL ACTUAL OUTCOME

The prompt question for step 4 is "How did the event come out for you?" Here, the actual outcome (AO) is pinpointed and described. Chronically depressed patients are rarely able to recognize the consequences of their behavior. Even if they do recall the outcome of some encounter, it is usually described reflexively and in a global manner (e.g., "Nothing ever works out for me"; "No one likes me," etc.). When one is unaware of the responses one evokes in others, one is perceptually disengaged from the environment in essential ways. Patients are made aware of the nature of their connection to others in Step 4, as they are asked to formulate the AO in behavioral terms. This step in SA is the beginning of learning to recognize consequences for behavior.

Therapist Rules for Administering Step 4

1. During the early sessions, the practitioner provides a rationale for the step before eliciting an AO sentence.

For example, the practitioner might say:

"Step 4 will be a description of how the situation came out—that is, the situational outcome. In SA we call it the '*actual outcome.*'

Being able to recognize outcomes is a crucial skill in assessing what effects you are having upon others. Learning to recognize situational outcomes accurately will play an essential role in helping you overcome your depression."

2. The therapist teaches patients to describe the AO in a time-anchored sentence that is framed in behavioral terms.

Step 4 is the "keystone" of the SA arch, as everything (cognitively and behaviorally) that has occurred up to now converges in the one-sentence description of the outcome. The remainder of the SA procedure depends upon the construction of a behaviorally formulated AO. The success or failure of the patient's situational behavior will subsequently be evaluated in light of the AO.

3. The therapist lets the patient do the work when constructing the AO sentence.

As stated in connection with earlier steps, the clinician should avoid paraphrasing, summarizing, editorializing, or otherwise doing the work for the patient. The patient must operationalize the endpoint of the event in behavioral terminology. The temptation is always present to expedite the process and construct the AO for the patient. As before, my advice is "Don't!" The patient needs to learn how to do it independently.

Avoiding Common Errors during Step 4

New therapists often make mistakes here that undercut or compromise the efficacy of SA. Five common errors that therapists make in administering Step 4 are as follows:

1. The AO is not anchored temporally.
2. The AO is formulated in emotional terms.
3. The AO is stated in ambiguous terms.
4. The clinician allows the patient to revise the AO in subsequent steps of SA.
5. The therapist works with multiple AOs.

1. *The AO is not anchored temporally.* If the endpoint of the event is not fixed firmly in time, the outcome will float temporally, and the

power of the consequence exercise will be compromised. Consider this example:

THERAPIST: How did the event come out for you?

PATIENT: Well, our agreement was never settled, and we talked again the next day and then had several more conversations after that. Nothing was ever decided. [The endpoint of the situation was not anchored in time.]

It is unlikely that this therapist will be able to demonstrate consequences for the patient's situational behavior, because the stopping point of the event was never established. The best stopping point would be at the end of the first conversation.

2. *The AO is formulated in emotional terms.* When therapists allow patients to construct their AOs in emotional terms—"I felt relieved," "I was upset," "I was really annoyed at the salesman,"—they are inadvertently precluding a focus on the environmental consequences by highlighting the patient's internal emotional state. I am not suggesting that emotional correlates don't accompany an AO, nor am I saying that patients should not be allowed to describe their emotional reactions when constructing their AOs. Rather, I am saying that *the AO must first be formulated in terms of an objective report of what happened at the end of the situation.* In essence, the AO must be articulated in such clear behavioral terms that an outside observer could confirm it.

3. *The AO is stated in ambiguous terms.* When the AO sentence is ill-defined, the outcome will not be clear to either the clinician or the patient. If the patient is to assimilate the full impact of the consequences of his/her behavior, the AO must be stated precisely. Another example will illustrate my point.

THERAPIST: How did the event come out for you?

PATIENT: Well, it ended up better than it had before. I sure felt that we had made some progress with the problem.

How should the psychotherapist respond?

THERAPIST: I'm not sure I understand how the event came out for you. Could you be more specific and state what you mean by it "ended up better" and "we had made some progress"? Try to say it in one sentence.

PATIENT: (Thinking) We settled our argument on Tuesday about who would wash the dishes, and we did it without yelling at each other.

THERAPIST: That's good. Now I understand how it came out.

4. *The clinician allows the patient to revise the AO in subsequent steps of SA.* Once stated, the AO must remain fixed; it is impossible to demonstrate the consequences of behavior when the AO is a "moving target." For example:

THERAPIST: How did the event come out for you?

PATIENT: Well, that's hard to say. On Monday, things didn't look good. Tuesday was a different story. Thursday, I thought the contract might work out. Friday, the deal fell through.

THERAPIST: Okay, looking back at how the event came out for you, choose which day's outcome you want to use for the AO.

PATIENT: I want to use Friday's outcome. I need to understand what went wrong.

Using Friday's perspective is fine; however, once the choice is made, it must remain fixed. The patient must make the call, and the therapist must hold the patient firmly to the decision. If the patient wants to go back and talk from Monday's perspective or Tuesday's perspective, or from some other perspective altogether, the therapist must impose limits if the SA exercise is to be effective.

This brings up an interesting point. The selection of an AO may seem artificial and dependent on *when* the person selects a "slice of time" to analyze. In any ongoing relationship, a particular conversation may continue over several hours, days, or weeks. How can anyone know which endpoint is more reflective of the interpersonal process than another? However, such questions can only arise from a formal operations thinker, who can generate numerous AOs to any interpersonal exchange. Since chronically depressed adults think about events in rigid and global ways, teaching them consequences for their behavior requires beginning with a problematical slice of time that has a beginning point and an ending point.

5. *The therapist works with multiple AOs.* Working with multiple AOs is a losing battle. When a patient reports more than one AO, the therapist must ask the patient to rank the AOs in order of importance and work only with the one in the first position.

Some patients, when they come to Step 4, have difficulty selecting just one outcome. These individuals behave as if they want "to keep their options open." Using only the first-ranked AO forces the person to make a decision and increases the probability that the individual will have to confront the consequences of his/her behavior.

Patient Performance Goal for Step 4

1. The patient learns to construct the AO in one sentence, using behavioral terminology.

Successful completion of Step 4 demonstrates that the individual is now able to focus on a discrete slice of time and to pinpoint an outcome for the occasion. Planful problem solving (Folkman & Lazarus, 1988) consists of focused efforts to alter problematic situations; combined with a cognitive-analytic approach, this approach leads to effective resolutions. This approach depends upon patients' being able to focus on the results of their behavior *at a given point in time* (D'Zurilla & Goldfried, 1971). Step 4 continues to challenge patients' preoperational worldview by requiring that they connect their cognitive and behavioral tactics with actual situational outcomes. Step 4 is another aspect of the "If this. . . then that" mismatching exercise, which requires a preoperational individual to think in formal operations terms.

STEP 5: SITUATIONAL DESIRED OUTCOME

The chronically depressed patient is now asked to do something he/she has probably not done before: think of specific possibilities and formulate a *desired outcome* (DO) for a particular event. When the clinician asks, "How did you want the situation to come out?", the attention of the patient is now focused upon the endpoint and the person must describe what outcome he/she wanted.

Step 5 is used in several ways:

- To motivate the patient to change
- To assess situational pathology
- To establish a marker by which the patient can assess the adequacy of his/her performance in a situation

- To help the patient develop goal-oriented thinking
- To prepare the individual to reap the rewards of successful living

Since individuals rarely achieve their DOs during the early sessions, discomfort is often produced when a patient is asked to compare and contrast, in the presence of the clinician, the DO with the AO. The intention, however, is to potentiate the discomfort level in this phase of SA, so that reduction of the distress occurs following more adaptive behavior. As discussed earlier, creating in-session distress sets the stage for the administration of negative reinforcement—which is a motivating event that leads to change.

Constructing the DO also establishes a standard of comparison against which both the therapist and patient can assess the patient's performance adequacy in the situation. If there is a discrepancy between what the patient produces (AO) and what he/she wants (DO), the crucial assessment question becomes "*Why* didn't you get what you wanted here?"

Identifying DOs helps individuals become goal-oriented in their thinking (Platt & Spivack, 1972, 1974, 1975; Platt, Siegel, & Spivack, 1975). Indeed, a significant change in treatment occurs when patients report spontaneously that they are constructing DOs on their own at the beginning of interpersonal encounters. Taking this kind of action indicates a developing goal-directed approach to living, and this marker is an early harbinger of change.

A final reason to have patients construct DOs is so that clinicians can prepare them to reap the rewards of interpersonal success when these do occur! When patients describe situations in therapy sessions where the AO = DO, it's time for celebration! The process of SA on these occasions makes it extremely difficult for the individual to avoid the fact of his/her success and accomplishment. Whenever AO = DO, the SA becomes a vehicle to highlight and strengthen those facilitative strategies that led to the successful outcome. The therapist is also in a position to use the AO-versus-DO comparison as a positive reinforcement tactic: The therapist's obvious delight and satisfaction over the patient's success serves as a powerful source of positive reinforcement. A cause-for-celebration moment is illustrated below:

THERAPIST: How did the situation come out for you [AO]?

PATIENT: I told my husband how much he had hurt me when he called me stupid. [The patient went on to say that her husband was very surprised and had no idea that his remarks had been hurtful. He also said that he would try not to say this sort of thing again.]

THERAPIST: How did you want the situation to come out [DO]?

PATIENT: I wanted to tell my husband how much he hurt me when he called me stupid.

THERAPIST: Did you get what you wanted in this situation [AO-versus-DO comparison]?

PATIENT: YES! I finally did it! I told him what I wanted to. I stood up to him for the first time! I've never done this before. It's unbelievable.

THERAPIST: *Why* do you think you got what you wanted here?

PATIENT: Because I finally asserted myself! It has taken me long enough, don't you think!

Therapist Rules for Administering Step 5

1. During the early sessions, the therapist provides the patient with a rationale for Step 5.

For example, the clinician might say:

"I am asking you to formulate a 'desired outcome' in SA to help you evaluate the adequacy of the actual outcome. Once you propose a goal for yourself, we can look carefully at whether or not you achieved it, and if you didn't, we can learn why not. We call the desired outcome the 'DO' in SA. It will play an important role in helping you change some things in your life that prevent you from obtaining the things you want."

2. The therapist teaches the patient to construct only one DO per situation, and to state it succinctly in behavioral terms.

Some patients propose multiple DOs for an event, as they do in AO construction. A patient who does this should be asked to rank the outcomes in terms of desirability, and then to work *only* with the DO ranked first. When several DOs are allowed to remain on the table, the SA exercise becomes unwieldy and confusing.

Another consideration to keep in mind is that patients should not be

allowed to construct nonbehavioral DOs. The error *always* becomes problematical as in the following example:

THERAPIST: How did you want the situation to come out [DO]?

PATIENT: I wanted to stop the art show plans before preparations went
any further. I also wanted to express myself to Mary, feeling confident.

THERAPIST: You've really got two desired outcomes here: that is, stopping the plans and expressing yourself to Mary, feeling confident. We
can use only one. Which one do you want to use? You choose the one
you want to go with.

PATIENT: I want to be able to express myself to Mary, feeling confident.

THERAPIST: Then we'll use expressing your feelings to Mary, feeling confident as your DO.

The therapist made one correct response when he had the patient
rank the two DOs and use only the first choice. What remains problematical is that the DO has been stated in emotional terms. It would be
acceptable to use the DO of "confidence" if the clinician had asked the
patient to operationalize the word by putting it into behavioral terms.
Perhaps saying something "with confidence" might be operationalized in
terms of "maintaining good eye contact," "stating my case in clear, concise sentences," and the like. However, since the DO is not operationalized behaviorally, the clinician is subtly programming the person to fail.
Why? Because this patient, like other chronic patients, usually does not
possess assertive skills and wouldn't have been able to assert herself to
Mary, feeling confident. Her first-choice DO assumes that assertive skills
are in place, and this was not the case. A more realistic DO might have
been simply telling Mary what she wanted to say. Ideally, emotional feelings such as confidence will hopefully come later, after assertive skills
have been developed.

Another reason why working with emotional DOs is discouraged is
because of the impossibility of producing specific emotional reactions in
difficult interpersonal encounters. Most events analyzed in sessions are
troublesome and problematical. It is easy as well as seductive to construct
a DO in terms of wanting to feel confident, bold, happy, satisfied, and
calm; to behave with grace and aplomb; and to leave the situation with a
forgiving attitude. The reality is that positive emotions usually follow the
mastery of difficult tasks or situations. Confidence, boldness, and so on,
rarely predate mastery experiences. This is particularly true with chroni-

cally depressed individuals. In situations where the DO is not obtained, the requisite behavioral skills will first have to be identified, then learned, and finally practiced until mastery is achieved. The skill deficits can then be remediated after they have been exposed.

3. The therapist teaches the patient to construct *attainable* and *realistic* DOs.

Remediation procedures for maladaptive DOs will not be described until Chapter 7, but for clarity's sake, the criteria for adaptive DOs will be briefly defined below.

Attainable Desired Outcomes

Two criteria must be kept in mind when patients construct desired outcomes. First, can the environment deliver what is desired? To say that a DO is "attainable" means that the environment is capable of delivering what the individual wants. In the interpersonal realm, this means evaluating the degree to which another person is willing or capable of providing what the patient wants.

Dealing with the attainability criterion is difficult for many chronically depressed adults. Many begin therapy poorly equipped to decide what can and cannot be obtained interpersonally. This comes, in large measure, from patients' inexperience with encounters where others went out of their way to extend respect or kindness. Therefore, it is not surprising that they have difficulty conceptualizing attainable interpersonal goals. Given their maltreatment history, the best most patients can do at first is to want another person to be different. Consider the example of "Anne":

THERAPIST: Anne, how would you have liked this situation to come out for you [DO]?

ANNE: I wanted my boyfriend to listen to what I said.

THERAPIST: Did you get what you wanted in this situation?

ANNE: Hell, no! He hit me and shoved me against the wall. I keep hoping he'll change. It's no use. He'll always be a jerk.

Anne has been living with "John" for five years. His behavior has remained consistent, and the clinician knows that John is unlikely to change. The DO is clearly *unattainable*—the environment will not deliver what Anne wants. Yet Anne keeps living with John, hoping that someday he will change. John's chronic and abusive reactions to Anne do not yet have a formative impact on her behavior. To date, she has not been able to consider seriously leaving John. The task of SA here is to highlight this unattainable DO during the remediation phase and to help Anne confront its destructive implications. During remediation, the therapist will continue to ask Anne how she will achieve her DO in these situations when her interpretations keep telling her she cannot. This scenario will probably be replayed several times before Anne will become able to accept the fact that John will never be the person she wants him to be. At that point, the patient will confront a major choice point: "If I want a man to listen to me and not hurt me, then I've got to find another man!"

Realistic Desired Outcomes

"Realistic" DOs are goals that the individual has the personal capability of producing. These goals may include behavioral skills, intellectual achievement, emotional reactions, athletic endeavors, etc. Examples of unrealistic DOs are wanting to play varsity football but having insufficient athletic ability; yearning to assert oneself with others without an assertive behavior repertoire; or desiring to love someone when the appropriate feelings are absent. In the first and last examples, the goals are unrealistic in an ultimate sense. The second involves a skill deficit that can be remedied.

Chronically depressed patients frequently propose unrealistic DOs for themselves. Their interpersonal rigidity and their limited social skills program these individuals to fail repeatedly in any social milieu. The pattern of failure will be maintained if the unrealistic DOs are not recognized and addressed.

Clinical practice provides numerous examples of unrealistic DOs. Here are some examples of individuals who expected the impossible from themselves:

1. "I wanted to obtain the job [when it is obvious the patient does not have the requisite skills]."
2. "I wanted to talk with my family about the effects their racial attitudes are having upon my friends and do it in an objective manner [when the bigotry of the family has led to uncontrollable rage outbursts toward the patient during many previous discussions]."

3. "I want to be able to talk to extremely rude customers with no emotional reaction [when a customer service job makes the patient take the brunt of frequent consumer attacks]."

4. "I want to pass the test [when the individual has not studied]."

5. "I don't want to be emotionally upset by the negative remarks my middle school math students make to me [God help all middle school teachers]."

6. "I want to be admitted into graduate school to study psychology [when the individual possesses a low-average level of intelligence]."

All these examples involve goals that are clearly unrealistic. In each case, the therapist must help the person modify his/her DO. Some of the examples illustrate situations in which the person desires things that are not achievable because of insufficient preparation (the job, the exam), while others are beyond the person's emotional capacity to produce (neutral reactions to bigoted family members, middle school students, and irate customers); finally, one individual did not have the intellectual ability to produce the desired goal (attending graduate school).

Most cases I see involve one or two major life areas where unattainable or unrealistic DOs are tacitly being lived out in repeated fashion, and remediating the one or two problem DOs has a generalized treatment effect on other life areas. One case in point involved a female patient who always played the dependent victim role with males. The patient learned how to be assertive with one male by telling him what she wanted and didn't want. The relationship quickly terminated, and the patient soon discovered that she was attracting a different type of man—males who were attracted to a previously dependent female suddenly found themselves without a partner.

Learning to strive for goals that are attainable while avoiding those that are not, and learning to have realistic expectations of oneself while eschewing unrealistic ones, are essential goals for patients in Step 5.

4. The therapist must understand every word the patient uses in the DO sentence.

Therapists must not guess at what patients mean by pet phrases, idiosyncratic expressions, or metaphorical descriptions. They should be asked to clarify their language so that the meaning of each word in each DO is clear, as in this example:

THERAPIST: How did you want the situation to come out for you [DO]?

PATIENT: I wanted him to "put his jack on the table."

THERAPIST: I'm not sure I follow you. Would you state this in another way?

PATIENT: I wanted Robert to tell me what he wanted.

THERAPIST: Now I understand the DO.

5. The therapist must not do the work of constructing the DO for the patient.

Once more, I state the obvious: Clinicians must teach patients to complete Step 5 without doing their work for them. As noted above, constructing a DO sentence is sometimes difficult, slow, and tedious. The temptation is always to give in to impatience and take over the task. Instead, a therapist should wait for a patient to work out the final sentence construction, even if it means repeatedly asking for revisions until the sentence meets the criterion stated in the second therapist rule (teaching the patient to construct only one DO that is stated in behavioral terms).

6. If the DO is achieved, but there is verbal or nonverbal distress evident in the patient (*or in the therapist*) concerning the DO, the DO should be revised.

These types of DOs occur on three occasions. First, some patients have difficulty saying no or setting limits on others, and their DOs often reflect a compliance theme that leaves them feeling dissatisfied or uncomfortable. What happens in Step 5 is that these individuals comply with the wishes of others (because they want to "be nice" or "help out"), and because of their compliance, they propose DOs that disturb them. Therapists should be sensitive to this problem when such DOs are achieved, especially when it becomes obvious that the person is uncomfortable with the achievement. Obtaining the DO is usually a positive event. When it is not, clinicians should question the patient about the desirability of what they wanted. For example:

PATIENT: I got what I wanted here [DO: I wanted to listen to my sister-in-law]. I was helpful to her when she started telling me about her marital difficulties with my brother. I really didn't want her to tell me these things, but I felt I should listen. [Patient gives both verbal and nonverbal indications of being upset.]

THERAPIST: There is something wrong here. Which goal did you want? Did you want to tell her not to disclose these things about your brother, or did you want to listen to her disclosures?

PATIENT: I could never tell anyone that I didn't want to hear something they wanted to tell me. I mean, what would I say to her: "Don't tell me these things" and just blow her off?

In this situation, a lack of assertion coupled with wanting to be helpful led to a DO that was undesirable. The therapist must put aside the SA procedure for a moment, address the behavioral deficit, and help the patient practice an appropriate way to set limits with her sister-in-law. Only then will the individual be ready to construct a truly "desirable" DO.

The second occasion arises when a patient constructs an aggressive DO designed to counteraggress a hurtful behavior initiated by another person. One clinician dealt with the problem this way. During the elicitation phase, a female patient described a situation in which her sister walked into the kitchen and began yelling at her because she had not washed the dishes or completed other chores. Both women yelled obscenities at each other and simultaneously left the room. The patient framed her AO this way: "I told my sister she was a bitch and walked out of the kitchen [counteraggressive behavior]." When asked how she wanted the situation to come out, she said, "I wanted to tell her just what I said!"

The patient's next comment, however, was a signal that there was a "problem" with the DO: "I left the room feeling mad, guilty and glad that I let her have it right back." The therapist decided to "step outside" the SA procedure to explore why the patient reacted this way. After asking the individual how her sister's behavior had affected her, as well as discussing several other similar incidents, the patient finally identified the reason for the counterattack: "She hurt me when she yelled at me. She always does—I wanted to hurt her back." Once the hurt feelings were brought into awareness, the clinician returned to the SA procedure and asked the patient to describe the situation once again; however, this time, to describe the event from the vantage point of having been hurt. Another DO was proposed: "I wanted to tell my sister how badly she hurt me."

A third type of problematic DO is seen when a patient expresses the desire to hurt someone deliberately. The therapist is usually uncomfortable with this goal, and for good reason. "I wanted to hurt my wife by tell-ing her what a damn bitch I think she is." Again, the most effective strat-egy is to put the SA procedure aside until the underlying hurt that is motivating the "revenge DO" is exposed. Focusing the person's attention on the painful cognitive-emotional interpretations of the spouse's behav-ior (e.g., "You hate me," "You go out of your way to put me down," "You delight in making me feel bad," etc.) is a productive tactic. As noted above, until the underlying pain and hurt are acknowledged and incorpo-rated into the situational description, no DO will resolve the interper-sonal conflict. Once this patient acknowledged the extent to which he had been hurt, he was able to propose a realistic DO: "I wanted my wife to know how badly she had hurt me when she said that."

The reason why dissatisfyingly compliant, counteraggressive, and vengeance-seeking DOs are unsatisfactory is because they cannot resolve the interpersonal problems present in the situation. DOs that inflame already existing interpersonal conflicts must be carefully scrutinized to expose the underlying issues.

Patient Performance Goals for Step 5

1. The patient learns to construct a one-sentence DO, using behav-ioral terminology.

Teaching patients to construct DOs that meet this criterion is well worth the effort. Now they have a standard against which to evaluate the quality of their situational performance. By the end of treatment, patients should be approaching all interpersonal encounters from a proactive, goal-directed perspective.

2. The patient learns to construct realistic and attainable DOs.

STEP 6: COMPARING THE ACTUAL OUTCOME TO THE DESIRED OUTCOME

The prompt question clinicians ask patients at the beginning of Step 6 is "Did you get what you wanted here?" The climax of the elicitation phase is precipitated by this question. Patients must now evaluate the adequacy of their situational behavior to assess whether or not they produced the DO. The answer to the question and the manner in which it is said often denote the degree of distress (or its absence) in an individual. *A therapist should not hurry a patient through this step.* Rather, the patient needs to examine directly the actual consequences of his/her behavior (AO) in relation to the DO. The AO-versus-DO comparison is likely to be the first time the patient has had to face his/her behavioral consequences. In the early stages of treatment, more often than not, the AO is not satisfying, the results are negative, and it is obvious that the DO was not obtained. By asking patients at these stages to compare their AOs to their DOs, clinicians are asking them to expose their own inadequate behavior—not a pleasant experience. The personal evaluation at this juncture directs the attention of preoperational patients to the cause-effect reality they have produced.

Step 6 is completed when a patient has provided some answer to the question. The practitioner does not spend much time examining the reasons; he/she is only interested in understanding the logic the patient offers for the perceived failure. The reasons patients give for not achieving their DOs will change significantly over the course of treatment. As patients become more adept behaviorally, their replies will reflect improvement in interpersonal functioning and a more acute awareness of the consequences of their behavior. Step 6 of SA represents a transition step leading directly into the remediation phase.

Therapist Rules for Administering Step 6

1. The therapist should state the AO-versus-DO question clearly and should not rush the patient through the step.

Therapists-in-training see the obvious and sometimes feel foolish asking patients whether they got what they wanted when it is clear they didn't. In such instances, therapists either make the comparison themselves or rush too rapidly through the AO-versus-DO comparison. In all likelihood, they are reducing their own anxiety and not focusing on the discomfort of their patients. A common response made by a novice therapist on such an occasion goes something like this: "It's obvious you didn't get what you wanted here. Why didn't you get it?" The patient is looking at the therapist's question from a radically different perspective. Reducing the therapist's anxiety is not the goal, and glossing over the question removes the opportunity for the individual to confront the consequences of his/her behavior.

> 2. The therapist asks the patient *why* he/she didn't achieve the DO *only after* allowing the patient sufficient time to make the AO-versus-DO comparison.

Again, therapists-in-training frequently spend too much time listening to the reasons given for failure or even suggesting additional reasons why their patients didn't obtain their DOs. As noted above, the "why" question is asked for assessment purposes only; that is, a clinician wants to see what causal sense a patient can make of the failure to achieve the DO. After the patient has given one or two reasons, the therapist should move directly into Step 1 of remediation. Optimally, there should be little or no therapist comment following the patient's expressed reasons. New therapists often get into lengthy discussions here concerning why the individual didn't produce the DO. I advise them, "Don't. Move on into the remediation phase."

Patient Performance Goal for Step 6

> 1. The patient learns to evaluate situational behavior, using the AO-versus-DO comparison.

Learning to self-evaluate one's own interpersonal behavior is one of the primary goals of the CBASP program. Situational focusing, self-evaluation, and goal-directed behavior are all primary didactic goals of the SA exercise. Over time, patients will increasingly develop improved self-evaluation skills, as demonstrated by the causal explanations they give to the "why" question. Two excerpts are provided below to illustrate the development of self-evaluation skills. The first was the patient's response during an early session, and the second during his final therapy session:

THERAPIST: Did you get what you wanted here?

PATIENT: No!

THERAPIST: *Why* didn't you get what you wanted?

PATIENT: It's the same old story. She said "no" to me because it's the story of my life. I should have known she wouldn't go out with me again. No woman will ever go out with me after the first date.

During the final session, the therapist asked the patient why he didn't obtain his DO. The outcome was similar to the one in the SA above in that the individual had been out on several dates with another woman and had asked her for a date on Saturday.

THERAPIST: Did you get what you wanted?

PATIENT: No, and I can tell you why. Sharon and I have been seeing each other for three weeks. She and I have some unresolvable differences. I have also thought about breaking it off, but I haven't had the courage to say it. Going against my better judgment, I asked her for a date Saturday. She told me what I really thought was best for us—that we shouldn't continue to date. Wish I had been able to say it first.

I will turn now to a description of the remediation phase of SA in which patients are taught to remedy the cognitive and behavioral errors that they made during the elicitation phase.

CHAPTER SEVEN

Remediation Phase of Situational Analysis

> ... the development of formal operational structures may be enhanced through therapeutic intervention ... formal operations opens up the hypothetical world for the individual such that reality becomes secondary to possibility.
>
> —D. E. GORDON (1988, p. 67, 56)

INTRODUCTION TO THE REMEDIATION PHASE

In Step 6 of the elicitation phase of SA, patients are asked *why* they didn't achieve the DO. This query inaugurates the remediation phase. Most beginning patients are unable to answer the question in a meaningful way because of a deficiency in causal reasoning. Typical answers to the "why" question are "No one likes me," "Things will never work out," "I just fail at everything I try to do," and "I'm stupid and no good." A preoperational view of the world is evident here. Once patients learn to evaluate their situational performance accurately, answers to the "why" question reflect perceptual shifts toward more sophisticated causal thinking. The answers will become more time-anchored and increasingly related to actual events that took place in the situation.

As the curtain goes up on the remediation phase, the therapist and patient have to address a situational conundrum that must be solved. The problem is determining what the patient must do differently to obtain the DO. SA gives the patient an opportunity to look back in time and "fix" a badly managed interpersonal event. As stated earlier, the exercise is not emotionally neutral. Not only is the patient scrutinizing highly personal information in the presence of the clinician, but also the event has probably been distressing because of the failure component. However, discomfort is a desirable state at this point because it is a necessary precursor to change.

Undertaking remediation in the absence of discomfort or when patients remain emotionally detached makes change unlikely. Sometimes chronic patients cannot identify an emotionally distressing situation, or they evince little or no emotion during SA. When these instances reflect trait patterns, the prognosis for a favorable treatment outcome is poor. Patients with comorbid schizoid personality disorder often pose such difficulties because of their extreme detachment in the interpersonal realm and their restricted range of emotional expression.

I turn now to a discussion of the four steps of remediation. For each step, I will include introductory comments followed by a delineation of administrative rules and patient performance goals.

STEP 1: REVISING IRRELEVANT AND INACCURATE INTERPRETATIONS

The importance of clearly operationalizing the AO and DO in behavioral terms becomes obvious in this first remedial step. The AO-versus-DO comparison serves as a constant reminder of the inefficacy of a patient's behavior. The DO, as the situational "bull's eye," focuses patients' attention on where they *want* to be. On the other hand, the AO, representing their initial attempt to hit the bull's eye, serves as a reminder of just how far off the mark they were. Clear behavioral definitions in both domains make the comparative process easier.

In Step 1 of remediation, the therapist focuses on each interpretation, one at a time, and asks the same question for each read,

"How does this interpretation contribute to your getting what you want?"

The question requires that the individual think in an "If this . . . then that" mode by evaluating the contribution each read makes to attainment of the DO. As discussed in Chapter 6, the adequacy of every interpretation is evaluated in terms of its *accuracy* and *relevancy*. Relevant reads anchor patients in a discrete "slice of time" and concentrate their efforts on the problem-at-hand. Accurate interpretations enable one to assess correctly *what is happening* in the unfolding interactive process, thus maximizing the possibility that the DO will be achieved. In short, relevant and accurate interpretations frequently result in planful problem focused action (Folkman & Lazarus, 1988) and attainment of the DO.

Many of the interpretive constructions of chronic patients have to be revised. Let's take a case example to illustrate how the remediation process works with irrelevant and inaccurate interpretations. The patient wanted to talk with "Bill," a colleague, about a disagreement they had had (DO). The AO—"we never discussed our disagreement, and I gave up"— was distressing to the patient.

THERAPIST: Look at your first interpretation and see what it contributed to your getting your DO. The first read you constructed was "I have failed once again." What you wanted [DO] was to discuss your disagreement with Bill. How did this interpretation contribute to your discussing your views with Bill? Help me see the connection between this interpretation and getting what you wanted.

PATIENT: I don't know. I don't suppose it contributed at all. It's just what goes on in my head whenever I face a difficult situation.

THERAPIST: Was the interpretation grounded in the situation? That is, was it *relevant*, and did it reflect something that was *actually happening* between you and Bill?

PATIENT: No. It's just a thought I have whenever I have a conflict with someone.

THERAPIST: Our goal here is to find an interpretation that plants your feet solidly in the event. This read obviously didn't do it. Let's see if we can revise the read to make it reflect what was actually going on between you and Bill.

PATIENT: I'll try: Bill said he was very busy and wanted to talk about the disagreement later.

THERAPIST: Now you're getting the hang of it. Is this read anchored to something that actually happened in the situation?

PATIENT: Yes.

THERAPIST: Does it accurately reflect what is happening between you and Bill?

PATIENT: Yes.

THERAPIST: If this is what is going on between you two, what does this say about your obtaining the DO? Think carefully about this.

PATIENT: It means he will not talk to me right now but he will later. [Revising the interpretation now makes the original DO unattainable.]

THERAPIST: Then what is a more attainable DO for you here?

PATIENT: To schedule a time when Bill and I can talk. [The DO is now attainable in light of the new interpretation.]

THERAPIST: You got it!

The revision of the first interpretation now exposes problems with the original DO of wanting to discuss the disagreement with Bill. How can the patient discuss the disagreement when Bill doesn't want to talk about it now? The environment (Bill) will not deliver what the patient wants and, therefore, the DO is currently unattainable.

In addition to attainability, DOs are evaluated from another perspective. Patients need to be able to produce what they want (a *realistic* DO). Sometimes patients cannot produce the DO; thus it will be unrealistic. Another excerpt illustrates the point:

THERAPIST: How did you want the situation to come out for you?

PATIENT: I wanted to feel real love for this woman [DO]. She's everything I've ever thought I wanted. I can't see why the feelings are not there. I should be able to love her.

There are two things wrong with this DO. First, it is not framed in behavioral terminology; second, and more importantly, it is an unrealistic goal. The man does not love the woman. He cannot produce the emotional feelings. Patients like this will frequently construct unrealistic goals, and as a result they express frequent disappointment in themselves.

DESIRED OUTCOME REVISION RULE: Whenever the desired DO is exposed as inadequate (unattainable or unrealistic) in Step 1 of remediation, the DO must be immediately revised and made to fit attainable or realistic criteria before continuing with further interpretation revision.

Returning to our first example, notice the way the inadequate DO will be revised and how the clinician used the revision process to teach the "If this . . . then that" perspective:

THERAPIST: You have revised your read. Bill wants to talk about the disagreement some other time. How does this relevant and accurate interpretation contribute to your getting what you want?

PATIENT: It doesn't. Bill didn't want to discuss our disagreement at that moment.

THERAPIST: This situation has got all sorts of learning possibilities for you. Look at what you want here. Is your desired outcome attainable in this situation?

PATIENT: No. He didn't want to discuss the matter then.

THERAPIST: The environment, or Bill, won't deliver what you want right now. That's clear. Now, what do we need to do about the DO to construct an attainable desired outcome for you, right now in this event?

PATIENT: (Long, thoughtful pause) I've got to come up with another goal. I could have asked Bill to schedule a time when we could talk.

THERAPIST: Fantastic! Now construct one sentence that expresses this newly formed DO.

PATIENT: To schedule a time when we could discuss the disagreement [an attainable DO].

THERAPIST: Is Bill likely to grant you your request? [The therapist is checking again for attainability since he does not know Bill—maybe Bill can't be counted on to do what he says he will.]

PATIENT: Yeah, he's really an okay guy.

THERAPIST: Then we've got a solid DO to work with now. Do you see how your revised interpretation led us to an achievable DO, given Bill's reaction to you? That's why it's so important that you learn to interpret situations relevantly and accurately.

PATIENT: Yeah, but I have trouble thinking that fast.

THERAPIST: We'll keep working on it—practice, practice, until you get it down. Let's go to your second interpretation to see how it might contribute to setting up a specific time to talk with Bill.

Chronically depressed patients generally need a great deal of practice with SA, as well as generous amounts of constant performance-based feedback (Bandura, 1977b), like that shown above, if interpretational mastery is to be achieved. Learning to modify interpretative behavior to obtain the DO while simultaneously interacting with another person requires a patient to remain focused during the encounter and to think in formal operations terms. The person must also learn to readjust the goal quickly when it becomes apparent that the original target is not attainable. Teaching patients to maintain their "aim" on the DO bull's eye is the first step.

It's easy to see why preoperational patients fail dismally in the social arena. The above example illustrates the self-centered, primitive thinking ("I have failed once again") so characteristic of this group. At first, the patient was unable to think of how to modify the outcome because he was unable to think in "If this ... then that" terms. The example also illustrates why the environmental consequences (the AO: "We did not discuss our disagreement") did not formatively influence the patient to schedule another time to talk; he was too busy concentrating on himself and not on the actual events as they unfolded. He had given up the desired goal of talking further about the disagreement because he had concluded (wrongly) that this was just another example of his ineptness. And, indeed, it turned out that surrender of personal goals, followed by long bouts of self-castigation, had been a long-standing pattern for him.

Successful Situational Management When AO = DO

The remediation phase also allows practitioners to highlight patients' successes when they achieve what they want—that is, when the AO = DO. As noted in Chapter 6, this is always a cause for celebration! It is a time to reinforce positively adaptive behavior and to inhibit any impulse to focus on mistakes that might have been made. The reactions of the clinician are crucial here. Interestingly, some patients are embarrassed by their success; others make light of it; some will attribute it to the fact that it wasn't raining and the sun was out ("People just feel better in pretty weather"). However, most patients are genuinely proud of themselves during these moments. The temporal focus of SA affords a wonderful opportunity to bring a patient's achievements to center stage. Just as SA blocks the attempted escape of patients who wish to avoid the specific reasons why they fail, SA also precludes escape from acknowledging the things they do right when they succeed. The opportunity for celebration must never be overlooked or hurried!

The following excerpt demonstrates how significant these first AO = DO successes can be.

PATIENT: I've got to tell you what happened! You know the SA we did last week when I was unable to tell my boyfriend how much what he said was hurting me and how much I wanted him to stop? It became clear to me that he had no idea what he was doing to me. You and I practiced what to say and how to say it. I left last session thinking I would never be able to do it. But I did it! I did it last night! And I got what I wanted! He stopped making sarcastic comments to me! It worked! He listened to me, probably for the first time since we've been dating!

THERAPIST: Take me through the SA. Don't leave out a thing. I want to hear it all. Wish I had some champagne. I'd break it out right now! First, tell me what happened in the situation. Let's go through the steps.

Such breakthroughs are wonderful and usually lead to increased motivation for change. This patient had demonstrated to herself, unmistakably, that *her behavior had consequences* (and, in this case, produced a desirable effect). The SA methodology strengthens the perceived connection between person and environment. Skinner (1953) was correct when he said that consequences formatively influence behavior—but only if we recognize the functional connection between ourselves and the effects we have on others.

Therapist Rules for Administering Step 1

1. Once again, the therapist should not do the work for the patient.
2. The therapist reviews each interpretation in the order that it was stated during the elicitation phase.

Some therapists have the mistaken notion that they should approach the remediation task by ranking the interpretations made in Step 2 of elicitation in terms of their importance to the patient. I advise such therapists, "Don't! Take each interpretation in the order it was stated." Interpretations should accurately describe the unfolding process of the interaction, thereby keeping the patient's attention focused on the situation. If interpretations are taken out of their temporal context, which happens when they are ranked, the patient's connection to the event will be compromised.

3. The therapist reviews each interpretation to determine its relevancy and accuracy, and then helps the patient see how the inter-

pretation either impeded or contributed to the achievement of the DO.

Begin slowly with preoperational thinkers and require that they ponder how they might move logically from an egocentric interpretation to a DO involving another person. Recall the previous SA above in which the patient wanted to discuss a disagreement with Bill. The patient's first interpretation was "I have failed once again." Given his DO (to talk with Bill about the disagreement), the first interpretation was irrelevant and did not reflect what Bill actually said ("Let's talk later"). Something new needed to be added to the preoperational construction. The innovation came by having the patient focus on Bill's behavior and then revising the first interpretation accordingly. Step 1 remedial work is slow and laborious, and patience on the part of the clinician is needed. The revision work is repeated many times, as the clinician methodically demonstrates the inadequacy of each interpretation to move the patient successfully toward the DO. Over time, however, patients acquire the ability to anchor their interpretations by focusing on what is actually going on between themselves and others.

4. The therapist should not separate the cognitive interpretation from its moorings within the situation or from the AO or DO.

Patients must be taught that their cognitive interpretations are always related to situational outcomes. Therapists trained in Beck's method (Beck et al., 1979) sometimes have difficulty with Step 1 because they naturally concentrate on the dysfunctional content of the interpretation per se. This excerpt was taken from a session of a Beckian therapist who was just learning to do SA:

THERAPIST: How did your first interpretation ["I can't stand up to my mother and let her know what I think"] contribute to your telling your mother that she was being rude to your wife [DO]?

PATIENT: It doesn't get me what I want.

THERAPIST: Haven't you had this thought in several situations? It's a rather automatic reaction to your mother. How does this thought leave you feeling?

PATIENT: Helpless and inadequate.

THERAPIST: What is another thought—let's call it "thought B"—that you could say to yourself, right here, that would give you another way to react to your mother?

PATIENT: I don't know.

THERAPIST: Try to come up with an alternative thought, a plan B thought that gives you more flexibility with your mother and doesn't lead to your feeling helpless.

PATIENT: I could say to myself: "I can tell her what I think."

THERAPIST: How would that thought leave you feeling?

PATIENT: A lot better, like I had a choice.

THERAPIST: Okay. Now you have a choice. You can do it the old way, or you can try out the plan B way. The choice is totally yours. Now let's look at your second interpretation and see how it contributed to your obtaining your DO.

This tactic subtly disengages cognitive behavior from the situational context as the focus is shifted from the environment to the patient's cognitive-emotional reaction. Focusing in this manner on the content of interpretations apart from the situational context has two ramifications: (1) Clinicians inadvertently wrest responsiblity for change from the hands of the patient and put it in their own court; and (2) they nudge the individual into the position of either complying or resisting—for, in such moments, it is up to the therapist to demonstrate the error of the patient's thinking, and the individual has no choice but to agree or disagree with the practitioner's logic.

Not only do behavioral consequences (the AO) become obscured in any disputational strategy, but the DO also loses its motivational power. The latter occurs because once behavior is separated from its environmental context, motivation for change is undercut. Whenever patients are allowed to relinquish a focus on the consequences of their behavior, it falls to the charisma and persuasive influence of practitioners to inspire change. Very few chronically depressed patients would overtly resist a clinicians's disputational maneuvers; instead, they would tend to agree with the conclusions and remain depressed.

Over the years and through trial and error, I have found this out the hard way: Letting chronic patients wrestle with the illogical consequences of their thinking and struggle to "fix" their situational interpretations in order to obtain the DO is the best way to modify preoperational cognitive structure. Step 1 has been designed to prevent the patient's escape from the illogical "hot seat." It also allows patients the opportunity to reduce their distress by constructing adequate interpretations.

> 5. Whenever a patient's problematic situations involve spouses, lov-ers, bosses, or friends, the therapist should proceed with caution before concluding that a DO is unattainable.

In Step 1 of remediation, therapists determine whether the DO is *attainable*. In the following example, "Sharon's" DO was getting her hus-band, "Tom," to help with the housecleaning. During previous SAs, Tom's refusal to cooperate with Sharon had led the therapist to conclude that he was unwilling to help his wife under any circumstances (thus making Sharon's DO unattainable). The attainability of the DO was a major con-cern in this SA.

THERAPIST: Let's assess the adequacy of your first interpretation to obtain what you wanted. How did interpreting your husband's behavior as "Tom's a lazy bastard" contribute to your getting his help with the cleaning?

SHARON: I'm not sure, but I know my interpretation is true.

THERAPIST: What part of the interaction does it describe?

SHARON: Well, when I asked him to help, he just looked at me and curled his lip. Then he told me that I'm an unpleasant lady.

COMMENT: Something is missing here that doesn't add up. The thera-pist knows that the patient has an abrasive and abrupt verbal style that, at times, sounds sarcastic and insensitive. He also knows that the patient obtains no cooperation from Tom in situations like this. The question of "verbal abrasiveness" is pursued to determine if Sharon's verbal style may be contributing to Tom's refusal to cooperate.

THERAPIST: Say to me what you said to Tom that morning, and try to say it in the same manner that you spoke it to Tom.

SHARON: "Stop what you're doing and help me clean the den! This is more important than shining your shoes." [Sharon's verbal style is abrupt, insensitive, and abrasive.]

THERAPIST: Now you be Tom and let's imagine that you are shining your shoes. I'll take your role and you be Tom. I'm going to ask you to help me the way you asked Tom. [The therapist makes the request, using Sharon's verbal and nonverbal style]. Now how did that come across?

SHARON: It sounds arrogant as hell.

THERAPIST: Had I asked you to do something for me and made the request this way, would you have done it?

SHARON: Probably not. Do you think this is why Tom doesn't want to help me?

THERAPIST: I'm not sure, but it's surely worth checking out. Why don't you talk to Tom about it? Now, given what you have learned about your verbal style today—and we don't know yet how widespread the effects are in your marriage—what interpretation would you add here to get some help from Tom in this situation?

SHARON: I've got to ask Tom to help me in a nicer way.

THERAPIST: We call this an "action read." It's a revised interpretation or read that *is added* to the situation that leads directly to the DO. Without the action read being added, your behavior doesn't change, and the chances of your getting his help don't look good.

In this case, where the therapist was able to pinpoint a feature of Sharon's verbal style through role play, Sharon became increasingly sensitive to her own stimulus value in such situations. After softening her requests for help, she reported more cooperation from Tom. As it turns out, Sharon's DO was attainable, but only when her verbal behavior changed. The example illustrates the danger of concluding that a DO is unattainable due to *others'* behavior. The therapist must investigate the patient's ability to behave in an appropriate manner before a DO is labeled unattainable.

In any instance where a patient may be inadvertently sabotaging his/her own efforts, a rule of thumb is for the therapist to be conservative and let the patient, over several SAs with a target individual, persuade you that the other person will not or cannot provide what he/she wants. If obtaining the DO from a spouse, friend, colleague, supervisor, or parent is demonstrated to be unattainable even when the patient behaves adaptively, then the DO is shown to be unattainable and must be revised.

6. The therapist teaches the patient to construct "action reads" while in stressful situations.

Patients must learn to construct action interpretations when, in trying to work something out with another person, they become aware that the present course of action is not working and that a more specific strategy will be required to move the interaction toward some goal. These interpretations are often precursors of assertive behavior, and as such, they play an important role in this first remediation step. Openness to learning this skill usually comes after the patient has begun to experience successes in the interpersonal arena. The following action interpretations made by patients illustrate their important role as precursors to assertive behavior.

"I've got to speak up or my agenda will be lost."

"I must tell Rachel how much she means to me—she doesn't think I care about her."

"Jumping on this assignment and doing it now is important—can't wait until Friday."

"We've been arguing long enough. I've got to remind Philip again of what I want."

"The meeting is drifting all over the place. I must express my concern that we are getting off task."

"My therapist is asking too much of me. I must tell her what effect she is having upon me by insisting that I do it her way."

"I must tell the couple sitting down the row that their talking is interfering with my listening to the concert."

Each one of these action interpretations prepares the individual for goal-directed proactive behavior that, if successful, leads directly to the possibility of DO achievement; however, this doesn't mean that the DO will always be obtained. It does mean that by using action reads, individuals place themselves in a much better position to obtain situational goals—if, in fact, they are attainable.

> 7. The therapist should never discard or revise a relevant and accurate interpretation, even when it does not contribute "*directly*" to achievement of a DO.

Good situational interpretations "ground" the person in the realities of the moment and focus energy and attention on the interactional process. These reads also help the person process the moment-to-moment exchanges that lead, finally, to some outcome. Not all adaptive interpretations are linearly related to the DO. The path of an interaction is sometimes circuitous, filled with twists and turns; there may be multiple points of agreement and disagreement until the situation ends at some point. Relevant and accurate interpretations focus the individual on the event as it unfolds from moment to moment, and they foster empathically responsive behavior.

For example, one patient wanted to achieve an agreement with a colleague concerning a marketing issue involving their company (DO). The discussion between the patient and colleague proceeded through several heated debates and disagreements. Agreement was ultimately achieved, but the path the dialogue took toward consensus was extremely circuitous. The patient's interpretations accurately tracked the route. These reads were eventually summarized as follows:

1. "There is severe disagreement at this juncture."
2. "The possibility of a compromise is at hand."
3. "Today's interaction exacerbates another strong disagreement."
4. "I've got to keep telling her what I want [action interpretation]."
5. "We agree on how to handle the problem—whew!"

The first three interpretations were relevant and accurate, though they did not lead directly to agreement. The crucial interpretation may have been the action read (4) wherein the patient said to himself, "I've got to keep telling her what I want." Interpretation 4 leads directly to the DO, while the other reads helped the person continue to react empathically with his colleague while, at the same time, press for consensus.

We want patients to learn to "hang in there" without surrendering the DO until it becomes obvious that it is unattainable. Accurately monitoring the ongoing process while concomitantly keeping one's aim on the bull's eye is the *only* way to do this.

8. The therapist should question the validity of a patient's SAs (a) when they are consistently unrelated to known problem areas, (b) when they are always constructed perfectly, or (c) when the DO is always obtained.

These cases will be the exceptions and not the rule, but when they occur, clinicians must make the SA *content* an issue. Some chronically depressed patients like to avoid major issues by reporting situations that are problem-free. For example, one man brought in SAs about going to Sears to buy a part for a lawn mower and going to the store and finding everything on the grocery list. The clinician knew that the patient's marital relationship was a major source of concern, and he encouraged him to construct SAs involving interactions with his spouse.

The individual who uses perfectionism as a shield has usually spent considerable time writing out the scenario, ensuring that all steps are perfectly constructed. Grammar, punctuation, sentence structure, and spelling will all be correct. What will be missing are the *sturm und drang* that usually accompany the elicitation and remediation work. If questioned, the person will usually say something like this: "I didn't want to burden you with my silly problems." Sensitive clinicians must address the person's approach to the SA assignment and encourage him/her in the beginning to "hang out the dirty laundry."

The third type involves individuals who only bring therapists successful SAs. Again, there will be a superficial quality to the AO = DO scenarios, because the problematical areas of living remain masked. Successful living is not what brought these individuals to therapy; however, the question that the clinician must raise is "Why are you hiding?" The problematical interpersonal issues that are not being exposed in these "successful" scenarios must be brought to light, so that future SAs can be utilized to address real problems.

9. When patient change does not occur and depression levels remain stable, the clinician must shift the focus of SA from interactions outside the session to in-session interactions between the therapist and patient.

Sometimes a patient does not change as long as the focus of the SA remains concentrated on interpersonal events that occur outside therapy. More often than not, clinicians will discover that interpersonal difficulties similar to those being reported about events outside therapy will be occurring within the session between the clinician and the patient. The problem can be tackled by having patients bring in SAs that focus on interactions involving the therapeutic dyad. Once the interpersonal obstacles are resolved between patient and clinician and change in behavior occurs, then the focus can return to interpersonal situations on the outside. One therapist handled the patient's lack of change in this manner:

THERAPIST: I've noticed that your BDI [Beck Depression Inventory] scores have remained stable over the past four weeks. You've brought in several SAs where you seem to reach a certain point with a friend, and then you cannot go any further. As you and I identified the difficulty, the point always seems to involve telling people about something they did that bothers you. Am I correct about this?

PATIENT: Yep. I never seem to be able to speak my mind when I need to.

THERAPIST: Let's shift our focus for the next few weeks with your SA homework. Think about some exchange that has gone on between you and me during the previous session—something that you wanted to say to me *but didn't*. Think you can do this?

PATIENT: I can already think of a situation that happened between us last week that concerned the session.

THERAPIST: Then let's take that "slice of time" and do an SA on it for this session. I think it may be relevant to some of the difficulties you are having with your friends.

The patient then talked about how the therapist asked her whether they could meet an hour earlier this week. Meeting at this time was inconvenient for her, but she simply said, "Okay." One of her SA interpretations was the following: "If I tell my therapist that I can't meet at that time, she will reject me or get mad." Predictably, the behavior described in the SA was compliant in nature; the AO was meeting today at an inconvenient time, while the DO was scheduling a more convenient time. When the therapist asked the patient why she didn't get what she wanted, the answer was predictable: "Because I didn't speak up."

The therapist next helped the patient revise the faulty interpretation and transform it into an action read: "I've got to tell Dr. Smith that this is a bad time to meet." After the exercise was completed and it had become clear that assertive behavior would have achieved the DO, the therapist wisely asked the patient to ask her now whether she would have gotten mad or rejected her. The patient did so, and now she confronted the reality of their relationship, which didn't involve either anger or rejection. This type of strategy is often effective with "stuck" patients. As stated above, once the barriers to change are resolved in the session, SA content can return to outside-the-session events.

10. The therapist teaches the patient to self-correct his/her interpretation errors without the therapist's assistance.

Therapy will not last forever. Progressively diminishing the performance-based feedback role is important here. As soon as patients understand the steps involved in remediating their interpretations, therapists should sit back and let them complete as much of the remediation work by themselves as they can.

Patient Performance Goal for Step 1

1. The patient learns to construct relevant and accurate interpretations and to self-correct the errors.

STEP 2: MODIFYING INAPPROPRIATE BEHAVIOR

By the time Step 2 has been completed, patients will have "fixed" the mismanaged situation. Now they can compare and contrast the original situational event with the revised version. When new behavioral strategies are discussed in Step 2, we often hear statements such as "I *could never* tell my husband what I really think"; or "I *will never be able* to confront my supervisor." Such comments should be taken seriously and without challenge. A clinician does *not* have to push for immediate action. There is a better way. If the patient wants to obtain the DO, behavior change is necessary. SA will have made this point explicit. The therapist can remind the individual of this on such occasions—for example, by saying:

"Well, if you get tired of your husband's hurtful comments, then you know what you have to do."

or

"If you grow weary of being penalized in the office because of your boss's unreasonable demands, then you know what has to be done." In short, "If you want to terminate the aversive situations you complain about in therapy, then you must change your behavior!"

Another problem that is often present when chronically depressed patients don't jump at the first opportunity to alter their behavior is their fear of change—especially when SA makes it apparent that a successful outcome is within reach. Suddenly patients are faced with knowing how to terminate their distress, and this knowledge can be emotionally over-whelming. Clinicians must remember that these persons have been depressed for a long time, and the sudden realization that life can be dif-ferent is sometimes inhibiting.

In training therapists, I dramatize this point about being patient with their chronic patients by talking about a national collaborative study of chronic depression in which I participated. In this study, 635 patients were treated at 12 outpatient sites (Keller, Harrison, et al., 1995). The *mean duration* of depression was 17.8 years (SD = 11.2 years). In other words, the average length of depression among these patients takes us back to the latter days of President Carter's administration! Chronic patients have often forgotten what feeling normal is like. When the opportunity for normalcy presents itself—that is, when the door to change opens (Sartre, 1961)—it's not unusual for them to hesitate or take their time before walking across the threshold. Sadly, some persons choose not to walk through the "open door."

When faced with statements to the effect that changing their behavior is impossible, therapists can decrease their patients' fears while concomit-antly highlighting the need for change by saying something like this:

> "You don't have to go home and do the things we talk about here.
> We can talk about solutions and practice resolving your problems
> in the safety of this office. No one else has to know. We just know
> that when you're ready to stop the pain, you can do it. Take your
> time."

Such statements create strong cognitive dissonance (Festinger, 1957). These patients now know how to stop the distress because the behavioral solution is available; they also know that they are prolonging their misery by inaction. Something has to give! When therapists act as if there is all the time in the world, patients frequently return the next session to report that they have tried out the new behavior. This strategy leaves the responsibility for change up to the patient; the clinician has carefully delineated the contingencies so that the patient knows what leads to what (Skinner, 1969).

Therapist Rules for Administering Step 2

1. The therapist teaches patients that their cognitive interpretations are functionally related to how they behave in situations.

It doesn't take long for patients to understand the functional connection between interpretations and behavior. Consider these examples: (1) "If I interpret the other person's behavior as rejection, then I withdraw or attack," (2) "If I interpret others as being uninterested in me, then I pout," and, (3) "If I interpret my thoughts, feelings, or actions as being unworthy or stupid, then I behave self-destructively." Patients also learn that the consequences for irrelevant or inaccurate interpretations are behaviors that preclude attainment of their DO.

After the interpretation errors have been corrected, a clinician can introduce Step 2 by saying the following:

> "Now that you have revised your interpretations, answer this question: If you had interpreted the situation this way, how would you have behaved to obtain what you wanted?"

The question contains the implication that cognitive interpretations and behavior are functionally connected. The stage is now set for patients to evaluate their behavior, as well as to target the behavioral responses that are necessary to obtain the DO.

2. The therapist and patient pinpoint the behaviors that contribute directly to DO achievement.

Patients must also understand that their behavior is connected directly to DO achievement. Here is an example of a beginning patient's bafflement after an SA has been successfully completed:

PATIENT: I'm not really sure why things are better. I guess I'm at a different place, but I'm not really sure what's different.

THERAPIST: It's important that you learn what contributes to your getting what you want. We will keep pinpointing and practicing until you are able to specify what leads to the desired outcome.

At first, the preoperational worldview of the individual makes it difficult to comprehend interpersonal causality. The therapist keeps the
patient's "nose to the grindstone" by practicing the exercises repeatedly
until the person learns to recognize the consequences of his/her behavior.

   3. The therapist and patient target the behaviors that need to be
      modified, as well as those that must be *added*, in order to obtain the
      DO.

    Step 2 will expose the areas of behavioral deficit. The first order of
business is to talk about *what must be changed* in the patient's existing
behavioral repertoire to achieve the DO. For example, a patient may have
to learn to soften her verbal requests, as Sharon did with Tom when she
needed his help around the house. In addition, certain behaviors may
need to be added to the situation to achieve the DO. A compliant patient
who finds it impossible to say "no" to the demands of others must add
assertive behavior to his/her skill repertoire.

   4. The therapist teaches new behavioral skills in the session only
      after the SA exercise is completed.

    Novel behavior that needs to be learned via training in assertiveness,
relaxation, interviewing, and empathy should be undertaken *after* the SA
exercise is completed. During Step 2, comparing the obvious association
between the revised interpretations and the requisite situational behaviors must be the primary focus.
    Once SA is completed, skill training can be initiated. Learning that
behavior has consequences—a central motif of SA—readies patients for
behavioral training. As long as patients maintain the fiction that it really
doesn't matter what they do, training and rehearsal strategies are likely to
fall on deaf ears (remember Ken in Chapter 1). Once individuals learn
that it *does* matter what they do, then, and only then, are they ready to
talk seriously about changing their behavior.

   5. The therapist teaches the patient to evaluate situational behavior
      in relation to the DO and to self-correct the problem behaviors.

    As stated above, patients must learn to monitor their behavior with
others while always keeping the DO in focus. Step 2 teaches them to pin-

point the problem behaviors and to recognize when new behavioral skills are needed. By the termination of treatment, patients should be able to accomplish this step independently.

Patient Performance Goals for Step 2

1. The patient learns to evaluate his/her situational behavior and self-correct the errors.

Expecting individuals to learn to enact effective behavior and to self-correct inappropriate behavior is one requirement for successful treatment. Once the problem behaviors have been targeted and revised during the early sessions, patients should be encouraged to do more of the self-corrective work themselves. One statement therapists might use to convey this point is the following:

"I expect you to learn how to self-correct your behavioral errors. I will assist you in the early going, but once you begin to see the same errors cropping up across SAs, then don't wait for me—take the initiative and resolve the Step 2 problem yourself."

2. The patient learns to enact the necessary behavioral skills that lead to the achievement of the DO.

This point has been stated above. Enacting the new behaviors, not just talking about possible solutions, is the ultimate performance goal for Step 2.

STEP 3: WRAP-UP AND SUMMARY OF SITUATIONAL ANALYSIS LEARNING

After completion of Step 2, the therapist asks the patient to summarize what has been learned in the exercise. The task is usually difficult for beginning patients, who may need several practice runs before they are able to recognize the similar cognitive and behavioral themes that are present across situational events. The Step 3 summaries underscore what changes in living must be instituted if the patient is to achieve the DO.

Therapist Rules for Administering Step 3

1. The therapist should sit back and allow the patient to assess what he/she has learned in the SA.

I advise therapists in training, "Don't hurry. Let the patient sum up and reflect upon the just completed SA. Follow the patient's lead to see what has been learned."

2. The therapist allows the patient to provide the summary review first.

Therapists must avoid telling patients what they have learned in this step. Not surprisingly, some clinicians have difficulty inhibiting the impulse to start talking and summarizing, and they reflexively highlight the salient points they believe their patients should remember. One eager trainee began the step by making the following comments:

> "We have covered a lot of ground in this SA. For example, you've learned how you tend to make global interpretations that don't contribute to your DO. Revising your interpretations and focusing on what you want are important. Then we added an action interpretation stating that you needed to speak up and tell your friend that you didn't want to go. Behaviorally, you also avoided telling her that you didn't want to go to the movie. You should see how assertiveness would have worked here."

Step 3, if used sensitively, provides a "window" into what the patient deems important about the just-completed SA. "Stop, look, and listen" is the rule of thumb for therapists here. Over the process of treatment, the content of these summaries will improve significantly. The same sort of improvement observed here is also evident in the answers given to the question in Step 6 of elicitation ("Why didn't you get what you wanted?"). Patients become as adept at targeting the most important behaviors in a just-completed SA as they do in evaluating their situational performance and assessing the causal parameters involved in DO attainment, or the lack thereof.

3. If the patient fails to mention aspects of the SA that the therapist deems important, *then and only then* should these behaviors be called to their attention.

For example, the therapist might say,

> "What about this part? It seemed that you asserted yourself when you felt uncomfortable with your boss's request. What can you learn here?"

Notice that the therapist's prompt comes in the form of interrogative sentences, not statements of "fact" about what are the "correct" or "important" aspects of the SA. Effective questioning such as "What about this part . . . ?" takes patients to the needed area of focus while simultaneously keeping the ball in their court. Answers to questions stated in this manner also provide information regarding whether or not the patient noticed the importance of some aspect of the analysis. If the individual missed a point, then the clinician can highlight it. Again, therapists should stop, look, and listen before telling patients anything; they should not do anything for submissive, chronic patients that they can do for themselves.

Patient Performance Goal for Step 3

1. The patient learns to focus on the relevant components of the SA exercise that have led to DO attainment.

Step 3 is a time for patients to step back from the situation and evaluate their performance, learn from their mistakes, digest the new learning, and celebrate when AO = DO. And, of course, evaluating a situational event in this manner requires formal operations thinking.

STEP 4: GENERALIZATION AND TRANSFER OF LEARNING

A crucial part of SA is teaching patients how to take what is learned and transfer it to similar incidents in their lives. The events may be past, present, or anticipated in the future. However, it is probably best to begin with past events because this allows patients to apply the new in-session learning to a similar situation that occurred during the recent past and then to revise any interpersonal behaviors that may have been problematical.

Being able to "fix" a difficult situation that happened in the past by identifying what went wrong and knowing the skills to manage such a situation more effectively in the future are empowering. Patients learn to recognize why they failed in the past, and they learn to reconstruct the past event in light of newly learned skills. Transfering these insights in Step 4 to other situations means that patients break the cycle of useless self-condemnation that has resulted from their mishandling of situations due to a lack of appropriate skills and behavior.

Therapist Rule for Administering Step 4

1. The therapist asks the patient to pinpoint other similar interpersonal events that are relevant to the SA situation.

The therapist might ask, for example,

"How does what you have learned here apply to other similar encounters with your colleagues? Describe a similar situation and discuss what you might have done based on what you learned here this morning."

Therapists must push for specificity to ensure that transfer of learning occurs. It is not enough for the patient to say, "What I have learned applies to my social life and to my job," because that entails nothing more than global thinking. Go one step further and request that the individual specifically describe another problem area and then transfer the new learning to a particular situation. Note how specific this patient's response is:

PATIENT: This situation is similar to what happened between me and my girlfriend Wednesday night. We were arguing again, and I withdrew and said nothing. We ended up going to a play that I didn't want to see. Taking what I've learned here, I must assert myself and let her know what I want. I also get into the same problems at work. Yesterday, my office mate turned on her radio and it messed up my concentration. I couldn't do my work. So, what did I do? I said nothing and just sulked. Telling her to turn it off or turn it down would have made such a difference. I see how I am messing myself up by just withdrawing and saying nothing.

THERAPIST: Now you are applying what you have learned in the SA in a constructive way.

Yet again, I note that effective generalization and transfer of learning from one situational context to other similar events require formal operations thinking.

Patient Performance Goal for Step 4

1. The patient learns to pinpoint other similar events outside of therapy where the skills learned in SA can be transferred and applied appropriately.

The more proficient patients become during Step 4 practice, the better equipped they are likely to be in managing daily stress. It is one thing to talk through a difficult interpersonal resolution strategy with the therapist present in the room. Being able to transfer in-session learning to "live" encounters with others is robust evidence that the work of therapy is having a generalized treatment effect on the person's life.

ADMINISTERING SITUATIONAL ANALYSIS FOR ANTICIPATED FUTURE EVENTS

Important upcoming events can be planned out and rehearsed by means of SA. A pending job interview, initiating an important discussion with one's spouse, or a scheduled date with a new romantic interest can all be processed through SA. The format for using SA for these anticipated events is a four-step one:

1. The patient pinpoints a DO (in behavioral terms) for the event.
2. The patient pinpoints the most likely AO (in behavioral terms) for the situation.
3. The patient delineates the behaviors that must be enacted in order to obtain the DO.
4. The patient identifies what interpretations (particularly "action reads") will probably be required to produce the DO.

One patient, "Lathan," constructed a future SA concerning a difficult appointment he had arranged with his department supervisor—an individual who was abrasive, sarcastic, and rude, and who frequently lost his temper with department employees. The patient wanted to ask the supervisor whether he could leave early the next Friday for a church retreat. The DO was "gaining permission to leave work two hours early the following Friday." The AO was "being granted permission to leave two hours early." However, the patient attached a caveat to the AO. The patient felt that he would gain permission *only* if he could avoid reacting hostilely to anything the supervisor might say about his request (e.g., "You church people are all alike; you're all hypocrites!"). The needed behaviors discussed were (1) saying clearly what he wanted, (2) talking slowly, (3) maintaining good eye contact, and (4) continuing to breathe normally throughout. The interpretations were largely action reads: (1) "Stay focused on the DO," (2) "Don't react to his sarcastic comments about my church by getting defensive," and (3) "Make sure he understands it's for next Friday at 3:00 P.M."

Patients who are able to complete a future-oriented SA in this manner should be well prepared to manage the event when it occurs. Lathan obtained his DO and went to the church retreat.

The next chapter describes the interpersonal dimensions of the CBASP program, detailing how therapists utilize a disciplined personal relationship with the patient to modify his/her behavior.

CHAPTER EIGHT

Using the Therapist-Patient Relationship to Modify Behavior

Furthermore, the only thing that will grasp the patient, and in the long run make it possible for her to change, is to experience fully and deeply that she is doing precisely this to a real person, myself, in this real moment.

—R. MAY (1960, p. 83)

INTRODUCTION

Chronically depressed adults, especially those who have maltreatment histories, are better served by clinicians who are willing to engage them with *disciplined personal involvement*. Such a relationship is informed by the transference hypotheses that target potential interpersonal "hot spots" (Chapter 5), and by the interpersonal style of the patient as measured by the Impact Message Inventory (IMI: Kiesler, 1987). Becoming personally involved with patients in a disciplined way also means that therapists must be willing to disclose both positive and negative personal feelings and reactions to the person without being invasive, becoming rude, or using him/her as an object to meet the therapist's needs. Personal involvement is a salubrious therapeutic tool when used wisely by clinicians who are emotionally mature and secure in their own self-definition.

Disciplined personal involvement adds several elements to the thera-

167

peutic process: (1) a clearly defined therapist role; (2) a channel by which hurtful past emotional experiences can be healed; (3) a variable that increases the change potential for patients, because it means that reinforcing consequences can be delivered directly to the patients; and (4) an interpersonal context within which patients can learn to generate empathy.

A verbatim example of the positive utilization of a male therapist's personal involvement with his patient ("Ben") is provided below. Ben was a 43-year-old double depression patient who had been depressed since early adolescence. During the Significant-Other history (see Chapter 5), Ben described his father as "cold and distant with me, and the sort of person who was fearful and passive around others." He reported that growing up around his dad had resulted in his lifelong habit of acting weak or inferior and playing down his strengths and accomplishments when around other males, particularly authority figures such as high school teachers, coaches, college professors, and work supervisors. The therapist constructed the following closeness/intimacy transference hypothesis after Session 2: "If I get close to Dr. Smith, then I will have to be a weak person, holding back and playing down my assets and strengths."

BEN: I have never been praised so much as I was last Monday by my CEO in the board meeting. Good God, he just wouldn't stop telling the board what great work I had done.

DR. SMITH: Fantastic! I'm thrilled to hear of your experience. [The therapist exhibits strong pleasure over Ben's success.] What's it like for you to tell me about your success at the board meeting?

BEN: I'm embarrassed telling you about it and feel like I've done something wrong.

DR. SMITH: Why? [The therapist knows that he is in a transference hot spot.]

BEN: I don't like talking to another guy about my successes or what I do at work.

DR. SMITH: How would your father have reacted to your success at the board meeting if you were able to tell him what you just told me? [Ben's father had died several years ago.]

BEN: He'd say, "That's nice," and then he'd walk off. I'd feel guilty for telling him, like I'd done something wrong and made him leave.

DR. SMITH: Describe my reactions to what you just told me.

BEN: You lit up like a Christmas tree. You asked for all the details. You were pleased that I had done so well and had been recognized for my work.

DR. SMITH: You're right. I reacted to you this way. So why the embarrassment and feeling like you've done something wrong by telling me?

BEN: Because I've always felt that way. Makes no sense, does it?

DR. SMITH: It makes a lot of sense to me. But given the fact that I'm really pleased by your success and that I haven't walked away, what are the implications for you here—right now, in this relationship with me.

BEN: I don't have to act like I'm weak any more. I can be a "strong me" with no apologies.

DR. SMITH: You've discovered some interpersonal possibilities with me that you never knew with your father. I'm not afraid of your success. Quite the contrary, I'm delighted.

BEN: Yes, I can see that.

DR. SMITH: Are you still embarrassed about telling me about your success at the board meeting?

BEN: Not as much.

Disciplined personal involvement characterized Dr. Smith's interaction with Ben during the exchange above. By personally reacting to Ben's success, the therapist proactively addressed an important transference issue as he compared his positive behavior toward Ben to the father's negative behavior. Consistent with the list presented above, three things were added to the therapist-patient interaction by the therapist's personal involvement: (1) The therapist defined his relationship with Ben (in the success situation) as being qualitatively different from the relationship Ben had had with his father; (2) the therapist, using his personal reactions in the IDE, directly modified the negative emotions Ben experienced when he was successful around his father; and (3) by highlighting his personal delight over Ben's success, the therapist positively reinforced Ben for talking about his accomplishments with a male.

Disciplined personal involvement also enhances empathic exchanges with patients. The following example shows one way a CBASP therapist used his personal involvement reactions to reinforce a patient's empathic behavior.

PATIENT: You look like you are frustrated with me for losing my temper with my wife and telling her what an imbecile I think she is.

THERAPIST: I am. [Personal disclosure of a felt negative reaction toward the patient.]

PATIENT: I reacted too strongly and said some things that made the argument much worse.

THERAPIST: I agree, but you certainly picked up on my frustration reactions toward you. How did you know how I was feeling?

PATIENT: It was the way you looked when I told you about what I had said to Jennifer. It was the look in your eyes.

THERAPIST: I like what you just did with me. You were sensitive to my reactions to you. How can you use what you have done with me the next time you and your wife have an argument?

PATIENT: I can watch how she reacts to what I say.

THERAPIST: I bet the more sensitive you become to how you affect her the more this will influence what you end up saying. Let me know what you observe the next time you two argue.

In summary, it is my strong opinion that therapists who become personally involved in a disciplined way with chronic patients will be more therapeutically effective than those who do not. Various ways in which personal involvement can be utilized in the session will be illustrated throughout this chapter. Chapter 12 will expound further upon this topic.

In Chapter 5, I discussed how CBASP therapists construct the transference hypotheses that help define one aspect of the therapist's interpersonal role with the patient. Now I will describe a second component that contributes to the construction of the therapist's role definition. The patient's "stimulus value" for the clinician (meaning the manner in which the practitioner is naturally inclined to respond to the patient's interpersonal style) must be identified following Session 2.

DETERMINING THE PATIENT'S
INTERPERSONAL "STIMULUS VALUE"

Kiesler's (1982, 1983, 1986a, 1986b, 1988, 1996; Kiesler & Schmidt, 1993) interpersonal research provides the framework and rationale for the recommended manner in which CBASP practitioners must determine the patient's stimulus value for them. A therapist completes Kiesler's IMI

(Kiesler & Schmidt, 1993) following the second interview. The IMI data constitute a major source of information about a patient's stimulus value for the clinician. The CBASP therapist role is designed on the basis of information from two sources: (1) the transference hypotheses (Chapter 5) and (2) the data obtained from the IMI.

The IMI is a self-report instrument that produces a type of conceptual stimulus value map graphically describing the covert reactions (emotional, cognitive, and behavioral) that one person "pulls" from another. Kiesler (1996) explains:

> The IMI was constructed on the assumption that the interpersonal or evoking style of Person (A) can be validly defined and measured by assessing the covert responses or "impact messages" of Person(s) (B) during interactions with or observations of A. (p. 28)

Multiple perspectives on interpersonal impacts (e.g., the patient's, the therapist's, an independent rater's, significant other's, etc.) can be graphically illustrated with the IMI. As noted, however, in CBASP we are mostly interested in graphing the patient's interpersonal impacts, or pulls, on the clinician. Identifying one's salient interpersonal impacts denotes the stimulus value one person is likely to have on another. One's stimulus value represents the most prominent interpersonal influence(s) he/she exerts upon another as well as predicts the usual way others respond to the patient. The IMI, by allowing therapists to identify the interpersonal domain(s) likely to exert the greatest influence, helps therapists anticipate how they must react so as to avoid the knee-jerk responses that will be destructive. For example, if therapists either inadvertently or deliberately express their natural and automatic response inclinations toward chronic patients by behaving in a dominant and/or hostile fashion, both of these knee-jerk responses will inhibit patient change. The IMI helps clinicians avoid these interpersonal "danger zones."

"Complementarity" is Kiesler's label describing our natural inclinations to behave in certain ways toward others, given specific interpersonal impacts or pulls. For example, submissive interpersonal styles naturally pull for dominant reactions; conversely, dominant interpersonal impacts pull for submissive behavior, hostility pulls for hostile counterreactions, and a friendly interpersonal style inclines others to reciprocate in a friendly manner. As noted above, the most natural reaction tendencies for therapists who encounter the prominent interpersonal impacts of chronically depressed patients are to respond by "doing the work of therapy for patients" (dominance) and by reacting to a patient's detached interpersonal style with hostility.

Examples of some of the interpersonal styles measured by the IMI (Kiesler & Schmidt, 1993), as well as their pulls for complementarity, were constructed specifically by Dr. Kiesler for use in this chapter. Kiesler has provided illustrative octant impact characterizations that are shown in Figure 8.1. Connotative verbal descriptors adjacent to each octant denote the prototypical "characterization" for that octant. The arrows in Figure 8.1 show the directions of the complementarity pulls, indicating how clinicians are naturally inclined to behave. As discussed in Chapter 4, chronic patients typically produce peak octant scores on the Submissive, Hostile-submissive, Hostile, and Friendly-submissive octants (McCullough et al., 1994b). Using the modal impact patterns of chronically depressed adults (McCullough et al., 1994b) and Kiesler's prototypical characterizations for these modal patterns (Figure 8.1), the natural reaction tendencies of most therapists toward their patients can be summarized this way:

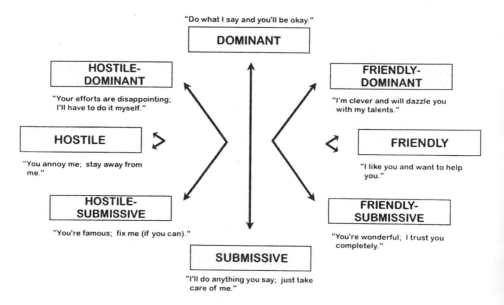

FIGURE 8.1. Octant complementary "pulls" of Kiesler's Interpersonal Circle.

- "Do what I say and you'll be okay." (*Dominant*)
- "Your efforts are disappointing; I'll have to do it myself." (*Hostile-dominant*)
- "You annoy me; stay away from me." (*Hostile*)
- "I'm clever and will dazzle you with my talents." (*Friendly-dominant*)

Avoiding these knee-jerk reaction tendencies during the therapy hour takes a considerable amount of discipline and constant work.

To continue with the description of the IMI, we see that the octant version (Kiesler & Schmidt, 1993) of the Interpersonal Circle (Kiesler, 1982) divides the circle into eight segments or radii, with each segment or radius representing one domain of interpersonal stimulus impact or field of action. Individually, each segment embodies the composite influence of two basic (orthogonal) relational variables that are present in all human interactions—namely, *control* and *affiliation*. The eight segments also maintain a "circular relationship" with one another (Kiesler, 1983, 1996), meaning that a segment is positively correlated with adjacent segments on the circumference, less positively correlated with segments further removed on the circumference, and negatively correlated with its opposite segment on the circumference (Gurtman, 1994; Kiesler, 1983, 1996).

The structural space on the Interpersonal Circle is defined or anchored by two major axes intersecting at right angles. Each major axis represents one of the two fundamental interpersonal dimensions: *control* (the vertical axis: a dominant-submissive continuum) and *affiliation* (the horizontal axis: a hostile-friendly continuum). Beginning from the top vertical segment (radius) and proceeding counterclockwise, we find the following interpersonal octants: Dominant (D), Hostile-dominant (HD), Hostile (H), Hostile-submissive (HS), Submissive (S), Friendly-submissive (FS), Friendly (F), and Friendly-dominant (FD). In another personal communication shown in Table 8.1, Kiesler has provided us with examples of items taken from each one of the eight octants to give us a flavor of the item content of the octants. Therapists rate patients on seven impact items within each octant (1, "not at all"; 2, "somewhat"; 3, "moderately so"; and, 4, "very much so") for a total of 56 items. After the clinician has completed the IMI, a mean impact score for each octant is computed. Then, an IMI Profile Summary Sheet (Kiesler, 1991) is used to plot the mean scores for each octant on the respective segments, each of which contains score designations ranging from 1.0 (center of the circle) to 4.0 (circumference of the circle). Octant

TABLE 8.1. Examples of Inventory Items for IMI Octants[1]

Octant	Sample IMI item
	"When I am with this person, he/she makes me feel . . .
D	bossed around."
HD	that I want to stay away from him/her."
H	distant from him/her."
HS	that I should tell him/her not to be so nervous around me."
S	in charge."
FS	that I could tell him/her anything and he/she would agree."
F	appreciated by him/her."
FD	that I could relax and he/she'd take charge."

D = dominant	S = submissive
HD = hostile-dominant	FS = friendly-submissive
H = hostile	F = friendly
HS = hostile-submissive	FD = friendly-dominant

[1] Personal Communication: Reproduced with permission from D. J. Kiesler (1993).

mean scores plotted the farthest from the center of the circle indicate the strongest impact domains. All eight plots are then connected, and the result is a circular graph of interpersonal impacts. The octants of most interest for therapists will be those with the highest (peak) scores.

To provide the reader with an example of how I use the IMI to identify the stimulus value of the patient, I completed an IMI on a chronic patient and her therapist following the fourth session. The rating was done for supervision purposes after I watched the videotaped session. The IMI Profile Summary Sheet is shown in Figure 8.2.[1] The figure illustrates a typical chronic patient profile, as well as an optimal therapist profile that I think is the most beneficial one for clinicians to strive to maintain. The peak octants for the patient are Hostile-submission, Friendly-submission, and Submission. Using the complementarity-pulls illustrated in Figure 8.1, the natural response inclinations of the therapist would be to react to the patient with Hostile-dominance, Friendly-dominance, and

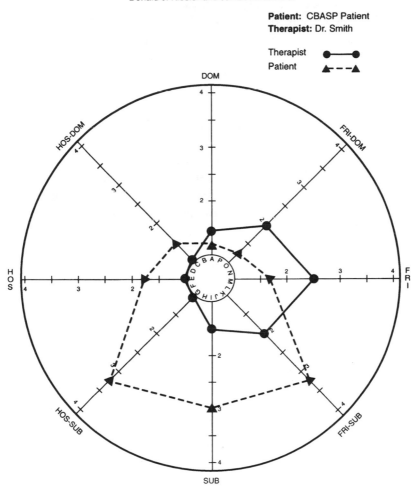

FIGURE 8.2. IMI profile on CBASP patient during Session 4 and "optimal" therapist IMI profile during the same session (both rated by JPM). Copyright © 1991 by Donald J. Kiesler. All rights reserved.

Dominant behavior. Instead, the disciplined therapist remained on the friendly side of the circle throughout the session and maintained a "moderate impact" score of 2 (equidistant plots on the Dominance-Submission axis and on the Friendly-dominant and Friendly-submission octants). He wisely remained task-focused during the session, requiring the patient to do the work while being friendly and facilitative.

THE OPTIMAL INTERPERSONAL STYLE
FOR THE THERAPIST

I've suggested what I think is the most beneficial interpersonal style for clinicians: staying on the friendly side of the circle, with moderate scores on the Dominant, Friendly, Friendly-dominant, and Friendly-submission octants. Therapists should try to avoid all response tendencies that pull them to the hostile side. The nondominant friendly stance will not be easy to achieve. In the beginning, the patient will "need" and work hard to elicit therapist dominance to allow the relationship to develop. Dominance is all they have known and experienced from others in the past. To a certain extent, therapists must allow themselves to be pulled into a dominant role in the beginning, but they must deliberately reduce the "directive" (dominant) maneuvers that are evident during the early sessions (e.g., taking the lead in deciding when to meet, directing the Significant-Other history procedure, instructing patients to read the *Patient Manual*, etc.) and gradually assume the optimal non-dominant friendly stance.

As noted throughout, dominance and hostility are "lethal" response tendencies for CBASP therapists because of the detrimental impact these behaviors have on patients. The complementarity pull for therapists who assume a dominant interpersonal stance is submissive behavior on the part of patients! The therapeutic goal is to weaken and extinguish submission patterns over time, not maintain them. My caveats in Chapters 6 and 7 not to do the work for the patient (the "dominance trap") are further grounded in Kiesler's research. The extreme submissive interpersonal style of most chronically depressed adults evokes a knee-jerk (and lethal) complementarity response of dominance from many mental health professionals. Avoiding the response pulls for dominance safeguards clinicians from repeating the destructive interpersonal patterns that these patients have experienced from significant-others. But even a conscious decision to avoid enacting a dominant role with a patient is not always successful. The decision to avoid taking over and doing the work must be made repeatedly, particularly when the patient is obviously waiting for the clinician's lead or makes statements such as "I can't," "I don't know how," "Please tell me what to do," or "You can't expect me to be able to do this!"

Additional IMI data substantiate my view concerning the optimal therapist style. The twelve-site psychotherapy supervisors in the Bristol-Myers Squibb (B-MS) National Chronic Depression Study (Keller et al., 1999, 2000; McCullough, Keller, et al., 1997; McCullough, Kornstein, et al., 1997) were monitored for CBASP procedural adherence (see Appendix B) bimonthly during the first six months of the study and monthly thereafter. All supervisors had been CBASP-certified by the author. Once the study began, adherence monitoring was carried out by using videotaped recordings of the therapy sessions. The supervisors sent their tapes to the study psychotherapy coordinator (Dr. McCullough) who would review the tapes, rate them for adherence, and return them to the site with recorded feedback. During the sixth month, Dr. McCullough randomly selected one videotaped therapy session from each supervisor and used the IMI to rate the 12 supervisors. All patients in the videotapes were in the acute phase of the study (first 12 weeks following enrollment). Octant means were calculated from the 12 IMIs and plotted on the Profile Summary Sheet. These data are shown in Figure 8.3. The supervisors' octant mean scores represent what I consider to be the optimal CBASP therapist IMI profile for the chronic patient. Figure 8.3 (like Figure 8.2) represents a task-focused interpersonal stance toward the patient that loads moderately on the friendly side of the circle.

DEALING WITH FRUSTRATION AND ANGER

It goes without saying that frustration and anger, in one form or another, are always part and parcel of a clinician's response to chronic depressives. Acting out these response tendencies in the therapy session potentiates the felt isolation of patients. What is the best way to manage the negative affect and mitigate the pull for hostile behavior? To answer the question, I will review my supervisory experiences with CBASP psychotherapists who treated over 400 chronically depressed patients in the recent multicenter B-MS study mentioned above (Keller et al., 1999, 2000; McCullough, Keller, et al., 1997). Most of the clinicians were experienced veterans, yet a majority of them continued to report difficulty managing their own frustration and anger. In videotaped sessions, I watched them react to their own negative affect in a variety of ways.

Profile Summary Sheet

IMPACT MESSAGE INVENTORY: FORM IIA OCTANT VERSION

Donald J. Kiesler and James A. Schmidt

Therapists: Twelve B-MS Site Supervisors

Rater: B-MS Psychotherapy Coordinator (JPM)

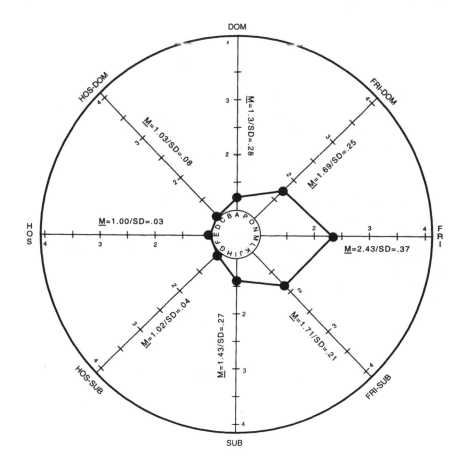

FIGURE 8.3. The "optimal" CBASP therapist IMI profile, based on mean data taken from JPM's ratings of the 12 site supervisors during the sixth month of the B-MS National Chronic Depression Study. Copyright ©1991 by Donald J. Kiesler. All rights reserved.

Some refused to deal with the affect and went on as if nothing had happened. Others admitted that they reflexively withdrew when patients expressed hostility toward them. Some felt a sense of pressure that pushed them to work harder to help the patient. Still others reported trying to be more accepting of whatever the patient was doing that was causing him/her to feel frustrated or angry. A final type of reaction was that of telling patients what to and not to do; on such occasions, clinicians did most of the talking and obviously took over the work of therapy. Regardless of the varied ways the clinicians' negative feelings were expressed, dealing with anger remained a problem for almost everyone. The question of how therapists can avoid moving over into the hostile side of the circle by acting out their anger is an important one. Since mitigating therapist dominance is easier to accomplish in CBASP supervision than managing therapist anger, one way anger can be addressed is discussed below.

My supervisory strategy for dealing with anger involves a stepwise procedure:

1. After listening to the clinician describe the situation (or watching the scenario on tape), I usually assure him/her that the reaction is not only normal but therapeutically useful:

"What you are feeling with this patient is normal and understandable. Learn to react to your anger as a signal that something important is going on between the two of you. Next, let's see if we can identify what that something is."

2. Then the clinician and I address his/her anger by beginning to construct a consequation plan of action, based on two principles that guide my supervision during such occasions:

Principle 1: Anger is usually a signal warning the therapist that the patient is perceptually disengaged from the therapist or is not aware of the interpersonal consequences of his/her hostile behavior.

I have encountered very few chronically depressed individuals who set out deliberately to hurt therapists. Usually patients are not aware of their stimulus value in the moment, nor will they be cognizant of the effects they are having upon the clinician.

The second principle is central to achieving a therapeutic outcome to the disconcerting experience of feeling anger toward the patient:

Principle 2: Try to avoid either withdrawing from or attacking the patient.

The usual reaction of most therapists is to ignore and avoid or (in rarer instances) to counter hostility with hostility, either passively or aggressively. Both types of reactions are counterproductive.

3. First, the therapist and I determine where the precipitating stimulus for the therapist's anger lies: Does the behavior that is producing the hostile reaction originate *inside* the therapy room or *outside*? Once the source is identified, supervision is directed towards formulating the details of a consequation plan.

4. If the problematic behavior is occurring in session, we try to pinpoint the cause of the anger. For example, I may try to ask the clinician,

> "Is it not taking what you say seriously? Deliberately avoiding any interpersonal cooperation or collaboration? Attacking what you say or subtly calling into question your professional competence? Procrastination? Overtly avoiding the work of therapy?"

In all these possible instances, the patient's behavior has left the practitioner feeling ignored, personally attacked, or incompetent. These effects frequently lead to frustration/anger reactions. As stated above, such patients are unaware that they are having a negative impact on the therapist.

5. I then help the clinician develop a specific plan to highlight the consequences of the patient's targeted problem behavior. I usually say something like this:

> "Assist the patient to see that 'If I do *this* with my therapist, *then* this is the *effect* I have on him/her.' The essential goal is helping the patient identify *why* he/she is treating you in this manner."

One way to catalyze this process for clinicians is to ask the patient, "Why do you want to treat me this way?" Clinicians accomplish four goals in this one question: (1) They verbalize their personal negative response to the patient; (2) they identify the specific behavior that has had a tangible impact on them; (3) they create an opportunity to teach the patient how to behave differently with them, so as not to produce these effects; and (4) they teach the patient the beginning step in the generation of *empathic behavior*—that is, they help the patient become aware of his/her impact on them. Approaching patient behavior in this manner undercuts any deflecting or minimizing the patient may attempt by saying, "I wasn't deliberately trying to do this to you," or "I didn't mean to do this," or "I'm not trying to give you a hard time." It also places the clinician in the position of making clear to the patient the troublesome consequences of his/her behavior.

This tactic is somewhat similar to the "metacommunication strategy" proposed by Kiesler (1988), whereby therapists feed back impact messages to patients during negative reaction moments. The CBASP maneuver differs from Kiesler's metacommunication strategy in the degree of personal involvement demonstrated by clinicians. Kieslerian metacommunication is conducted in a more detached or objective fashion. CBASP therapists first make patients aware of their behavior and its negative impact by asking, "Why do you want to treat *me* this way?" Wording the question in this way personalizes the therapist's inquiry, softens the impact on the patient, and designates the therapist as the recipient target (consequence) of the patient's action, yet leaves the problem squarely in the patient's corner.

When the patient's stimulus value for the therapist produces hostility, the clinician is in an optimal position to make explicit the interpersonal consequences in a safe environment. Personalizing the effects of the patient's behavior avoids the other alternative, which is just "talking about" the effects one has on others. Consider the effects of saying,

"When you behave this way, it leaves me feeling frustrated and upset with you,"

Versus

"Why do you want to make me feel frustrated and upset with you?"

The first comment allows the patient to "talk about" the consequences from an observer perspective. The second personalizes the consequences by nudging the patient toward a recognition that it is he/she who is upsetting the clinician. Patients who learn to be sensitive to how they affect their therapists eventually learn how to interact empathically. Therapists who are willing to engage patients on a personal basis facilitate the development of these crucial empathic skills.

6. In a similar vein, I help the clinician manage anger that stems from events occurring *outside* the therapy room by identifing the troublesome behavior and formulating a specific consequation plan. Often, a therapist's frustration/anger reactions are associated with issues in the patient's life that have been repeatedly addressed in past sessions but still remain problematical. A common one involves a patient who has used previous SAs to describe a destructive relationship with a lover. The AOs typically involve getting emotionally hurt, verbally attacked, and/or physically abused. Such patients, even though they will have remediated their past SAs in the session, continue to maintain contact with the malevolent individual. Careful questioning will reveal that these individuals often engage in a particular type of wishful thinking about the lover: "Maybe one day John/Mary will change and treat me right." It will be a foregone conclusion to the therapist that the lover is not and will never be a suitable partner. Then the patient comes in reporting that he/she "did it again"; that is, he/she either agreed to go out again with the person, actually went out, or otherwise initiated contact. If contact occurred, not surprisingly, he/she will report being hurt again. Many of these patients are the kind who complain frequently that nothing ever works out for them. The knee-jerk (though silent) reaction of the clinician probably goes something like this:

> "You stupid idiot! You knew what would happen; I knew what would happen; your friends have told you countless times to get rid of the bum/witch; yet you keep going back and getting hurt! When will you ever learn!?"

The problem here is that the consequences (getting hurt) have not yet modified the patient's behavior. Instead, the patient is still hoping for a different outcome (based on wishful thinking), and an implicit unattainable DO still drives the approach behavior.

Once the behavior of the patient is targeted as the cause of the therapist's frustration/anger, the supervisor must help him/her channel the hostility into a consequation strategy. I frequently encourage clinicians to use a chalkboard, eraserboard, or sheet of paper in order to review the behavior and consequences both verbally and visually with the patient. I suggest printing something like this on the writing surface:

Jane encounters Bob (*behavior*) ⟶ ends up emotionally hurt/verbally attacked/physically abused (*consequence*).

Then the patient is asked to articulate *what behavior* led to the hurtful outcome (e.g., making contact), and that phrase is added to the board. Once the individual has noted the obvious, the clinician can ask another question with an obvious answer: "Jane, what was the consequence of your behavior?" After the patient has verbalized the consequence once again, the clinician can follow up with more questions that highlight the refractory pattern even more. Here are some examples:

"Why do you suppose Bob treats you this way?", "Why doesn't he treat you differently?", "Why can't you make him treat you differently?", "If you go out later this week, what will be the likely outcome?"

Using this method, clinicians give patients additional practice in discriminating reality from wishful thinking. To put it another way, they help patients discriminate attainable DOs from unattainable ones. When the exercise is complete, the therapist might say the following:

"From what you have told me, we know clearly how to get you hurt—just go out with Bob. But if you get tired of getting hurt, then you will have to do something else. I really cringe when you come in and tell me that you have been hurt. But if you want to keep getting yourself hurt, we certainly know the best way for you to do it."

Leaving the responsibility for change up to the patient is not always easy. The goal of this consequation exercise is to place the individual at a "choice point" that includes the option of behaving in a more adaptive manner (in this case, refusing to contact or see Bob again). This exercise will probably have to be repeated several times with these patients before they begin to seek other companionship.

ACTUALIZING THE CLINICIAN'S ROLE

The CBASP program offers practitioners two highly specific interpersonal contexts within which to implement their therapeutic role with patients. The first occurs during the SA (Chapters 6 and 7), and the second during the IDE (Chapter 5). In discussing how the interpersonal role of the therapist can be actualized in each context, I will use additional data from C. H.'s case, which introduced in Chapter 5.

In Chapter 3 I stated that the ultimate goal of interpersonal development is to be able to enter into empathic encounter with others—a skill that chronically depressed patients do not possess. Therapists begin Session 3 with the tools needed to assist patients in moving toward this goal. For example, by using the IMI, clinicians will have identified the stimulus value patients have for them, and constructing the transference hypotheses will have sensitized them to their potentially negative stimulus value for particular patients. Identifying the potential "hot spots" with the transference hypotheses helps clinicians to maneuver themselves into position to expose patients to new interpersonal vistas.

Situational Analysis

I will now illustrate how this is done in the context of SA. First, Figure 8.4 illustrates the IMI data plotted for my patient, C. H., following Session 2. C. H. peaked on the Submissive, Hostile-submissive, and Friendly octants. The peak score on the submission octant makes it apparent that she wants me to "be in charge." Her extremely compliant stance with me is one that I expect she universally enacts with everyone. Her compliance also places the "responsibility for change" in my court, and there is a strong pull for me to take over and do the work for her. C. H. augments her compliance with a facade of sociability (on the friendly octant) that leaves me feeling that I am important to her. Peak scores on the friendly octant usually signal that the individual desires a relationship. However, I am struck by her obvious nervousness during our sessions. I suspect that her discomfort stems from her ambivalence towards me (concomitant hostile and friendly pulls), as evidenced by her score on the Hostile-submissive octant. The particular configuration of peak scores on the Friendly and Hostile-submissive octants causes me to be wary and cautious in any encounter with C. H. The peak scores on these two octants leave me feeling "interpersonally confused" about where I really stand with this patient. Her ambivalence is a prominent feature of the therapeutic relationship at the outset.

How is the therapeutic role enacted during SA? Role enactment is conceptualized in terms of how I should react to the patient during SA. I will procede slowly with C. H.—that is, remaining on the friendly side of

Profile Summary Sheet
IMPACT MESSAGE INVENTORY: FORM IIA OCTANT VERSION
Donald J. Kiesler and James A. Schmidt

Patient: C. H.
Therapist: JPM
Date: Post Session 2

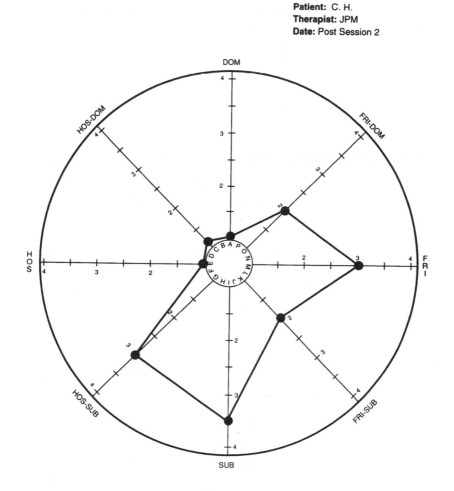

FIGURE 8.4. IMI profile on C. H. following Session 2 as rated by JPM. Copyright © 1991 by Donald J. Kiesler. All rights reserved.

the circle while avoiding the strong pull to take over (i.e., responding with dominance in the face of her submissive behavior). I will strive to be patient with her, perhaps more than I normally would during the administration of SA. I will let C. H. struggle with the difficult steps in SA, providing assistance only when it becomes obvious that she is really stuck. Compliance will be met with task-focused encouragement to do the work herself. In terms of her ambivalence (concomitant hostile and friendly pulls), I will also go slowly and assume that nothing positive has happened between C. H. and myself until my assumptions have been explicitly checked out and confirmed by her.

Interpersonal Discrimination Exercise

The second way the friendly, task-focused therapeutic role is enacted with C. H. will occur in relation to the two transference hypotheses that were identified for this patient in Chapter 5:

1. "*If* I get close to Dr. McCullough, *then* he will want something from me (i.e., I'll have to serve him, take care of him, and end up getting hurt)."
2. "*If* I am really honest with Dr. McCullough and let him know how I feel, *then* he will 'pooh-pooh' what I say (i.e., make me feel that I am wrong or a bad person)."

During the sessions, I will look for openings to administer the IDE. I will shift C. H.'s attention to the therapist-patient relationship by means of the IDE.

An opportunity to address the second transference hypothesis arose during the fourth week of treatment, when C. H. called me on the phone and told me that she did not want to come to the session at a particular time because she was fearful of being alone with me in the office. She and I had originally scheduled the meeting at a time when there would be a minimum of staff personnel in the clinic. I had foreseen no problem with this arrangement. Two hours before the appointment, she called and said she did not want to meet; she stated further that she was afraid to be in the office suite with me when my secretary was not at her desk. We scheduled another time to meet. I realized while talking with her that she had just disclosed personal, honest feelings with me, and that we might be in an interpersonal "hot spot."

The next time we met, I asked C. H. to describe what it had been like to call me on the phone and reschedule the appointment. She responded with a litany of incidents in which she had been punished or made to feel stupid for telling someone what she felt and wanted. It was obvious that she had expected me to react hostilely when she asked to reschedule. She also disclosed that she thought that I wouldn't want to see her again as a result.

Following the procedure described in Chapter 5, I first asked C. H. what her mother would have done had she disclosed such personal feelings. Next I inquired about her father's reactions in such instances, and then what her ex-husband would have done. Displaying hurt feelings and tears, she recalled several incidents in which significant others had told her that she was either overreacting, stupid, or selfish. No one had ever taken her wishes seriously.

Shifting C. H.'s attention from the maltreatment reactions of significant-others to my own response to her, I asked her to describe, as best she could, my reactions to the request. She stated that I had taken her seriously and had respected the fact that she was scared. She also mentioned that I had not judged her negatively, had not "pooh-poohed" what she said, and had accommodated her wishes. We discussed the implications of her relationship with me in the present therapy context and contrasted it to those with significant others. She verbalized a new (though tentative) perspective. She said, "Maybe, with you, I don't need to hide my feelings any more—maybe."

We also talked about the meaning of listening to one another from an empathic perspective. She said that she had experienced my concern over the phone; then she remarked that during this present session, she felt that I was proud of what she had done. I confirmed that she had read me right on both occasions, and I explicitly highlighted both of her empathic reads.

The use of transference hypotheses in the IDE allows the clinician to highlight new interpersonal realities that are being offered to the patient. For C. H., this moment took on power and significance once the new experience in therapy was compared and contrasted with older encounters involving maltreatment. The logic of the IDE becomes clear to the patient: "This is the way you behaved in the past with significant-others (hiding, keeping your feelings/opinions to yourself, withdrawing); this is the way you have behaved with me (assertion); and these are the consequences—changing the outcome of a frightening situation!"

Staying in an interrogative mode during the exercise with C. H. kept me from telling her what had just happened between us. C. H. lived through the hurt of the previous memories that were activated during the recall. The hurt was mitigated somewhat by the excitement of the relational possibilities being offered in the present moment. After the dust had settled from the emotional shift from one of hurt to relief and energy, I helped her discuss the implications of what it might be like if she let others know what she feels and wants. In this manner, disciplined personal involvement can be enacted in both the SA as well as in the IDE contexts.

DISCIPLINED PERSONAL INVOLVEMENT WITH PATIENTS

As stated at the beginning of the chapter, disciplined personal involvement with patients is an important aspect of the CBASP therapist role. Encouraging clinicians to interact personally with chronically depressed patients is warranted for three reasons:

1. Clinicians cannot teach patients how to relate to them empathically unless they themselves are willing to reveal their personal feelings and reactions.
2. The therapists' personal reactions to the patient must serve as the discriminating criteria when comparing and contrasing the quality of the dyadic relationship to patients' earlier maltreatment relationships.
3. When patients continually behave in a primitive, hostile, or destructive manner, therapists can teach them to become aware of the hurtful effects they are having by disclosing their personal reactions to patients.

Making one's personal feelings and reactions available to patients can be done easily and naturally. Consider the response of one CBASP clinician, who had very little difficulty using his personal involvement as a change variable.

PATIENT: You look like you are tired today.

THERAPIST: What gave you that idea?

PATIENT: It's the look in your face, in your eyes. You seem like you are worn out.

THERAPIST: You read me right, and I appreciate your taking note of my fatigue. It's been a long day. But I've got to tell you something. Hearing you say that has just given me a shot of energy.

PATIENT: What do you mean?

THERAPIST: You are expanding your horizons by becoming aware of *my* feelings. A fantastic change in you!

PATIENT: You're right. And I'm also becoming aware of a lot of things in other people that I never observed before.

The therapist's reaction was consistent with the CBASP goal of teaching empathic behavior. It both confirmed and affirmed the empathic nonverbal read of the patient. Contrast this response to the way I learned to react to patients during my clinical training days:

PATIENT: You look like you are tired today.

DR. MCCULLOUGH: We're not here to talk about me. Where would you like to begin today?

I refused to participate personally (and honestly) in a reciprocal dialogue with the patient, because I had learned that the appropriate "therapeutic response" was to say something to move the conversation back to a focus on the patient. Without my realizing it, my earlier strategies were extinguishing the empathic behavior of my patients.

The ability to engage in empathic encounters when one uses language to understand and be understood is a major goal of interpersonal development, as noted earlier. The willingness of clinicians to become personally involved with patients, rather than involving themselves only in unilateral ways where the focus is always upon the patient, potentiates interpersonal giving and receiving—which are the sine qua non of empathic responsiveness.

In employing the IDE, CBASP therapists are encouraged to "put on the table" both their positive and negative reactions toward patients. That is, therapists must be willing to allow patients to experience and examine their positive feelings of acceptance, caring, and concern, as well as the manner in which they handle and express the negative reactions they have toward patients. Once the therapist's responses are disclosed, they can then be compared and contrasted with the negative responses of significant-others in handling such exchanges. The ability of the patient to discriminate between the healthy responses of the therapist and the destructive patterns of significant others is enhanced when he/she is exposed to a wide variety of personal reactions from the therapist. Indeed, the greater the range of reciprocal emotional exchange between therapist and patient, the more material the patient has to draw from in making interpersonal discriminations between the therapist and significant others.

Some discrimination opportunities come to mind:

- The therapist might ask the patient how the therapist's emotional expressions change from moment to moment, compared to those of a significant-other who never disclosed any affect while with the patient.
- The therapist can have the person compare the accepting quality of his/her voice to the harsh, shrill, and rejecting tone of a significant other.
- The therapist might ask the patient to contrast his/her warm, accepting words and the detached demeanor of a significant-other.
- During periods of stress, it may help if the therapist asks the patient to recall his/her encouraging words and then compare that response to the punitive and rejecting verbal criticisms that occurred during similar stressful periods when the person was younger.

Finally, disciplined personal involvement is essential to socialize hostile and primitive patients. Patients who display Hostile or Hostile-dominant behavior (see Figure 8.1) are extremely difficult to work with and are almost universally disliked in clinical settings. I have observed these patients systematically isolate themselves from everyone on a clinic's staff, including the pharmacotherapist, nursing personnel, secretaries, and receptionists. Such individuals *are* verbally and nonverbally bombastic and hurtful. Most importantly, they are usually oblivious to their negative effects upon the staff.

What is the best way to approach treatment in such cases? I usually encourage CBASP therapists to "become a problem for the patient." This means focusing the patient's attention on the effects his/her behavior is having upon the clinician. I will illustrate the point with a verbatim exchange I observed in a videotaped therapy session.

PATIENT: I'm sure this therapy thing, meeting with you, is going to be a waste of my time.

THERAPIST: You sure do know how to hurt a guy.

PATIENT: What is that supposed to mean?

THERAPIST: What do you think I mean? When do people say that sort of thing to someone?

PATIENT: I guess when they've been hurt.

THERAPIST: Why do you think I reacted this way to you?

PATIENT: I guess I hurt you by what I just said.

THERAPIST: You're right. Now, I've got to ask you another question. Why would you want to walk into my office and hurt me like this? I've got to know the answer before we go any further.

PATIENT: I don't know, but you must be pretty thin-skinned if you let me hurt you.

THERAPIST: Why do you say that? You don't feel you have the capacity to hurt me by what you say?

PATIENT: Yes, I guess I do.

THERAPIST: Then, if you know it, I'm going to ask you again. Why would you want to hurt me this way?

Using this tactic (and it can be implemented in several ways), the clinician becomes "a problem" or "an interpersonal obstacle" that the patient must learn to deal with over time. From an interpersonal point of view (Kiesler, 1983), this strategy rejects the complementarity pulls to be hostile (push away) and dominant (take control) (see Figure 8.1). It is the interpersonal equivalent of saying to the patient, "To hell with your attempt to get me to behave like you want. Deal with *me*!" Many hostile individuals, like the one in the preceding excerpt, can learn alternative interpersonal strategies if clinicians are willing to interact personally with them and thereby to socialize them. Socialization is achieved by gently *consequating* hostile behavior: Patients learn to use the therapist's honest reactions as indices with which to monitor their own barbs, slights, and outright hostile comments. Many hostile patients eventually make a common observation that, in essence, "No one ever stayed around long enough to teach me how to behave differently." Clinicians who have difficulty revealing personal emotions to patients will probably have problems dealing effectively with overtly hostile patients.

Requisites for Personal Involvement

I only recommend the implementation of disciplined personal involvement with chronically depressed patients to highly mature professionals who have had extensive experience conducting psychotherapy. de Jong et al., (1986) made a similar point when they discouraged novice or inexperienced clinicians from treating chronically depressed patients. I concur with this view. Inexperienced therapists may not have had the time to develop the necessary personal discipline as well as the requisite interpersonal skills to tackle one of the most difficult types of outpatients we see in clinical settings.

Needless to say, the disciplined personal involvement I recommend prohibits any type of sexual contact or innuendo with patients. Patient growth and development flourish within an intimate but nonsexual and empathic relationship.

Difficulties with Disciplined Personal Involvement

Most readers will be unable to recall supervisors, attendings, or workshop/ conference leaders in their training histories, past or present, who have encouraged them to use personal involvement to change human behavior. In fact, personal involvement with patients has long been discouraged in our field. It is well known that the relationship variable is a controversial and difficult dimension to deal with when training therapists (Lambert, 1983). Unfortunately, I know of many clinical supervisors who simply refuse to discuss this aspect of psychotherapy.

Freud (1917/1950, 1917/1960, 1933, 1963) argued that personal involvement interferes with the essential goals of treatment. During training, analysts underwent a personal analysis to "neutralize" potential countertransference issues (personal matters or perspectives) that might compromise their analytic effectiveness in functioning as a "blank screen" onto which patients project their associations.

Carl Rogers (1942, 1957, 1959) inadvertently maintained the personal involvement taboo in clinical training, in spite of his novel emphasis upon the need for therapist empathy. Rogers' empathic approach to personal involvement has influenced clinical training for over 40 years. Personal involvement was acceptable, according to Rogers, as long as clinicians maintained the "proper therapist attitude," which meant offering patients a continuous serving of "unconditional positive regard." His ideal attitude for clinicians is captured in the following quote:

> If the self-experiences of another are perceived by me in such a way that no self-experience can be discriminated as more or less worthy of positive regard than any other, then I am experiencing positive regard to this individual. (Rogers, 1959, p. 208)

Not only is the attitudinal stance of ubiquitous unconditional positive regard impossible for most psychotherapists (or anyone) to maintain, to do so with chronically depressed adults precludes their learning the *consequences* of their behavior—which is essential for modifying their behavior.

Either Freud's negative views or Rogers' unrealistic ones concerning personal involvement have dominated clinical and psychiatric training programs throughout most of the 20th century. The only serious challenge to the therapist role definitions conceptualized by either Freud or Rogers comes from the interpersonal psychotherapy (IPT) movement (Anchin & Kiesler, 1982; Andrews, 1991; Kiesler, 1988, 1996; Safran, 1990a, 1990b; Safran & Segal, 1990). In the IPT approach, therapists are encouraged to disclose feelings and provide personal feedback in order to teach patients how they impact others. As noted earlier, Kiesler (1988) labels one of these change techniques "metacommunication":

> . . . metacommunicative feedback refers to any instance in which the therapist provides to the patient verbal feedback that targets the central, recurrent, and thematic relationship issues occurring between them in the therapy session. (p. 39)

Metacommunication moves therapists toward potential personal involvement. The strategy can also be used to enhance patients' expressions of empathy. That is, clinicians can also encourage their patients to reciprocate in kind, by metacommunicating with their therapists.

An example of reciprocal patient-to-therapist metacommunicative feedback might go something like this:

THERAPIST: Why don't you give me an example of when you last felt that way when you were with your wife?

PATIENT: You always push me too hard! You know I don't know how to do this stuff. I get scared when you ask me to do this, and I can't think of anything to say on the spur of the moment. You really frustrate me when you ask me to give you specific examples. I don't want to talk about this any more.

THERAPIST: Let me give you some feedback on what you have just done to me.

PATIENT: I don't understand.

THERAPIST: You became angry with me when I asked for your help to work on the problem with your wife. I feel that any time I ask for your help to work on a problem, you tell me, "Butt out!" or "Back off!" That makes me feel that the only safe thing for me to do with you is not to ask you to do anything—you want to go it alone, and you want me to keep my distance.

In this dialogue, the final response of the therapist "feeds back" to the patient the negative impact or effect the person is having upon the practitioner. The message is clear: *Whenever the therapist asks for the patient's assistance to work on some problem, the individual becomes scared, frustrated, and angry, and then verbally withdraws.*

CBASP therapists would be encouraged to focus on another aspect of this hypothetical exchange. The exchange has a healthy, bi-directional quality to it, in which the consequences of each person's behavior are immediately fed back to the other. The therapist *asks* → the patient becomes scared, frustrated, and angry. The patient expresses fear, frustration, and a desire to withdraw → the therapist feels pushed away. The reciprocal components are seen clearly in the clinician's and patient's reactions to each other, though the patient may not be fully aware of the implications. Not only can the therapist teach more adaptable behavior to the patient when the individual is actually feeling afraid in the moment, but the patient can also learn to recognize the effects he/she is having on the therapist and the effects that both interactants are having on each other. When the respective consequences for each interactant are made explicit during the exercise, the patient gains empathic knowledge.

DON'T DOWNPLAY THE THERAPIST'S ROLE

Most psychotherapists I know are very genuine and caring human beings who strive to offer a rich and sensitive relationship to patients. Given that, I have often wondered why my colleagues are so reluctant to make explicit to their patients the significant contributions they make to patients' lives. The answer I usually receive is that calling attention to oneself is narcissistic, braggadocio, or "tooting one's horn" as if to say, "Look how *great* I am." Such reactions miss an essential point and overlook the serious, ongoing interpersonal issues between therapists and chronic patients. I have found repeatedly that chronically depressed patients whose therapists extend kindness, warmth, continual support, and caring feedback almost always fail to recognize these wonderful behaviors. They also usually fail to understand the implications these positive reactions have for them and for the way they relate to others. The reason for the oversight is not surprising: A person must have a *precedent emotional experience* of receiving such positive relational gifts before he/she can recognize the gifts when they are offered. The current misery of patients precludes the recognition of these positive reactions. Even more to the point, many patients report histories in which facilitative relationships were absent—there is *no* precedent for recognizing the gifts of relationship that therapists extend. When questioned about the healthy quality of the therapeutic relationship, most patients will admit never having had such a positive interpersonal experience. Some chronic patients are unable to recall even one positive relationship over an entire lifetime! All too often, these adult children simply wait quietly for the therapist's hammer of rejection to fall upon them, despite all the clinician's positive interpersonal maneuvers. *The positive interpersonal reality between therapist and chronic patients must be made explicit repeatedly, or the new reality will go unrecognized.*

During the IDE, when chronic patients are proactively assisted in seeing that the therapist is not a cold manipulative mother, an abusive alcoholic father, or a rejecting spouse, an interpersonal revolution can take place! Clinicians are simply helping patients to recognize the obvious—that is, who the therapist actually *is*: a caring human being who is deeply committed to their well-being. The CBASP interpersonal methodology works to ensure that the patient will terminate therapy with an accurate perception of *who* the therapist is; *what* the patient's stimulus value for the therapist has been; *what* the therapist has done for the patient within the confines of the relationship; and, finally, *what impact* the therapeutic relationship (compared and contrasted with the negative significant-other relationships) has had upon his/her current functioning.

In the next chapter, I will show the way CBASP has been operationalized so that patient change can be empirically measured and described.

CHAPTER 9

Measuring Acquisition Learning and Generalized Treatment Effects

> The overall psychotherapy process theoretically depicts a series of ideal antecedent-consequent conditions designed to enact change . . . The various shifts in the patient's behavior and the rules that facilitate these shifts comprise the stage account of a particular psychotherapy, i.e., the system's "process."
> —S. CASHDAN (1973, p. 5)

Something must be added to the psychological repertoire of chronically depressed patients if they are to overthrow their entrapment in the depressive experience (McCullough & Carr, 1987). Said another way, in order for chronically depressed adults to achieve remission status, they must acquire certain perceptual and behavioral skills they did not possess before treatment began. Measuring the acquisition of novel learning and assessing its generalized treatment effects (GTEs) in CBASP is the subject of this chapter.

The essential CBASP goal is for patients to learn to self-administer the entire SA procedure correctly. SA is the "active ingredient" in this therapy; it shows patients how to resolve their interpersonal problems by using cognitive-analytic and empathic-behavioral skills. Being able to self-administer SA "to criterion" (self-administering SA twice in succession without assistance from the clinician) also implies that patients are devel-

196

oping an awareness that their behavior has environmental consequences. In my view, acquiring the ability to self-administer SA is so essential to successful treatment that clinicians should monitor the acquisition learning task by measuring the degree to which patients learn to perform it.

MEASURING TWO TYPES
OF DEPENDENT VARIABLES

In the CBASP program there are two types of dependent variables: performance learning (involving SA) and GTEs. The performance learning variable reflects how much of the SA protocol the patient has acquired. The ability to perform SA acts as a "mediator variable" (Baron & Kenny, 1986; Holmbeck, 1997) influencing treatment outcome. The instrument used to assess learning of SA is the Patient Performance Rating Form (PPRF: McCullough, 1995b). More will be said about rating and scoring the PPRF in a moment.

The second type of dependent variable, GTEs, is mediated by the degree of SA learning and includes such measures as changes in symptom intensity, perceived locus of control, psychosocial adjustment and functioning, coping style, attributional style, and interpersonal functioning. Another GTE indicator that ultimately reflects the effects of learning to self-administer SA is the *DSM-IV* diagnostic status of the patient at the end of treatment. I am assuming a causal (mediating), not a correlational, relationship between learning to self-administer SA and modification of the GTE variables.

Instruments in CBASP used to assess changes in the GTEs include the Beck Depression Inventory (BDI: Beck et al., 1979), the Hamilton Depression Rating Scale (HAM-D: Hamilton, 1967), the Rotter Internal-External Locus of Control Scale (I-E Scale: Rotter, 1966), the Social Adjustment Scale: Self-Report (SAS-SR: Weissman, 1975; Weissman & Bothwell, 1976), the *DSM-IV* Global Assessment of Functioning Scale (GAF Scale: APA, 1994), the Ways of Coping Questionnaire (WCQ: Folkman & Lazarus, 1988), the Attributional Style Questionnaire (ASQ: Peterson et al., 1982), and finally the *DSM* structured diagnostic interview such as the Structured Clinical Interview for *DSM-III-R*: Patient Edition (SCID-P: Spitzer, Williams, Gibbon, & First, 1990).

There is certainly nothing new about measuring the GTEs of psychotherapy using data collected from instruments such as the ones mentioned above. What is new in CBASP, however, is the operationalization of its active ingredient technique—SA—so that one can empirically demonstrate the extent to which the patient has learned the "subject matter" of therapy.

HISTORY OF THE CURRENT CBASP METHOD

I proposed an acquisition model of psychotherapy several years ago (McCullough, 1984a, 1991; McCullough & Carr, 1987), in which measuring patient learning of the "subject matter" of treatment was an essential feature. The methodology was similar to that of the current program, and the target patient population was similar (i.e., chronically depressed adults). Progress in learning SA was rated similarly, but scoring the SA performance of patients involved a 6-step Patient Performance Rating Form (PPRF) instead of the current 5-step form. An original PPRF step that was later removed was a probe asking patients to pinpoint the most salient emotion experienced during the situation. When I realized that emotional pinpointing did not contribute to the acquisition of perceived functionality, I deleted this step both from the SA procedure *and* from the PPRF rating form. Another slight difference between the earlier and later versions of the model is the fact that the earlier rendition of CBASP divided the therapy process into discrete operationalized stages. Following an initial baseline stage in which patient data were collected before change techniques were implemented, cognitive and behavioral training stages were conducted. Before patients were shifted from one stage to another, they had to meet preset stage criteria. For example, in Stage 2 (cognitive training), patients were taught the SA procedure but could not move into Stage 3 (behavioral training) until the six SA steps had been performed to criterion (i.e., SA had been performed at least twice in succession without any remedial assistance from the clinician).

Behavioral training in CBASP was administered in the third stage. Using Goal Attainment Scaling (Kiresuk & Sherman, 1968), the Stage 3 criterion for patients was also preset: Behavioral performance (usually involving assertive behavior in one to three target situations or with specific individuals) was required to meet an operationalized "expected outcome level." The behavioral goals were defined in terms of the frequency of occurrence of the target behavior over some unit of time (e.g., asserting oneself to an inconsiderate boss at least three times during a one-week period). Stage 3 ended and CBASP therapy was terminated when the behavioral performance criterion was reached.

AN IMPORTANT DISTINCTION BETWEEN ADMINISTERING SITUATIONAL ANALYSIS AND RATING THE PATIENT'S PERFORMANCE USING THE PPRF

Throughout the book, SA has been described as a multistep procedure requiring 6 administration steps in the elicitation phase (Chapter 6) and 4 administration steps in the remediation phase (Chapter 7). Following the end of a therapy session, clinicians use the PPRF to rate the SA performance of the patient. The reader must make a distinction here between rating SA performance with the PPRF and administering SA, because at first glance the two tasks may appear to be discrepant. For example, there is no point-to-point (step-to-step) correspondence between the 5-point PPRF rating scale and the 10 SA administration steps (if we count the total number of steps in both the elicitation and remediation phases). Why does a discrepancy exist between the total number of administration steps and the number of performance steps rated in the PPRF? More will be said about this later, but a quick explanation is that the PPRF describes the patient's ability to self-administer correctly and without assistance most (but not all) of the steps that are included in *both* the elicitation and remediation phases. Excluded in the PPRF scoring procedure are Steps 3 and 4 in the remediation phase (the wrap-up/summary and the generalization steps).

As noted above, the 5-point PPRF score reflects the extent to which the patient can go through the entire SA exercise by himself/herself, correct any step error(s) that may have been made during the elicitation phase, and complete the remediation procedure, meeting the performance criteria for each step. The PPRF scoring steps include producing a situational description that meets criterion (Step 1), producing relevant and accurate interpretations (Step 2), describing behavior that was appropriately related to the DO (Step 3), stating an AO in behavioral terms (Step 4) and formulating a realistic and/or attainable DO (Step 5). I will now describe the PPRF in greater detail.

THE PATIENT PERFORMANCE RATING FORM

As noted above, the PPRF is used to assess how well the patient has learned SA. The rating format is presented in Table 9.1. As discussed in Chapter 6, patients fill out a Coping Survey Questionnaire (CSQ) (see

TABLE 9.1. Patient Performance Rating Form Using SA

Instructions: After the therapy session has ended, rate the SA performance of the patient, using the scale below. The only situations that should be rated will be the ones actually covered during the therapy hour. Ratings must be based upon the actual verbal performance of the patient.

Scoring: A rating of "yes" is given only if the patient required *no corrective feedback* from the therapist for the step or if the patient self-corrected his/her error(s) with no assistance from the therapist.

Circle the correct answer:		Yes	No
1. Step 1.	Situational event relevant to a *significantly stressful* situation, with a beginning point and endpoint demarcated.	1	0
2. Step 2.	Patient produced relevant and accurate interpretations of event.	1	0
3. Step 3.	Behavior was appropriately related to desired outcome.	1	0
4. Step 4.	Patient pinpointed in behavioral terms an actual outcome (or the "endpoint" in the situation).	1	0
5. Step 5.	Patient pinpointed in behavioral terms a realistic and/or attainable desired outcome.	1	0
6. Total Score (add the number of "yes" scores, divide by 5, and convert to a % score for the exercise).		Example: 2/5	40%
7. Did the actual outcome = desired outome? (circle one)		Yes	No
8. If not, why not? _____			

Table 6.1) prior to each session. SA is then conducted using the homework CSQ. Following the session, the clinician rates the individual's SA performance using the PPRF.

The in-session goal of teaching SA can be described this way:

> The therapist must finally be able to sit back, fold his/ her arms together, and assume the attitude, "All right, now, you go through the SA and do it for me."

The ultimate SA training goal is for patients to self-administer the entire procedure with no assistance from therapists. SA is operationally considered learned to criterion when patients can perform SA successfully twice in succession. PPRF rating instructions to therapists follow.

The object of scoring is to rate what patients have been able to do by them-selves during the session. A perfect self-elicitation phase *and* a perfect self-remediation phase mean that patients meet all criteria for each step, as well as self-correct all step errors without the clinician's assistance. Therapist raters are urged to be conservative in their scoring of the patient's SA performance. Each step is rated 1 for correctness and 0 for incorrectness. Obviously, patients may earn a total of 5 points or 0 points or any number in between.

If the therapist has to do any significant prompting or correcting, the patient should not receive credit for that or any other related step.

Guidelines for rating each step:

Step 1

The situation must be crisply described in time and will ordinarily unfold over a short period of time (e.g., minutes or hours; in some instances, however, a situation may continue over one or two days). The situational endpoint must be specified clearly. Patients must not "edito-rialize" during this step, such as providing reasons why they did this or that or speculating upon the motives of others.

Step 2

Interpretations must be *accurate* and must accurately track the process flow of the unfolding event. Interpretations must also be *relevant* to or grounded in the actual event, as well as tied to the specific behaviors ongoing between the interactants. All interpretation sentences must be understandable to a therapist.

Note: Sometimes interpretations are accurate and relevant, even though the patient did not achieve the DO. As long as an interpretation is accurate and relevant, the patient can receive credit for the interpreta-tion even though it might not contribute directly to the achievement of the DO. The rule for scoring an interpretation is that it must describe accurately some portion of the interactive event.

Step 3

Scoring of this step *presupposes* that the patient has identified a realistic and/or attainable DO during either the elicitation or the remediation phase. *Credit will be given only if the patient also receives credit for Step 5 (DO step).* If credit is given for Step 5, scoring of this step is contingent on the patient's showing that he/she produced behavior that was instru-mental in realizing the DO *or* he/she produced alternative behavioral options during remediation that might have been more effective.

Step 4

Rating this step presupposes that the patient has identified a clear end-point for the situation. The corresponding AO must be stated in one sentence and framed in *behavioral terminology* (not as a feeling state or in emotional terms). It is acceptable, however, if the patient describes the feelings that are attached to an AO.

Step 5

Rating this step presupposes that the patient has identified a clear end-point for the situation. The DO must be stated in one sentence and be framed in *behavioral terminology* (not in emotional terms) that is realistic and attainable. The patient can receive credit if an inadequate DO is revised correctly during the remediation phase.

Generating SA Performance Curves with the PPRF

Rating SA performance with the PPRF at the end of each session will generate an acquisition learning curve over the course of psychotherapy. The session numbers can be plotted on the horizontal axis and the total number of correct SA steps on the vertical axis. One performance curve, taken from the older CBASP model (McCullough, 1984a), is shown in Figure 9.1 because it illustrates so clearly the acquisition of SA over therapy sessions. The acquisition curves produced by most CBASP patients are rarely this efficient. Again, it must be noted that the six PPRF scored steps shown in the figure stem from the older CBASP model.

Relationship of SA Performance to Therapeutic Outcome

As noted, the extent to which patients learn to self-administer SA substantively affects changes in the GTEs and is also related to the achieved level of therapeutic outcome. It follows that patients who do not learn to self-administer SA should benefit less from CBASP treatment than those who do. Thus, SA mastery ought to produce greater improvement in GTE scores as well as a better overall therapeutic response than inadequate SA learning.

Partial support for this hypothesis comes from the 5-point PPRF performance data taken from the all twelve sites participating in the B-MS study (Keller, McCullough, et al., 1999; McCullough, Keller, Hirschfeld, et al., 1997; McCullough, Kornstein, Klein, et al., 1997). The SA performances of all psychotherapy patients were rated at the end of each ther-

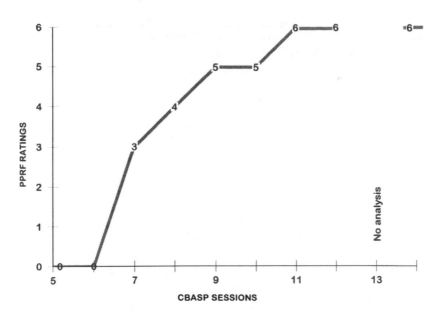

FIGURE 9.1. A CBASP patient's PPRF scores over fourteen therapy sessions.

apy session. Using the PPRF data scored over the last three sessions in which SA was administered during the Acute Phase allows us to compare the degree of SA mastery to three levels of treatment response.

Completing patients at all twelve sites who participated in the Psychothrerapy-only (n = 165) and the Combined (n = 177) Treatment Groups were divided into three "within subjects" outcome groups. Each treatment outcome group was organized based on patients who completed the Acute Phase and whose HAM-D scores during the last month of the study placed them in one of three response categories. Response to treatment in the B-MS Study was operationalized as follows: (1) *Full Response* (FR): HAM-D score of ≤ 8 on two of the last three ratings during the acute phase; (2) *Partial Response* (PR): HAM-D score of > 8 and ≤ 15 and a ≥ 50% decrease from the baseline score on two of the last three ratings; (3) *Nonresponse* (NR): those patients who did not meet criteria for full or partial response.

A summary of the within treatment comparisons on the average PPRF scores (for the last three sessions) for the Psychotherapy-only and Combination Treatment Groups is show in Table 9.2. A trend for a significant level of response main effect for the Psychotherapy-only Group was

TABLE 9.2. Within Group Comparisons of the Average 5-Point PPRF Score for the Last Three SAs Conducted during the Acute Phase Organized by Three Levels of Therapeutic Outcome

	CBASP-only (n = 165)		Combination (n = 177)	
	M/SD	N	M/SD	N
Full Response	3.88/.92[a]	39	3.95/1.07[a]	74
Partial Response	3.64/1.19[a, b]	48	3.46/1.27[a]	77
Nonresponse	3.38/1.11[b]	78	3.15/1.30[b]	26

Note. A total of 8 completing patients from the Psychotherapy-only Group and 2 patients from the Combination Group were dropped from the analyses due to missing data.

Means within the groups in the same column that do not share superscripts differ at $p < .05$.

obtained with ANOVA (F [2, 162] = 2.84, $p < .06$). Paired comparisons using Least Significant Difference (LSD) tests were run. The FR Group (M = 3.88) differed significantly from the NR Group (M = 3.38). No differences were obtained between the PR (M = 3.64) and NR Groups. A second ANOVA was conducted to compare the mean PPRF scores across 3 levels of outcome within the Combination Group, and a significant overall main effect for level of response was reported (F [2, 174] = 5.52, $p < .01$). To identify which combination groups might differ from one another, LSD paired comparisons were run, and the FR (M = 3.95) and PR (M = 3.46) Groups differed significantly from the NR Group (M = 3.15) but not from each other.

The hypothesis that degree of mastery of SA is related to levels of therapeutic outcome is supported by data obtained from the Combination Treatment Group and mildly supported by data reported from the Psychotherapy-only Treatment Group. In the Combination Group, both the FR and PR groups differed significantly from the NR group, with their respective mean values falling in the predicted sequential directions (i.e., FR ranked first, PR ranked second, and NR ranked third). In the Psychotherapy-only Group, the overall within group comparison almost reached significance ($p < .06$), again with the three outcome level PPRF averages falling in predicted directions. As expected, the highest PPRF mastery scores in both CBASP treatment conditions were obtained by both FR Groups; the next highest scores, by the two PR Groups.

Rater Reliability with the PPRF

It is important to know whether different therapists can reliably rate PPRF performance, including step-by-step agreement as well as total

PPRF sum score agreement. Data collected during the B-MS study (Keller et al., 1999, 2000; McCullough, Keller, et al., 1997) from 162 psychotherapy patients in the intent-to-treat sample (37% of all psychotherapy patient subjects) allowed us to calculate interrater agreement. For the purposes of the reliability analyses, each patient's performance on the PPRF was rated twice—once by the treating psychotherapist at the end of the session, and once by the reliability rater after viewing a videotape of the therapy session. The reliability raters included myself (the study psychotherapy coordinator) for the supervisor-study coordinator comparisons, and the site supervisors for the site psychotherapist-supervisor comparisons. For each of the two cohorts of judges (supervisor-coordinator and psychotherapist-supervisor), the ratings were collapsed across raters and sites. Several indices of agreement were obtained: (1) kappa (Cohen, 1960) as well as percent agreement for PPRF steps 1–5 (nominal variables); (2) intraclass correlation coefficient (ICC: Shrout & Fleiss, 1979) for PPRF sum of steps 1–5 (continuous variable ranging from 0–5: total number of steps correctly performed); and (3) calculated kappas and percent agreements on the PPRF sum by dichotomizing this variable. Specifically, a "perfect" overall PPRF performance score of "5" was recoded as 1, whereas an overall summary score of less than 5 was recoded as 0. Consistent with one use of the PPRF in the B-MS study (viz., a patient would obtain an "additional" therapy session during a week if he/she did not obtain a perfect PPRF score for that week's session), the dichotomized scores were examined in order to examine the reliability of PPRF overall scoring when used as a criterion of the patient's performance/progress. The PPRF interrater reliability data are shown in Table 9.3.

    The overall findings indicate that the PPRF is a fairly reliable clinical rating scale for use in CBASP. With regard to the reliability of the 5 PPRF steps, interrater agreement on the individual steps ranged from fair to substantial for the coordinator-supervisor ratings and from fair to moderate for the psychotherapist-supervisor ratings. Agreement problems arose with Steps 1 (situational description) and 4 (situational AO). Lower kappas were reported between the coordinator (myself) and the supervisors, though percent agreement for the two steps remained in a satisfactory range (76% and 72%, respectively). It seems that rating disagreement arose in part because I applied the PPRF rating criteria more stringently than did the supervisors, consistently rating their patients' performances lower than they did. For example, an issue in Step 1 involved disagreement concerning when "assistance" was given. I interpreted the rule of "no assistance" literally, while some supervisors rated their patients' per-

TABLE 9.3. PPRF Interrater Agreement Ratings on the Five-Step PPRF Scale

	Kappa[1]	% Agreement	ICC
Study coordinator versus site supervisors (n = 67 patients across sites)			
PPRF Sum Ratings			
(rating 0–5)	—	—	.65
(rating 0, 1)	.70 (substantial)	90%	—
PPRF Steps			
Step 1 of SA			
(0, 1)	.51 (moderate)	76%	—
Step 2 of SA			
(0, 1)	.63 (substantial)	82%	—
Step 3 of SA			
(0, 1)	.73 (substantial)	87%	—
Step 4 of SA			
(0, 1)	.35 (fair)	72%	—
Step 5 of SA			
(0, 1)	.53 (moderate)	76%	—
Site psychotherapists versus site supervisors (n = 95 patients across sites)			
PPRF Sum Ratings			
(rating 0–5)	—	—	.62
(rating 0, 1)	.73 (substantial)	92%	—
PPRF Steps			
Step 1 of SA			
(0, 1)	.26 (fair)	63%	—
Step 2 of SA			
(0, 1)	.59 (moderate)	81%	—
Step 3 of SA			
(0, 1)	.54 (moderate)	77%	—
Step 4 of SA			
(0, 1)	.40 (fair)	73%	—
Step 5 of SA			
(0, 1)	.44 (moderate)	72%	—

Note. Appreciation is expressed to Dr. Dina Vivian, research associate professor, SUNY at Stony Brook, for conducting the above analyses.
[1] Interpretation of kappa values according to Landis and Koch (1977).

formances using a liberal interpretation; that is, they rated Step 1 as being correctly performed even though they provided some assistance. Lower agreement was also found with Step 4. The conservative versus liberal rating styles again appeared to account for the lower kappa.

Similar kappa trends were obtained for the psychotherapist-supervisor site ratings when the PPRF steps were scored. Steps 1 and 4 (kappas of .26 and .40, respectively) mirror the above-described issues between the supervisors and myself. Psychotherapist-supervisor percent rating agreement for the two steps was 63% and 73%, respectively. The same conservative versus liberal rating patterns were present when the data were further examined. The supervisors were more conservative than their therapists, who gave their patients credit for the step even though they had provided some assistance. Finally, with regard to the overall PPRF sum score (perfect performance versus less than perfect performance), there was substantial agreement among raters for both cohorts of judges.

These above data strongly suggest that PPRF performance can be reliably scored. More stringent (literal) adherence to the PPRF scoring criteria (Table 9.1) by all rating participants would probably have resulted in higher rating agreement across all reliability domains.

MEASURING ACQUISITION OF PERCEIVED FUNCTIONALITY

In Chapters 2 and 3, I defined perceived functionality as a general cognitive set in which an individual perceives that his/her behavior has specific consequences in the environment. Perceived functional thinking requires formal thinking in that patients are viewing their behavior in causal or contingent terms. When examined in terms of the goal of interpersonal development (the ability to interact empathically with others), perceived functionality describes the fact that people are cognitively aware of their interpersonal effects upon others and of others' effects on them. A social learning construct that closely resembles the CBASP concept of perceived functionality is Julian Rotter's construct of "internal locus of control" (Rotter, 1954, 1966, 1978). Rotter's I-E Scale (Rotter, 1966) is older than other instruments used in CBASP, yet his external and internal locus of control constructs well describe the CBASP cognitive variables targeted for change. For example, Rotter (1990) defines the "contingency" dimension of internality as the degree to which individuals expect that reinforcement, or some behavioral consequence, is contingent upon what they have done or results from their own personal characteristics. This description of internality is synonymous with CBASP's definition of perceived functionality.

As stated frequently throughout this book, the preoperational dilemma of the beginning patient is marked by repeated complaints of feeling helpless and hopeless. The patient's general lack of felt empowerment is summarized nicely by Rotter's (1978) description of the individual who has an external locus of control and who faces a problem-solving task:

> If a person feels that he or she is only the passive victim of luck, fate, or powerful others, or even that he or she cannot comprehend, let alone change, the world around him or her, it is unlikely that that person will successfully be able to cope with personal problems, no matter what technique of therapy is used. (p. 4)

In order to find an empirical construct to measure the acquisiton of perceived functionality and the movement away from an external locus of control orientation, I began to use Rotter's I-E Scale (1966).

Data are now available concerning the locus of control orientation of chronically depressed adults. My colleagues and I (McCullough et al., 1988, 1994a, 1994b) found that the external locus of control scores among untreated chronically depressed adults who were studied longitudinally remained stable over time and did not change. Mean scores ranged from 12.5 (SD = 4.5) to 13.9 (SD = 4.3) at baseline, and the mean score at the end of the study was 12.5 (SD = 3.8). I (McCullough 1984a, 1991; McCullough & Carr, 1987) also noted that CBASP psychotherapy typically obtained external locus of control scores between 11 and 15 at baseline. These same patients produced lower externality scores (M = 5–7) by the end of treatment, signaling shifts in orientation from external to internal sources of perceived control.

I encourage clinicians to administer the I-E Scale at least three times during treatment: at baseline, following the mid-point of treatment, and after the final session. When the mid-point externality score shows little or no change when compared to baseline, the clinician should take that as an indication that the patient has not made changes in his/her perceived functionality set. Scores at midpoint serve as a "temperature read," signaling that either patients are moving in the right direction or that more assiduous attention must be given to helping them recognize their contingent relationship to the environment.

The mediating effects that learning to perform SA to criterion has on the GTEs are exemplified in the case history of B. F.

CASE EXAMPLE OF B. F.

B.F. is a 37-year-old, divorced African-American man who works for a newspaper as a reporter. In the first meeting he stated he had been depressed for the past 24 years. The patient currently lives alone and has been dating a woman for 10 months; they are thinking about getting married. The patient was diagnosed as having double depression at the screening interview. The onset of his dysthymia occurred when he was 13 years old and in the 7th grade. His developmental history was traumatic; he lived with a verbally abusive mother and a physically abusive and alcoholic father. He stated, however, that he always made better than average grades and his college academic record placed him in the top 10% of his class. He graduated from a large university and majored in journalism. He said that his first marriage was difficult and that his wife had "finally left me." The couple had had no children. He blamed the marital problems on his depression. He reported recurrent major depressive episodes that seemed to be exacerbated by problems at work. He has continued to have work-related problems for the past few years, due mainly to a newly assigned editor who gives him reporting assignments at the last minute. The editor complains loudly whenever he misses a deadline for a story. The relationship with the editor has deteriorated so badly in the recent past that he was fearful that he might lose his job. He came into therapy worried that being fired was a distinct possibility. From all the therapist could determine, his employment concerns were valid.

B. F. was screened by a "blind" rater who diagnosed him using the SCID-P and then administered a 24-item version of the HAM-D. He was also rated on the *DSM-IV* GAF Scale (Axis V) and was given a psychosocial functioning score of 53. Following screening at our clinic, the patient completed the Rotter I-E Scale and the WCQ, providing us with GTE baseline scores. The same rater continued to administer HAM-Ds to the patient throughout treatment which consisted of 22 sessions. Beginning with the third session, a PPRF was completed on his SA performance. I also completed an IMI (see Chapter 8) on B. F. following Session 3 and at the end of therapy (Session 22). His PPRF scores over the course of treatment, as well as the HAM-D and Rotter I-E scores, are shown in Figure 9.2. Figure 9.3 illustrates another GTE, by showing B. F.'s pre- and

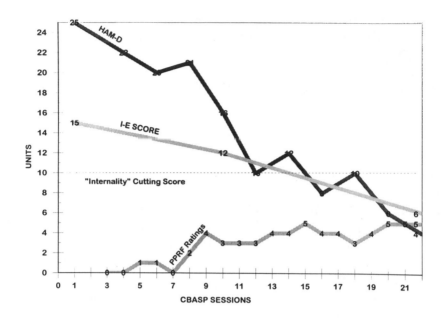

FIGURE 9.2. B. F.'s HAM-D, I-E Scale, and PPRF scores over 22 sessions of CBASP therapy.

post-treatment IMI profiles. B. F.'s pre- and post-treatment "relative" coping scale scores obtained from the WCQ are shown in Table 9.4.

Learning SA to Criterion

B. F. learned SA to criterion, meaning that he performed SA perfectly (5 hits/5 PPRF steps) during Sessions 20, 21, and 22 (see Figure 9.2). The mediating effects of learning SA are illustrated by the decreases in his HAM-D scores, which reached nondepression levels by session 20. B. F.'s GAF rating at baseline was 53, improving to a level of 82 at treatment termination. Another GTE change was reflected in his I-E scores. B. F. was administered the I-E Scale prior to the Session 10 (the midpoint) and obtained an externality score of 12, which I interpreted to mean that since B. F. had not yet learned to self-administer SA to criterion, his behavior was not yet being influenced by behavioral consequences. I highlighted these perceived functionality issues during the remaining SA exercises by focusing his attention on the situational outcomes he

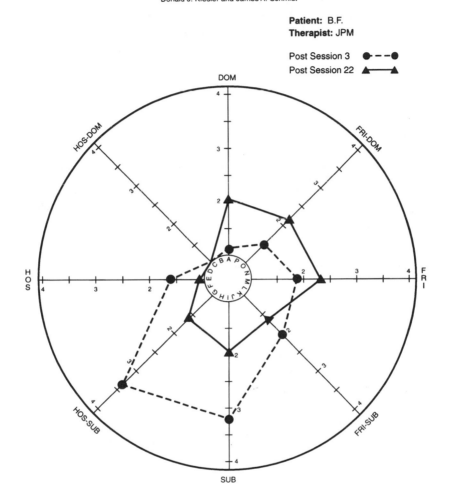

FIGURE 9.3. IMI profiles on B. F. as rated by JPM following Sessions 3 and 22. Copyright © by Donald J. Kiesler. All rights reserved.

TABLE 9.4. Comparison of B. F.'s Pre- and Post-treatment "Relative" Coping Scale Scores Using the WCQ

Pre-session 1 scores	Relative scores	Post-session 22	Relative scores
Accepting responsibility	.21	Planful problem solving	.22
Escape-avoidance	.19	Seeking social support	.16
Self-controlling	.17	Accepting responsibility	.15
Confrontive	.12	Distancing	.14
Distancing	.10	Positive reappraisal	.10
Planful problem solving	.09	Escape-avoidance	.10
Seeking social support	.09	Self-controlling	.09
Positive reappraisal	.03	Confrontive	.04

Note. "Relative" scores on the WCQ illustrate the contribution of each coping scale relative to all of the scales combined. Computing relative scores controls for the unequal numbers of items in the various scales and for individual differences in response rates (Folkman & Lazarus, 1988).

reported. The I-E Scale was readministered at Session 22, and an internality score of 6 was reported. The decreases in externality were paralleled by improved PPRF ratings. As noted above, by the final sessions of treatment, B. F. reached the SA performance criterion.

The peak scores on B. F.'s IMI profiles at the beginning (post Session 3) and end of treatment (post Session 22) also illustrate positive GTE changes in relation to his interpersonal behavior with his therapist. The most dramatic IMI changes occurred in "peak" (highest octant score) to "nadir" (octant directly opposite the peak octant) shifts (Kiesler, 1966) in the Hostile-submissive to Friendly-dominant and Submission to Dominant domains. The nadir shifts in the Friendly-dominant and Dominant octants were comparable. The combination of detached, nervous, hostile, and extremely submissive behaviors evidenced by B. F. at the outset of treatment shifted in a salubrious direction. When the IMI profile following Session 22 was compared to that following Session 3, several conclusions regarding his interpersonal skills (based on my case notes) were apparent:

- B. F.'s overall demeanor is friendlier now. As evidenced by the decrease in the Hostile-submissive octant, his attempts at friendliness and intimacy are more verbally and nonverbally congruent.
- By the 15th session, humor plays a significant role in our relation-

ship. I am more apt to "chide or tease" B. F. without fear that he will perceive me as rejecting (Friendly octant increase; Friendly-dominant octant increase).

- B. F. is taking the lead in the sessions now. He no longer waits for me to suggest directions of focus (Dominant octant increase; Friendly-dominant octant increase; decrease in Submission octant).
- B. F. exhibits more confidence when he talks about himself in relation to others (Friendly octant increase; Friendly-dominant octant increase; decrease in Submission octant).
- B. F. makes me feel that he trusts me more, though there is still a small amount of holding back (Friendly octant increase; note the remaining Hostile-submission octant score on the post-treatment IMI: He is still somewhat detached and nervous around me).
- B. F. is becoming more assertive with me, his colleagues, his editor, his fiancee, and with friends (Dominant octant increase; Friendly-dominant octant increase; decreased score on Submission octant).

The final GTE change was seen in his pre- to post-treatment "relative" coping scale scores taken from the WCQ. The most notable change was the increase in planful problem solving coping (deliberate problem-focused coping with a cognitive-analytic component) that moved this particular coping style in rank (relative to the other scales) from 6th to 1st place. The escape-avoidance (wishful thinking and efforts to avoid or escape the problem), self-controlling (efforts needed to regulate one's feelings and behavior within the stress situation), and confrontive (aggressive action to alter the problem, with some degree of hostility and interpersonal risk-taking present) styles of coping evidenced lower rankings when compared to their rankings at pretreatment. Escape-avoidance maneuvers had fallen to 6th place, self-controlling efforts to 7th place, and confrontive coping style to last place. In summary, by the end of treatment, the negative coping styles had been replaced in rank by problem-focused coping (planful problem solving) and seeking social support (exerting effort to obtain more information and tangible support from others). These gains in coping abilities mirror the peak-to-nadir shifts on the IMI. By the end of Session 22, B. F. was friendlier and more assertive in his dealings with others; in addition, he approached daily stressors more directly and with greater coping effectiveness. Finally, as noted above, his GAF psychosocial functioning score changed from 53 at screening to 82 at termination, reflecting improved psychosocial functioning. The case of B. F. demonstrates how *learning to perform SA to criterion has benefical generalized treatment effects that are measurable*.

The final section of this book, Part III, includes a description of the emergence of the CBASP program on the national scene (Chapter 10), training procedures for CBASP therapists (Chapter 11), a comparison of CBASP to Aaron Beck's CT and Gerald Klerman's IPT (Chapter 12), and a discussion of several intervention strategies useful in managing patient problems and crises (Chapter 13).

PART THREE

HISTORY AND OTHER ASPECTS OF CBASP

CHAPTER TEN

CBASP Emergence on the National Scene

Psychotherapy rests on a very simple but fundamental
assumption, i.e., human behavior is modifiable through
psychological procedures.

—A. BANDURA (1961, p. 143)

A brief history of CBASP was presented in Chapter 9. A recent nation-wide investigative study, the B-MS National Chronic Depression Study, has become part of this history. The B-MS study has been mentioned in Chapters 8 and 9, but it is described in greater detail in this chapter because it is the most stringent acute-phase treatment efficacy test for CBASP that has been conducted to date.

Until October 1994, CBASP had been administered mainly to chronically depressed patients and research subjects at VCU. Psychotherapists had included myself, a few clinical colleagues, and my clinical psychology doctoral students. During the fall of 1994, CBASP was selected by a group of 12 clinical researchers to be used in a combined drug and psychotherapy national study sponsored by B-MS (Keller et al., 1999; McCullough, Keller, et al., 1997; McCullough, Kornstein, et al., 1997). Plans called for enrolling 665 subjects (approximately 55–60 subjects per site). The B-MS investigation was the largest pharmacotherapy and psychotherapy study ever undertaken in psychiatry as well as the first investigation of its kind involving chronically depressed outpatients. It seems safe to say that the B-MS study

217

launched CBASP onto the national scene. Since the commencement of this research project in January 1996, approximately 70 certified CBASP psychotherapists have administered CBASP to over 400 chronic patients. CBASP treatment was administered to patients either alone or in combination with nefazodone (Serzone).

Three psychotherapy models were considered for use in the B-MS project: IPT (Klerman et al., 1984), CT (Beck et al., 1979), and CBASP. In late October 1994, a majority of the principal investigators selected CBASP over IPT and CT, primarily because CBASP was the only model specifically designed to treat the chronically depressed patient.

In the next sections, there will be a detailed description of the training, supervision, and certification procedures in the B-MS study. This is followed by a summary of the acute-phase results.

THE PSYCHOTHERAPY ARM OF THE BRISTOL-MYERS SQUIBB STUDY

Psychotherapy training for the professional clinicians participating in the B-MS collaborative study began with a four-day workshop held in Richmond, Virginia, during March 1995. The overriding goal of the workshop was to teach CBASP methodology so that participants would be able to take their workshop learning experience back to their sites and recreate a similar type of learning environment when they began to treat chronic patients. No one in the workshop had ever heard of CBASP before coming to Richmond.

The workshop was sponsored by the Center for Psychological Services and Development and the Unipolar Mood Disorders Institute (UMDI), both part of the Department of Psychology at VCU. I am the executive director of the UMDI and was the leader of the workshop. Five of my graduate students (Dr. Sue Caldwell-Sledge, Dr. Arthur L. Kaye, Dr. J. Kim Penberthy, Ms. Anmarie Hess, and Mr. Chris Roberts), as well as the staff of the UMDI (Ms. Laurie Burke, Ms. Sarah Norris, and Dr. Susan Kornstein), assisted in all phases of the training. The psychotherapists represented a variety of theoretical backgrounds and persuasions and were organized into two groups: the 12 site psychotherapy supervisors (each of whom had been appointed by the site principal investigator) and 4 or 5 psychotherapists from each site. Because of attrition during the three-and-one-half-year study, approximately 13 new clinicians had to be certified in CBASP after the study began; 2 of these were site supervisors.

Specific outcome goals were set for the training workshop:

1. To teach participants how CBASP has been constructed to address the idiosyncratic pathology of chronically depressed patients.
2. To demonstrate CBASP techniques, using patients who were currently being seen in treatment.
3. To provide the clinicians with hands-on experience in using the methodology.
4. To ensure that participants were familiar with the overall experimental design of the B-MS study.

Psychotherapist Selection Requirements

The 12 supervisors included individuals with psychiatric, psychological, and social work credentials, and all had had previous experience in supervising psychotherapists. Psychiatric and psychology supervisors were required to have had seven years of experience following their psychiatric residency or doctoral degree; and the MSW supervisors, 10 years. The selection criteria for the site psychotherapists were as follows: psychiatrists and PhD psychotherapists had to have two years of experience post residency following their training or degree; and the MSW therapists, five years. In addition, it was preferred that clinicians selected to participate in the study have some previous psychotherapy experience treating chronically depressed patients; however, many did not.

The overall B-MS supervision and certification plan called for me to act as the study psychotherapy coordinator. This meant that I would supervise and certify the psychotherapy supervisors as they conducted 16 sessions of psychotherapy with two chronically depressed patients as pilot cases. Following certification in CBASP, the supervisors then supervised to certification the site psychotherapists, who also conducted psychotherapy with two pilot patients at the site. Throughout the B-MS study, I continued to monitor the supervisors' adherence to the study protocol; they, in turn, monitored the adherence of their site psychotherapists.

I am most indebted to the 12 site supervisors who participated with me in holding weekly teleconference calls for almost four years. Their robust enthusiasm, encouragement, and assistance gave me the opportunity to clarify and expand my thinking concerning CBASP. The supervisors are listed in Table 10.1. In essential ways, this book has grown out of our many conversations and group problem-solving efforts as we struggled together to administer the study.

TABLE 10.1. CBASP Psychotherapy Supervisors in the Bristol-Myers Squibb National Chronic Depression Study

Supervisor	Site
Dr. Bruce Arnow	Stanford University
Dr. Steve Bishop	Brown University
Dr. Janice A. Blalock	University of Texas Medical Branch at Galveston
Dr. John E. Carr	University of Washington
Dr. David C. Clark	Rush Presbyterian-St. Luke's Medical Center (Chicago)
Dr. Greg Eaves	University of Texas Southwestern Medical Center at Dallas
Dr. Baruch Fishman	Cornell University
Dr. Rachel Manber	University of Arizona
Dr. Larry Pacoe	University of Pittsburgh
Dr. Barbara O. Rothbaum	Emory University
Dr. Dina Vivian	SUNY at Stony Brook
Ms. M. Paige Young	VCU

Hours Expended to Prepare for the B-MS Study

It is interesting to note that the time expenditure it took me, the supervisors, and the psychotherapists to train to administer the psychotherapy arm of the B-MS study was immense. Several of us estimated the total amount of time that our group accrued over the one-year training period. The estimate was based on data taken from time worksheets used at the sites to track the hours individual faculty members spent on the project. The hour count included my work hours and the total supervisor and psychotherapist work hours (entailing teleconference calls, supervision time, patient contacts, project staff planning meetings with psychotherapy personnel, and weekly psychotherapy team meetings). The total hour count was approximately 16,410 hours. When the total was reduced to 8-hour work days, the number was 2,051 work days or over 8 work years.

ACUTE-PHASE STUDY RESULTS

The acute-phase data from the B-MS study (Keller et al., 1999, 2000) are now briefly summarized. A total of 681 patients meeting *DSM-IV* criteria for chronic depression (≥ 2 years duration)—that is, chronic major depression; major depressive disorder superimposed on antecedent dysthymic disorder (double depression); or recurrent major depressive disorder with incomplete interepisode recovery—were enrolled. Patients were randomly assigned to receive 12 weeks of acute-phase treatment under one of the following conditions: nefazodone monotherapy, CBASP monotherapy, or combined nefazodone and CBASP treatment. Responders to the acute-phase treatment then received 16 weeks of continuation-phase treatment. Nonresponders to CBASP monotherapy or nefazodone monotherapy were crossed over to 12 weeks of the alternative treatment. Continuation-phase responders entered a one-year double-blind maintenance phase, in which patients on nefazodone or combination treatment were randomly assigned to either a nefazodone or placebo group, and CBASP monotherapy patients were randomly assigned to either maintenance CBASP or assessment only.

A brief summary of the patient variables indicate the female-to-male ratio was 65% to 35%; mean age was 43 years (SD = 10.7 years); 91% were Caucasian; 43% were either married or cohabitating, 27% were single, and 28% were divorced/separated; the mean duration of the current major depressive episode was 7.8 years (SD = 9.6 years) and at baseline, the mean for the 24-item HAM-D was 26.8 (SD = .32).

Among completers of the study, the results of the acute-phase demonstrated that nefazodone and CBASP monotherapy were equally and satisfactorily efficacious at week 12 (55% and 52% response rates, respectively). However, the combination therapy response rate not only was significantly more effective (85%) than either monotherapy but also resulted in higher rates of response and remission among acute-phase completers than any previously reported treatments for chronic depression. *These data strongly suggest that combination treatment represents the optimal therapy regimen for chronically depressed outpatients.*

Another 12-week, acute-phase national study conducted with 635 chronically depressed outpatients at 12 sites (Keller et al., 1998) showed that medication response rates for patients who completed the phase were as follows: sertraline 58%, [full remission = 36%], and imipramine 61%, [full remission = 40%]. Given these outcome rates for medication alone, the effect of CBASP when combined with medication, looks highly promising. The B-MS study data on the combination treatment protocol stand in stark contrast to the fact that, to date, no single study of depressed patients has ever reported a significant advantage for combination treatment over monotherapy (e.g., Conte, Plutchik, Wild &

Karasu, 1986; Manning, Markowitz, & Frances, 1990; Roth, Fonagy, Parry, Target & Woods, 1996; Rush & Thase, 1999). The B-MS combination response rates also robustly support the American Psychiatric Association's (1993) practice guideline that recommends combination treatment for major depressive disorder. In light of the B-MS combination data, the guideline, while it might not be applicable to patients with episodic/acute major depression, is certainly applicable to chronically depressed patients.

CHAPTER ELEVEN

Training CBASP Psychotherapists

Practice, practice, practice makes perfect.
—ANONYMOUS

THE CBASP TRAINING WORKSHOP

The best format for therapists to learn to administer CBASP therapy is a small-group setting, wherein each participant has multiple opportunities to practice the exercises and receive feedback. Given CBASP's strong emphasis on disciplined personal contact with patients, including addressing the behavioral effects patients have on therapists, small-group training sessions afford the most effective medium to model and teach these skills. Experiential small-group training goals are twofold. First, participants must observe and experience with their trainers the interpersonal qualities needed to conduct CBASP (e.g., empathy, sensitivity, the ability to give facilitative support, and emotional "tracking skills," whereby trainees experience *themselves* being emotionally "heard" and their reactions personally acknowledged by their trainers). We want trainees to have the type of interpersonal experience with their trainers that we feel is important for them to "recreate" (at their home sites) with their chronically depressed patients. Second, participants must observe and experience how to arrange contingencies so that learning is enhanced. The trainers organize the small-group learning experiences into achievable (shaping) steps, so that "reinforcement" for correct performance is given frequently. For example, SA is difficult for even the most experienced clinicians to master. CBASP trainers deliberately construct the training procedures so that participants will experience, first-hand, just how difficult it is to master SA. The first time veteran practitioners try their hand at doing SA in a small-group setting, they make multiple mistakes, apologize profusely for their mistakes, and say they feel clumsy, stupid, and embarrased. *The trainers know that in the beginning, CBASP patients will feel exactly the same way!* The task for the trainers is to transform this "mistake-ridden" and embarrassing experience for the trainees into one of improved performance by teaching them to become more proficient in administering SA. We also want the training experience to end on a positive note, with the trainee feeling that it is okay (and safe) to make mistakes while learning SA. Constant encouragement, constructive feedback when mistakes are made, and then positive reinforcement for correct performance are frequently given during the practice sessions. The termination of distress (negative reinforcement) that results when trainees cease to make mistakes is also in evidence during the latter stages of the small-group training sessions. Again, we want the training clinicians to be able to recreate the same kind of interpersonal learning environment with chronic patients that they have experienced with their trainers during the workshop. Therapists who are "SA learners" first and who experience the same difficulties CBASP patients will encounter make the best CBASP therapists/teachers.

Didactic Phase of Training

Just as the beginning phase (Sessions 1-2) of CBASP is didactic, in that the treatment rationale is explained and discussed with patients, the training workshop begins with a didactic lecture and discussion period in large-group sessions. The program outline for these didactic sessions is listed below:

- Review of the psychopathology of the chronically depressed adult.
- Comparison of the CBASP program to CT, IPT, Rogerian psychotherapy, and short-term psychoanalytic therapy to clarify its unique features.
- The role of the CBASP therapist/teacher as an arranger of contingencies to facilitate patient learning and change.
- Introduction to disciplined personal involvement of the therapist with the patient.
- Introduction to measuring patient learning during therapy.

Patient Psychopathology

The patient's psychopathology is the beginning point for training new therapists to administer CBASP (Chapters 3 and 4). The trainees are shown how the model is designed to address the unique problems of the patient and how it cannot be understood apart from the patient's psychopathology.

Uniqueness of the CBASP Program

Trainees are encouraged to put their favorite techniques and therapeutic biases "on the shelf" as much as possible. To facilitate this shift, a detailed explanation of the uniqueness of the CBASP program compared to other existing therapeutic programs (Chapter 12) is provided. CBASP's uniqueness is best demonstrated by showing how the technique addresses the idiosyncratic pathology of the chronically depressed patient (Chapter 3). No other therapy system describes this type of patient in a similar manner.

Introducing the CBASP Contingency
Arranging Techniques

SA (Chapters 6 and 7) and the IDE (Chapter 5) are now reviewed. The fact that both techniques involve arranging contingencies in order to modify the behavior of the patient is stressed. This point is highlighted and discussed repeatedly in all the training sessions.

Disciplined Personal Involvement with Patients

Introducing practitioners to the CBASP goals of disciplined personal involvement is next on the agenda (Chapter 8). A number of questions always arise here, because, as noted earlier, personal involvement with patients is likely to have been discouraged by previous clinical supervisors and attendings. The usual concerns about personal involvement will be aired (the risks of therapists dating patients, engaging in sexual acts, taking patients to lunch or otherwise scheduling contacts outside the therapy hour, etc.). After all the concerns surrounding the personal involvement issue have been stated and listed on a chalkboard, the CBASP goals for disciplined personal involvement are again reviewed and discussed further.

It is important that all the negative reactions concerning personal involvement be resolved, and that all the participants' questions be fully answered. The immediate danger for a workshop participant, if he/she continues to have lingering unanswered concerns and/or questions, is that he/she may withdraw from participating further—if not by actually leaving the workshop early, then by psychologically "tuning out" the rest of the training proceedings.

Measuring Patient Learning and the GTEs

The trainees are then introduced to the way CBASP therapists assess patient learning of the "subject matter" of therapy and measure the GTEs (Chapter 9). Assessment is defined as continually taking a "temperature read" of the patient's progress. Administering the CBASP program by "flying by the seat of one's pants" (conducting therapy without systematic measurement of the patient's progress) is energetically discouraged.

The didactic phase of the program usually takes a full day. All sessions are interactive, with a strong emphasis placed on audience participation. The large group is then divided into small training cells (each cell is led by a certified CBASP trainer) where intensive practice in administering the therapeutic techniques is conducted. Before the workshop ends, participants will also be exposed to all the measurement instruments employed by CBASP and instructed in their use.

Practice Phase of the CBASP Workshops

Several days are spent practicing the CBASP techniques in the small groups. The agenda includes the following practice exercises:

- Administering SA
- Administering the Significant-Other history and constructing the transference hypotheses.
- Administering the IDE.
- Exposure to CBASP measurement instruments and procedures.

CERTIFICATION OF CBASP PSYCHOTHERAPISTS

The only formal certification training program for CBASP therapists took place during the B-MS National Chronic Depression Study (Keller et al.,

1999, 2000; McCullough, Keller, et al., 1997). To be certified, a training clinician, following the workshop, was required to administer 16 sessons of videotaped CBASP to two chronically depressed outpatients under the intense guidance of a certified CBASP supervisor. After each session, the supervisor viewed the tape and provided performance feedback in an individual supervisory session, as well as by rating the clinician on the B-MS adherence rating instrument: Rating Scales for Adherence Monitoring and for Evaluating the Quality of the Interpersonal Relationship (see Appendix B). CBASP certification criteria require that the supervisor give the clinician a rating of 4 or above on every item of the adherence instrument during the final three sessions of each case. Future certification of CBASP therapists will follow the same general training procedures.

I turn now to a brief discussion of the optimal therapist qualities that I advocate for CBASP psychotherapists.

OPTIMAL CBASP THERAPIST QUALITIES AND ABILITIES

Optimal general characteristics for CBASP therapists include these:

- A stable self-identity
- Motivated to help others in need
- Sensitive to the verbal and nonverbal emotional expressions of others
- An ability to convey a supportive interpersonal demeanor
- Willing to adhere to a structured therapy plan over time

Optimal capacity for emotional awareness of oneself and others includes the following specific abilities:

- Emotional openness to oneself and others (i.e., ability to interact empathically)
- Able to "track" the moment-to-moment emotional reactions of another person
- Able to "track" the moment-to-moment emotional reactions in oneself and to use one's emotions in facilitative ways
- Able to tolerate periods of moderate to severe negative affect in oneself and others

Optimal interpersonal qualities and abilities are as follows:

- Able to conceptualize an interpersonal relationship from a historical-process perspective
- Willing and able to set interpersonal limits on patients
- Able to arrange in-session contingencies to modify behavior
- Willing and able to use empirical measurement to monitor patient learning and change

No one possesses all of these qualities and abilities in full measure. Each quality or ability can be thought of as existing on a continuum ranging from the attribute's not being present to its being maximally present. Supervisors training new CBASP clinicians can rate the degree of presence of each quality and ability on this scale: Rating the Presence of Optimal CBASP Therapist Qualities and Abilities (see Appendix C). I recommend that supervisors administer the scale several times during the training period (and discuss the results with the trainee) so that practitioners can observe the progressive changes they make over time in these crucial therapeutic areas.

A clinician's weak area(s) can usually be strengthened by a supervisor who provides personal feedback that targets specific problems, and who then works with the trainee to ameliorate the weakness(es). Many of the performance domains listed above will improve simply as a function of rigorous CBASP training. I will discuss each optimal quality and ability briefly and show its relevance to the CBASP program.

1. *Stable self-identity.* CBASP therapists will need a stable identity in order to work with chronically depressed patients. Because these patients typically begin treatment with an unstable identity characterized by four deficient areas—they are unsure of who they are; they grossly misinterpret their assets and limitations; they are unaware of their stimulus value for others; and they are oblivious to their contribution to their own dysphoric state—these are the particular components of a stable identity that the CBASP therapist emphasizes in creating a base of operations for the beginning patient.

2. *Motivated to help others.* Most CBASP psychotherapists I have trained and supervised are heavily endowed with this quality. The motivation to assist others is usually manifested in an obvious attitudinal willingness to help others. This motivational drive often translates into a type of energy during treatment that enables a clinician to "hang in there" when

the going gets difficult and the impulse to withdraw from a patient is strong. Therapists who do not feel a deep-seated motivation to help others will soon find that treating chronic patients becomes a burdensome chore.

3. *Sensitive to the verbal and nonverbal emotional expressions of others.* I have listed this optimal characteristic separately, though it is usually present in individuals who possess the first two characteristics. Being sensitive to the emotional needs of others means being willing to express that sensitivity and doing it in a disciplined and enlightened manner. Disciplined sensitivity will be needed during the IDE as well as during moments when it is important that therapists recognize the particular emotional needs patients have.

4. *Ability to convey a supportive interpersonal demeanor.* All of us have known individuals who exuded supportive reinforcement and encouragement; the interpersonal experience with such individuals is usually a facilitative one. This quality is highly desirable for CBASP therapists. The attribute is often present among persons who are motivated to help others (see the second item above). This type of interpersonal style easily generates hope and encouragement among patients. Supportive therapists are the kind of persons who, even when they don't verbalize encouragement, communicate an "I know you can do it" message to others. Chronically depressed patients, with their knee-jerk conclusions of hopelessness, will need all the interpersonal support and encouragement they can get.

5. *Willing to adhere to a structured therapy plan.* Some therapists cannot or will not follow a prescribed therapeutic plan of action. Obviously, these individuals will not be viable candidates for CBASP training. Failure to adhere to the CBASP program usually means that the patient's behavior is not consequated on a regular basis and hence cannot be modified. This means that these practitioners are often "checkmated" by the behavior of chronic patients. In addition, a therapist's inability or unwillingness to comply with the CBASP program severely limits the collaborative goals that are part and parcel of this specialized methodology. A patient cannot learn to collaborate if there are no rules or guidelines by which to abide!

6. *Emotionally open to oneself and others.* This characteristic is a vital one for CBASP psychotherapists. Openness to new experiences, whatever they might be, requires a tendency to be creative, behaviorally flexible, and nondogmatic in one's attitudes and values (Costa & McCrae, 1992). Emotional openness to oneself and others also enables a therapist

to generate empathic encounters with a patient. Empathy is an important interpersonal goal for patients in CBASP, and teaching empathic responsivity is easier when the therapist is a naturally empathic person. Being emotionally open also conveys a willingness to accept novel or different emotional experiences in others without judging their behavior. Such individuals are usually highly motivated to understand the other person and to make themselves understood and succeed at these two tasks, using both verbal and nonverbal forms of communication.

7. *Being able to "track" other's moment-to-moment emotional reactions.* This optimal therapist characteristic is part and parcel of the attribute of emotional openness. I have differentiated it here in order to identify the more specific behaviors that comprise emotional openness. Being able to follow and recall the emotional path a patient has taken during the session, as well as being able to assess sudden emotional shifts as they occur (e.g., relief moments), are highly desirable "tracking" skills. Most expert psychotherapists, regardless of their theroretical persuasion, possess these skills. CBASP becomes more effective, particularly during relief moments when patients verbally or nonverbally exhibit signs of assuagement, when therapists can track these shifts in distress and call patients attention to the fact that they are feeling better—then explore what brought about the shift.

8. *Being able to "track" one's own moment-to-moment emotional reactions.* Again, this item is a further elaboration of emotional openness. Being aware of and able to monitor one's own fluctuating emotional states is crucial to discerning what is occurring between the therapist and patient. For example, clincians who know how they feel in various interpersonal situations often work back from this knowledge in order to identify and confirm what is presently going on between themselves and a patient. In this way, emotional openness to oneself becomes a sort of "guide" or "marker" clarifying the moment-to-moment interactional events that are ongoing during the hour. During a single session, a chronic patient often evokes emotional reactions from a therapist that run the gamut from compassion to outright hostility. It is not always immediately clear to the therapist what the patient has done to elicit these covert emotional responses. Without ever having responded to either the pull to give assistance or the impulse to push back, the wise therapist, skilled at tracking his/her ongoing emotional reactions, soon observes what the patient has done to make him/her feel this way or that. Now the therapist can make an enlightened decision concerning what he/she wants to do, if anything, about the patient's behavior that is evoking these reactions.

9. *Able to tolerate negative affect in oneself and others.* Tolerance of pain and distress in oneself and in others without feeling compelled to decrease the discomfort is a necessary attribute for CBASP therapists to develop. Using a negative reinforcement paradigm to change behavior requires that one be able to tolerate negative affect. As mentioned earlier, CBASP therapists want their patients to experience discomfort *in order to be able to experience the cessation of the distress* (relief moments) when more appropriate behavior is emitted. Behaviors that reduce distress tend to be strengthened. Tolerating discomfort also means that the clinician will be able to adhere to the CBASP program of helping the patient identify those behavioral strategies that reduce negative affect. Making people feel better is not the primary goal of CBASP. Rather, teaching patients to recognize behaviors that terminate their own discomfort is the primary goal.

10. *Able to generate a historical-process view of a relationship.* Stepping back from any interaction in the present moment and being able to see where the relationship began, to visualize the path it has taken up to the present time, and then to focus on a future goal is a highly developed formal operations skill. Therapists need to be able to conceptualize the process of treatment from this point of view. To say that a patient has developed insight into himself/herself is to say that the individual is able to take a process view of his/her behavior, situation, and/or relationship. Inherent in insight are the "before" and "after" ramifications of the event or process that the patient suddenly has "sight into." Such gains also signifiy a loosening of a preoperational view of reality. CBASP encourages patients to develop these formal operations skills when it asks them to generalize their learning in SA or requires that they make interpersonal discriminations between their therapists and significant others. It goes without saying that therapists must possess these formal qualities before they can teach these skills to patients.

11. *Willing to set limits on patients.* I have known CBASP trainees who were unable to administer SA because they could not keep patients on track or teach them to remain focused on one event at a time. In short, these individuals were very permissive, and they let patients do pretty much what they wanted to do during the therapy hour. CBASP goals are sacrificed when therapists act in this manner. Clinicians who feel that they must maintain a nondirective or supportive stance with patients at all times will not make effective CBASP therapists.

Interestingly, the inability or unwillingness to develop the therapist characteristics described in this point and the next has resulted in the termination of training for several individuals seeking CBASP certification.

The administration of CBASP represented a therapeutic approach that was "foreign" to the way they naturally worked with patients.

12. *Able to arrange contingencies to modify behavior.* Klerman et al. (1984) state, "Although the therapist is active, the ultimate responsibility for change lies with the patient" (p. 216). In the CBASP perspective, the interaction of the person *and* the environment is the sine qua non of behavior change. Neither the therapist nor the patient is solely responsible for behavior change; *both* are responsible, because the two are inextricably bound together in the change process of psychotherapy.

The crucial role of the CBASP therapist in changing patient behavior is to arrange (by directing the focus of the individual) behavioral contingencies so that behavior modification can occur. The degree to which this is accomplished is the degree to which behavior change occurs. The CBASP change paradigm explicitly identifies therapists as central partners in regard to any changes patients make.

If one requires a more specific answer to the question of who or what is responsible for patient change in CBASP therapy, the answer must finally be *behavioral consequences.* But who teaches a patient to perceive the consequences of his/her behavior? It is the clinician who focuses attention on the contingencies and who shoulders the greatest responsibility for instigating the change process at the outset of treatment. Once perceived functionality is acquired by the patient, the responsibility for change necessarily shifts from the clinician to the patient.

13. *Willingness to utilize empirical measurement to monitor progress.* In Chapter 9 I have shown how measuring the degree to which patients learn the subject matter of therapy is one way to assess the teaching efficacy of practitioners. Knowing where patients are in relation to the goals of treatment is important in CBASP and can be measured. As noted in Chapter 9, the PPRF is a reliable indicator of in-session learning, and the Rotter I-E Scale is a process measure of the acquisition of perceived functionality. Both of these instruments, as well as others mentioned in Chapter 9, help practitioners assess essential patient learning and progress. Therapists who do not implement psychometric measurement in psychotherapy are "flying blind" and remain unable to monitor the effectiveness of their therapeutic efforts and interventions.

CHAPTER TWELVE

Comparison of CBASP to Beck's Cognitive Therapy and Klerman's Interpersonal Psychotherapy Models

> Whatever happened to coping and the environment?
> —J. C. COYNE & I. GOTLIB (1986, p. 703)

I have selected Beck et al.'s (1979) and Klerman et al.'s (1984) programs of psychotherapy as comparison counterpoints because both programs have been used extensively to treat depression (Elkin et al., 1989; Haaga, Dyck, & Ernst, 1991; Sotsky et al., 1991; Klerman & Weissman, 1993; Weissman & Markowitz, 1994) and because both are widely known and highly recognizable.

I initially thought that contrasting the techniques advocated by each model would be the most effective means of pointing out the distinct features of CBASP. This would mean discussing the tactics that are or are not employed by each system. Several clinicians have discussed differences (Strupp & Bergin, 1969; Frank, 1973; Klerman et al., 1984) or similarities (Goldfried, 1980) among psychotherapy systems by proceeding in this manner. Klerman et al. (1984) argue that the basic differences between many therapy models boil down to the fact that some models use certain techniques while others do not. Other approaches seek to identify technique similarities rather than distinctions (Goldfried, 1980). One such "similarity" method uses in-session foci (e.g., a therapist-manipulated content focus on the thoughts and/or emotions of the patient; a focus on the linkage a patient makes between his/her actions and those of others; a time-frame focus concerning past, present, or future issues, events, or individuals; etc.) and the degree to which various models manipulate patient foci similarly as basic measures of likeness between programs (Goldfried, Castonguay, Hayes, Drozd, & Shapiro, 1997; Goldfried, Raue, & Castonguay, 1998).

The technique comparison approach, while somewhat informative about what differences or similarities exist between models, is insufficient when used alone. Focusing only on techniques tends to obscure substantive differences that involve assumptions about etiology and psychopathology. Another problem that arises with the technique comparison approach is that it glosses over and obscures the reasons why certain behaviors are targeted for change while others are excluded. Analyses that focus upon differences/similarities in technique also tend to downplay the treatment goals of the respective models. Finally, technique comparison approaches highlight the middle phase of a therapy paradigm, while frequently overlooking the beginning phase of identifying etiology and pathological functioning and the end/goal phase of resolving the psychopathology. To avoid these limitations, I compare the way that CBASP, cognitive therapy (CT), and interpersonal psychotherapy (IPT) conceptualize etiological and pathological issues, and then I contrast the manner in which the models describe what it means when the pathology is resolved. It is only after defining the beginning and end/goal phases of a psychotherapy program that we can fully understand why particular techniques are selected.

Comparing CBASP to CT and IPT will be undertaken in the following manner. Using the Beck et al. (1979) and Klerman et al. (1984) texts as my comparison yardsticks, I will organize each section below by first defining the CBASP position, followed by the CT and IPT positions. Each section concludes with a brief discussion highlighting the main distinctions between CBASP and the other two models.

BEGINNING PHASE DISTINCTIONS

Etiology/Psychopathology: CBASP

The position of CBASP regarding etiology and psychopathology is based on the "person × environment" assumption (discussed in Chapter 2).

That is, chronic depression is assumed to result from coping failures that lead to an essential breakdown in one's perceived relationship with the environment. The prototypic chronic patient is perceptually disconnected from the environment—meaning that he/she is not influenced by environmental contingencies or feedback.

This cognitive-emotional-behavioral *disengagement* of the person from others typically coincides with an early developmental history of maltreatment (early-onset disorder). In such instances, cognitive-emotional development is derailed, and the young child remains stuck at a preoperational level of social-interpersonal development. Inability to cope effectively during late childhood and/or adolescence because of the structural retardation leads to entrapment in the withdrawal phase of the depressive experience (see Figure 2.1).

Perceptual disengagement from the environment also occurs among young adults who fail to cope effectively with stress and who do not recover from a late-onset major depressive episode. Such a person's inability to terminate the depressive episode leads to an intense state of helplessness and hopelessness that results in a deterioration of cognitive functioning. Faced with an inescapable affective dilemma, the individual regresses to primitive, preoperational functioning. As with the early-onset individual, the overwhelming and pernicious effects of an unresolved depressive episode during adulthood lead the late-onset patient to entrapment in the withdrawal phase of depression. Primitive structural functioning is thus proposed as the etiological reason all chronic patients become entrapped in the withdrawal phase of the depression experience.

Etiology/Psychopathology: CT

Before I describe Beck et al.'s position regarding etiology and psychopathology, it is important to remember that CT was first proposed in 1979, a year before *DSM-III* was published. The diagnostic criteria for depression in the *DSM-II* (APA, 1968) lacked specificity, and the chronic affective conditions were considered to be personality disorders. CBASP and CT have been proposed in two different clinical eras, and the two systems are separated by three editions of the *DSM* as well as by 20 years of clinical research. It should not be surprising, then, that clear differences exist between the two therapy models.

Turning to the etiological origins of depression from the CT point of view, I find it difficult from a reading of the text to determine exactly how or why depression originates. Beck et al. (1979) state:

As mentioned previously, the cognitive model, however, does not address itself to the question of the possible *ultimate etiology* or cause of unipolar depression: for example, hereditary disposition, faulty learning, brain damage, biochemical abnormalities, etc., or any combination of these. (p. 19; emphasis in original)

Comments made in other sections of the book allude to hypotheses regarding a predisposition to depression. Early negative experiences are posited as the developmental precursors for global negative schemas regarding the self, ongoing experiences, and the future. The onset of depression seems to be "triggered" by later-in-life experiences that activate certain latent negative schemas with origins in an earlier time. Activation of the negative schemas in the present distorts one's perceptual "intrapsychic" view of reality. I would paraphrase the etiological position of CT as follows: Some individuals are more prone to reacting to stress with depression because they have been previously traumatized or sensitized by certain classes of negative life events during their developmental years. When they are stressed by similar classes of events during later life, their hypersensitivity to these situations sometimes leads to depressive disorder.

The weakness in CT's etiological position is the fact that the environment's role in causing depression remains somewhat obscure. In the absence of a conceptual description that would ground the etiology (as well as a current description of depressive pathology) within a "person × environment" interaction, it appears that Beck and colleagues are saying that "cognitions cause depression." Haaga et al. (1991) go to great lengths to deny that Beck et al. are, in fact, assigning the weight of the etiology to faulty cognitions. However, when one reads the Beck et al. book closely, the only well-developed concept left on the pathological playing field is the dysfunctional cognition—how it originated is not clear.

In a similar vein, the role of the environment is not made clear when Beck et al. discuss current cognitive pathology. Depressive pathology denotes perceptual distortions of reality that are maintained by negative schemas—but Beck et al.'s intrapsychic definition of pathology makes it easy to conclude that cognitive functioning operates in isolation from environmental interaction (Coyne & Gotlib, 1986). Beck et al. (1979) write:

. . . we have arrived at the position that we should look for the primary psychopathology in the peculiar way the individual views himself, his experiences, and his future (the "cognitive triad") and his idiosyncratic way of processing information (arbitrary inference, selective recall, overgeneralization, etc.). (p. 19)

To put this another way, in CT the primary pathology does not involve a perceptual disengagement in the relationship the person has with the environment. Rather, primary pathology is assumed to originate *within the psyche* of the individual.

Another feature of Beck's approach to pathology is seen in the subtle assumption that negative schemas are somehow nonrepresentative of reality—they distort reality. But what about instances where negative schemas *are* representative constructions of actual events or environmental realities that characterized a patient's earlier life? Even though the dysfunctional cognitions distort *current realities*, they are maintained by a prepotent and all-too-real earlier developmental history. This point suggests two assumptions: First, cognitive-emotive organizations or schemas involving the self and others *may* reflect actual environmental experiences in the past; and second, when this is the case, the earlier developmental perceptions of the individual's environment must become a central concern of the psychotherapist in assessing cognitive psychopathology in the present.

Etiology/Psychopathology: IPT

"IPT has been designed for ambulatory patients who meet the medical criteria for major depression" (Klerman et al., 1984, p. 18). Klerman et al's text was published four years after the publication of *DSM-III*; as such, it appeared during a new era in psychiatry, in which the utilization of more stringent diagnostic criteria was reorganizing the affective disorder sphere. Beckian psychology uses the generic term "depression" to denote CT's target population; the mental health field during 1984 required more diagnostic specificity when the recipients of pharmacologic and psychotherapeutic interventions were described. To IPT's credit, since the original text was published in 1984, the model has been adapted to treat a number of other diagnostic populations, including chronic depressives (Klerman & Weissman, 1993; Markowitz, 1993a, 1993b, 1994; Weissman & Markowitz, 1994). However, comparisons of CBASP and IPT will be based upon Klerman et al.'s text. I don't feel that substantial theoretical revisions have been made in IPT since 1984 that would significantly modify the positions taken in the original Klerman et al. text.

Determining IPT's view of etiology and pathological functioning is made difficult because of a theoretical conundrum in Klerman et al.'s conceptualization. On the one hand, these authors view depression as a medical illness and describe the patient as being "ill/sick." On the other hand, the authors write that depression arises from interpersonal origins involving social role conflict. How the illness of the patient and the social origins of the illness/disease are related is never satisfactorily explicated. IPT never integrates the biological/medical and psychological/social role conflict domains into one etiological construct, as does Kiesler's (1999) biopsychosocial model of behavior. Thus we are left with the (unexplained) etiological conclusion that patients with major depression are "ill/sick" because they are having interpersonal conflicts with others.

Klerman et al.'s reliance on a medical-disease etiological model is the source of the problem. For example, the authors write:

> The first step in using IPT successfully is to recognize just what depression is: the distinction between normal and clinical depression; the social, biological, and medical antecedents of clinical depression as diagnosed through the use of the medical model. (p. 6)

Two further quotes illustrate the problem:

> The interpersonal approach, however, views disturbances in interpersonal relations as antecedents to mental illness. (p. 48)

> The basic approach upon which IPT has been developed, both theoretically and therapeutically, begins with the conviction that the patient has a disorder, that this disorder is diagnosable, and that it is therapeutically to the patient's benefit to be labeled as such (rediagnosed), so that the assumption of the "sick role" becomes legitimate. (p. 38)

IPT's description of etiology becomes much clearer when the authors begin to pinpoint the psychological sources for depression. Klerman et al. target four interpersonal problem categories as precursors of a depressive disorder: (1) grief over the death of a loved one; (2) interpersonal dispute between intimates (e.g., marital conflict); (3) role transition (e.g., taking a new job); and (4) faulty social learning (e.g., social skill deficits).

Treating current psychopathology is also described in psychological terms. The psychological focus of IPT is apparent when the authors state

that this form of psychotherapy modifies problematical interpersonal relationships in the present or immediate past:

> ... IPT, on the other hand, intervenes with symptom formation and social
> adjustment/interpersonal relations, working predominantly on *current* prob-
> lems and at conscious and preconscious levels. (p. 7)

In short, the treatment of major depression consists of teaching patients
to resolve current perturbations in social role functioning. The reader is
still left with an unresolved riddle: How does the resolution of interpersonal problems serve as a remedy for the depressive illness/disease?

Further theoretical problems are apparent with IPT's "sick role" construct and the manner in which IPT therapists, at the outset of therapy,
deliberately encourage patients to assume the sick role (Parsons, 1951).
Patients are told, in essence, "Your symptoms stem from an illness that has
made you sick. Your illness does not, in any way, reflect on who you are as
a person." This communication neatly disengages the patient's behavior
from environmental consequences and from the distress that necessarily
accrues from maladaptive living. Yet, at the same time, patients are held
responsible for behavior change: "Although the therapist is active, the
ultimate responsibility for change lies with the patient" (Klerman et al.,
1984, p. 216). How can a patient be both not responsible for his/her problems *and* responsible for making changes at the same time?

Klerman et al. contend that exempting individuals from normal
social obligations and interpersonal pressures and responsibilities as well
as assuring them that they are not responsible for their social maladjustment facilitate the treatment process. The sick role strategy, proposed
within a system of psychotherapy, has obvious "person × environment"
implications that don't appear to have been taken into account. On the
one hand, IPT defines depression as a medical-disease entity and advo-
cates a sick role of nonresponsibility for patients; on the other hand, the
treatment for this medical disease is placed squarely in the psychological
domain, wherein patients are taught to change their behavior—which
they aren't responsible for—in order to terminate the disease.

Distinctions: CBASP versus CT and IPT

The paramount distinction among CBASP, CT, and IPT regarding the
etiology and psychopathology of depression is the fact that CBASP (1) is
based upon a biopsychosocial model of psychopathology and health, and

(2) presupposes that depression arises from faulty coping, which results in perceptual disengagement of the individual from his/her environment. In contrast, CT endorses cognitive distortion of reality as the etiological variable, while IPT describes etiology and psychopathology in both medical-disease and psychosocial (interpersonal problems) terms.

END/GOAL PHASE DISTINCTIONS

Treatment Goals: CBASP

Behavior change, personal empowerment, and the amelioration of emotional dysregulation result from patients' learning to view their problems in living from a "person × environment" (perceived functionality) perspective. This is a reiteration of the second CBASP assumption discussed in Chapter 2. CBASP patients who learn to use SA, as well as to think contingently in terms of what leads to what (i.e., "If this ... then that ... " thinking), learn a social problem-solving strategy (D'Zurilla and Maydeu-Olivares, 1995).

Perceived functionality implies, first, that one can decide upon and implement a solution strategy when confronted with an interpersonal problem situation. Second, it implies a rational problem-solving approach to resolving stressful situations (Logan, 1988) that is based upon a specific algorithm (i.e., the SA procedure).

Another major goal of CBASP is teaching patients how to interact empathically with others. Empathic responsiveness has been described in earlier chapters as the marker of the highest level of interpersonal encounter. Empathic behavior means that one is using verbal and nonverbal communication to understand another person as well as to make oneself understood.

The final goal of CBASP is to make certain that patients learn the "actual" behaviors (e.g., assertive behavior skills, interviewing skills, parenting skills, resolving interpersonal conflict skills, etc.) required to produce desirable interpersonal outcomes. Patients are no longer shackled by the symptoms of helplessness and hopelessness, once they learn to guide interpersonal outcomes in positive directions.

In summary, the primary goals of CBASP are (1) to help patients acquire an outlook of perceived functionality, (2) to teach patients to interact empathically with others, and (3) to help them master the requisite behavioral skills in order to enhance interpersonal relationships.

Treatment Goals: CT

CT techniques are designed to identify and revise the cognitive distortions underlying the patient's depression by subjecting the awry cognitions to reality-testing precedures that highlight the thinking errors. Patients then begin to learn how to tackle behavioral problems equipped with realistic perspectives. This realistic thinking is believed to facilitate the development of more adaptive behavior, which leads to a reduction in depressive symptoms. Beck et al. (1979) describe their treatment goal in the following manner:

> We propose, furthermore, that when the patient's personal paradigm is reversed and realigned with reality (a kind of "counter-revolution") his depression starts to disappear. (p. 21)

Treatment Goals: IPT

The general goal of IPT is to improve the social adjustment of the patient (e.g., Weissman & Bothwell, 1976) and thereby to alleviate the symptoms of depression. This means that successfully treated patients are able to solve their own interpersonal problems and pursue their own life goals, free of the disorder that brought them to therapy. More specific IPT outcome goals are linked to the four interpersonal problem areas (grief, interpersonal conflict, role transition, and interpersonal deficits) that can be targeted for modification, depending on the particular case. The interpersonal target areas are agreed upon by the therapist and patient during the first few sessions. For example, if one interpersonal problem area turns out to be *grief* over the death of a loved one, the goals for that area are twofold: (1) facilitating the mourning process and (2) assisting the individual in reestablishing interests and relationships that will ultimately function as a substitute for the lost relationship. Goals for *interpersonal dispute* involve (1) identifying the nature of the dispute, (2) deciding on a plan of remedial action, and (3) modifying the patient's expectations for the interpersonal conflict or altering his/her problematical communication patterns in order to resolve the conflict.

Treatment goals of the third target area, *role transition*, are realized when (1) the individual has successfully mourned and accepted the loss of the old role; (2) the patient is beginning to regard the new role in a more positive light; and (3) self-esteem is restored, following progressive mastery of the demands of the new role. The final set of goals addresses a group of difficult patients who present with *interpersonal deficits*. With these individuals, IPT therapists seek to (1) reduce their social isolation and (2) assist them in establishing new relationships.

Distinctions: CBASP versus CT and IPT

1. CBASP differs from CT and IPT in regard to the way it empirically evaluates the degree to which patients have learned the subject matter of therapy.

Evaluating the degree to which patients learn the subject matter of treatment is not discussed in either the Beck et al. (1979) or Klerman et al. (1984) texts. In CBASP, the PPRF (see Chapter 9) is utilized to assess the extent to which patients have learned to perform the SA procedure. When patients reach the stage of performing SA to criterion, mastery is typically accompanied by a new perspective of perceived functionality, salubrious gains in interpersonal relationships, emergence from entrapment in the withdrawal phase of the depressive experience, and reduced depression symptomatology—culminating in a move toward remission of the depressive disorder.

2. CBASP can be distinguished from CT and IPT in terms of how it measures the GTEs that accrue from learning the subject matter of therapy.

GTEs (see Chapter 9) are not discussed specifically by either Beck et al. or Klerman et al. CBASP predicts several psychometric shifts that should accompany successful treatment outcome. First, the acquisition of perceived functionality will be represented by lower externality scores on the Rotter I-E Scale during the latter stages of treatment. The usual trend is reflected in scores that begin in the externality range and shift downward toward an internal locus of control expectancy set. In addition, successful outcome should also be accompanied by predictable changes in the IMI—specifically, lower scores on the Submission and Hostile octants and higher scores on the Dominant and Friendly octants. More specifically, we look for decreasing scores on the Hostile and Hostile-submission octants and increasing scores on the Friendly-dominant and Friendly octants.

3. CBASP conceptualizes cognitive-emotive, behavioral, and interpersonal functioning within a "person × environment" perspective.

Improved functioning in any one domain necessarily affects the quality of functioning in the other domains, as well as the contingent relationship one has with the environment. This latter outcome results in change in one's perceived connection to the environment. Unlike in CT or IPT, CBASP views the cognitive-emotive, behavioral, and interpersonal domains as being equally important. They must all be seen, understood, and treated as part and parcel of the individual's total response to environmental demands. A particular domain is focused on only to the degree that it contributes to a discrete situational outcome and *only* when such an awareness will help the person perceive his/her contingent relationship with the environment.

4. CBASP describes successful treatment as involving the ability to engage in formal operations thinking. More specifically, this means being able to engage in empathic behavior with the therapist and to perform SA to criterion.

Empathic encounter and criterion performance of SA both indicate that the patient has the ability to think in formal operations terms. Neither of these end/goal phase abilities serves as an outcome-of-treatment aim for either CT or IPT. In CBASP, preoperational thinking is seen as the identifying characteristic of beginning phase chronically depressed patients: this immature cognitive-emotive perceptual level precludes both problem solving and empathic behavior. Successful treatment must overthrow the preoperational dilemma and replace it with formal operations thought patterns, which open up the perceptual gate to effective problem solving and empathic encounters.

MIDDLE PHASE DISTINCTIONS

In evaluating the three models in relation to the middle phase of therapy, I will focus on the therapist's role, the use of transference, the use of motivational variables to facilitate change, and perceptual focus and behavior change techniques.

Therapist Role

Therapist Role: CBASP

The CBASP role for the therapist is characterized by (1) disciplined personal involvement; (2) the generation of empathic give-and-take between clinician and patient; (3) a specific focus on inhibiting the evoked tendency in the therapist to be interpersonally dominant and/or hostile; and (4) an emphasis on functioning as a teacher who continually arranges contingencies so that patients learn.

Disciplined personal involvement on the part of psychotherapists is advocated by CBASP because of the developmental histories of maltreatment reported by many chronically depressed patients. During the IDE, a therapist uses his/her salubrious relationship with a patient as a standard of interpersonal interaction to underscore the fact that the patient is participating in a positive and novel relationship. It is expected that the personal involvement style of the clinician will stand in stark contrast to that of significant others who traumatized the patient in the past. The clinician must also prevent the individual from overlooking these differences. Old behavioral patterns and transference expectancies are exposed as inadequate and then revised in light of the new interpersonal realities existing between patient and therapist. "Revision," as it is used here, means that the patient learns new ways to behave with the clinician.

Several personal involvement tactics are particularly suited to teaching empathic behavior through modeling and to facilitating empathic give-and-take during therapy process.

In addition, CBASP therapists are specifically trained to be on the alert for the strong pulls for interpersonal dominance and hostility that are universally characteristic of working with chronically depressed patients. Learning to rely on the CBASP methodology to change patient behavior helps prevent practitioners from assuming a take-charge role or reacting with hostility to patients' provoking behavior.

Finally, CBASP therapists function as teachers who continually choreograph the perspective of patients by arranging contingencies during the session so that patients confront the consequences of their behavior.

Therapist Role: CT

Extending interpersonal warmth to patients, generating empathic responses, and interacting with genuine honesty with patients are universally desirable therapist characteristics. Thus it is not surprising that these qualities are also espoused by Beck et al. as desirable attributes for CT psychotherapists.

In addition to warmth, empathy, and genuineness, Beck et al. (1979) describe collaboration and giving guidance as aspects of the therapist's role:

> In contrast to "supportive" or "relationship" therapy, the therapeutic relationship is used not simply as *the* instrument to alleviate suffering but as a vehicle to facilitate a common effort in carrying out specific goals. In this sense, the therapist and patient form a "team" ... The patient's unique contribution to this collaborative effort is to provide the *raw data* for this inquiry—namely, to report his thoughts, feelings, and wishes. The therapist's special contribution is to guide the patient about what data to collect and how to utilize these data therapeutically. (p. 54)

In other words, the CT therapist functions as a collaborative team member who encourages the individual throughout the process of treatment (using warmth, empathy, and genuineness, etc.) and as a guide who counsels the individual about what data to bring to the session and how to use the data to modify his/her behavior.

Beck et al. also encourage therapists to ask patients for feedback to discern how well they understand the clinician's explanations and suggestions. It turns out that there is a secondary gain in addition to clarity. Beck et al. note:

> We have found that patients generally respond favorably to the elicitation of feedback and presentation of capsule summaries. Many of them have remarked that these procedures make them feel closer to the therapist. In analysis of videotaped interviews, we have concrete evidence that the development of empathy and warmth is facilitated by these techniques. (p. 84)

Thus teaching empathic behavior to patients, while not a primary goal of CT, is nevertheless a desirable generalized treatment effect that accrues from asking patients to provide clinicians with feedback.

Beck et al. also encourage therapists to avoid responding hostilely when confronted by angry or resistant patients. According to these authors, "interpersonal sensitivity" that avoids the interpersonal trap of intrusiveness or detachment is always desirable. Offering "accurate empathy" (meaning empathy that is circumscribed by the intellectual and emotional objectivity of the therapist) and *not* responding with "sympathy" (meaning expressing compassion and reciprocally sharing in the feelings of the patient) will maintain the prescribed therapeutic role. Finally, the CT therapist's predominant role as guide focuses the patient's attention on the primary pathological target of negative beliefs and attitudes, in order to help him/her "think and act more realistically and adaptively about his psychological problems and thus reduce symptoms" (p. 4).

Therapist Role: IPT

Many similarities exist between CT and IPT when it comes to delineating desirable therapist role features. Again, the role advocated by Klerman et al. (1984) is a two-part task: The clinician functions both as a facilitative and encouraging ally and as a didactic guide. Facilitative behaviors include communicating optimistically to patients that their problems can be resolved and being generally supportive, helpful, and reassuring.

A little more personal in-session latitude is advocated for IPT therapists than for CT clinicians. IPT therapists may be self-revealing and freely discuss a number of topics in their interactions with patients. When the patient's issues at any given point in time are relevant to problems the therapist may have had to address, practitioners may express personal opinions or give examples of how they dealt with the difficulties. However, a caveat is wisely stated by Klerman et al. regarding these dyadic disclosures: The therapeutic relationship is not a friendship. In other words, there are boundaries in the relationship that must be communicated to each patient and adhered to. These boundaries include refraining from having social contact with patients or engaging in extratreatment business relationships.

The didactic role, similar to this role in both CT and CBASP, is enacted by active manipulation of the patient's attention so that the in-session focus remains on the primary pathology—that being the emotional, cognitive, and behavioral problems contributing to conflicts in interpersonal roles.

Distinctions: CBASP versus CT and IPT

All three models endorse similar personal qualities and interpersonal skills as desirable therapist attributes. The therapist role distinctions existing between CBASP and the other models arise largely because of the particular characteristics chronically depressed patients bring to psychotherapy. Their cognitive-emotional and behavioral primitivism, combined with the refractory nature of the disorder, require therapists to behave in ways that are not discussed by either Beck et al. or Klerman et al. For example, patients may be asked to focus on the behavior of the therapist during the session. The therapist's personal reactions to patients are highlighted and discussed, in order to compare and contrast them with those of negative significant others.

The more prominent therapist role distinctions among CBASP, CT, and IPT are as follows. First, disciplined personal involvement on the part of therapists is advocated in CBASP and used to modify the depressive pathology of patients, whereas personal involvement is generally discouraged by Beck et al. and Klerman et al. Both CT and IPT therapists try to maintain an in-session focus on the patient and not on the therapist-patient relationship. Second, CBASP therapists are trained to avoid the lethal pulls for interpersonal dominance that usually lead to doing the work of therapy for patients. Beckian clinicians, on the other hand, are traditionally directive and leading; hence, the role enacted by CT therapists is one usually characterized by dominance. I am not aware of any specific warnings in the Klerman et al. text that discourage therapists from assuming a dominant role with depressed patients. However, interpersonal dominance issues are addressed by IPT therapists when they pertain to "dominant others" in patients' lives. Klerman et al. (1984) write:

> Once the therapist has gathered enough information, the relationship with the dominant other must be interpreted to the patient. The therapist also clarifies the need to live for oneself rather than conforming to the wishes of others by denying one's own wishes (p. 13).

The IPT therapist inadvertently enacts a dominant role on this occasion while simultaneously encouraging the patient to overthrow the submissive stance he/she has assumed toward others.

Use of Transference

Use of Transference: CBASP

The second session of CBASP treatment is spent eliciting the Significant-Other history. Transference hypotheses regarding intimacy, emotional need, failure, and negative affect are formulated to identify negative interpersonal material that may bias the therapeutic relationship from the patient's perspective. Transference hypothesis construction also enables therapists to modify, in a proactive way, patients' negative interpersonal expectancies by helping them become aware of the fact that they are participating in a novel and facilitative interpersonal relationship.

Use of Transference: CT

When there are "transference problems," Beck et al. (1979) urge therapists to shift the focus to interpersonal issues existing between the clinician and patient. The focus is present-centered and tied to maladaptive beliefs. For example, a patient may view the practitioner as being too old, too young, the wrong sex, not experienced enough, rejecting, not interested in the patient, or the like. Once these ideas and beliefs are reality-tested, a valuable lesson can be learned about the impact of distorted beliefs. Each time the patient's unreasonable beliefs about the therapist are exposed, he/she learns how distorted thinking negatively affects interpersonal functioning.

Unrealistic positive transference beliefs, according to Beck et al., may also impede progress, and these are dealt with in a similar manner. If individuals think of their therapists as "saviors," their high expectations may result in decreased motivational drive when life events don't go well or when progress is slow. Again, the task here is to make the distorted beliefs explicit by exposing them to the light of reality. The overriding CT rule in handling problematic transference problems is to remain focused on the negative beliefs underlying the interpersonal distortions. Utilizing reactive strategies, such as personal involvement or sympathetic behavior, to modify transference issues is discouraged. Once any transference problems become obvious, CT therapists react by focusing on and discussing the patient's distorted beliefs that involve the clinician.

Use of Transference: IPT

In order to avoid any psychoanalytic overtones, Klerman et al. (1979) encourage clinicians to ignore positive transference strivings by not interpreting or exploring their origins. The only time an IPT therapist addresses a transference issue is when a patient's feelings or behaviors toward the clinician interfere with treatment progress; these instances usually involve cases of negative transference enactment. Expressed negative transference is handled by focusing the person's attention on the way he/she is behaving toward the therapist. The patient is then assisted to look at how the same interpersonal behaviors might be interfering with interpersonal relationships outside of therapy. Next, alternative behaviors are instituted to resolve the conflict not only with the clinician but also with significant others in the patient's life.

Interestingly, Klerman et al. (1974) state that the "therapeutic relationship is not a manifestation of transference" (p. 214); the therapeutic dyad, they contend, cannot be viewed as a condition in which a patient reenacts or acts out his/her previous interpersonal learning history. But if transference is defined as behaving toward people in the present the way one has learned to behave with significant others in the past (I happen to believe that this is a more accurate definition), then Klerman et al.'s approach to the manifestation of transference in the session is too limited. My position is that all interpersonal behavior has autobiographical meaning and that one's interactions with others reflect earlier and/or current learning concerning how one should behave.

Distinctions: CBASP versus CT and IPT

The refractory interpersonal behavior of chronic patients requires CBASP therapists to focus on how patients manage the relationship. Interpersonal "land mines" that have a deleterious effect on the therapeutic alliance are myriad among the chronically depressed population. Therefore, proactive assessment and management of the transference problems are central features in the CBASP program.

Major differences between CBASP on the one hand, CT and IPT on the other, in the approach to transference involve the following. First, disciplined personal involvement of CBASP therapists with patients makes the management of both negative and positive transference a central aspect of CBASP. Focusing on transference issues is discouraged in CT and IPT except on those occasions when transference interferes with a patient's progress. Second, CBASP targets likely transference problems in four interpersonal areas: intimacy, emotional need, failure, and negative affect. Specification of transference content is not attempted by either CT or IPT. Finally, CBASP proactively addresses the transference issues of the patient, while CT and IPT assume a reactive posture toward transference.

Use of Motivational Variables to Facilitate Change

Use of Motivational Variables: CBASP

One of the most powerful motivating events occurring in psychotherapy is the moment when patients discover the means to end their suffering. It is my opinion that negative reinforcement, present in situations where distress is reduced following the emittance of some behavior, is a more powerful change event than instances in which positive reinforcement is delivered. Suffering and subjective distress are unsettling and painful, and behavior that leads to a termination of the aversive state is easy to remember.

SA is designed to elicit a patient's pathology as well as any corresponding discomfort that was present in the situation. CBASP *wants* the patient to be in distress in the session and in fact choreographs the therapy hour so that discomfort is inextricably connected with undesirable behavioral outcomes. For example, when discomfort arises from not attaining the DO, the patient is aided in reducing the discomfort by constructing a behavioral strategy that will succeed. When termination of the distress becomes obvious through the individual's verbal or nonverbal behavior, the positive shift is highlighted by the practitioner.

Paradoxically, patients who learn to understand, through the SA exercise, how they contribute to their own misery often report feeling a ray of hope. Feeling hopeless and helpless is difficult to maintain once individuals realize that their personal despair is directly related to the way they live. Similar negative reinforcement strategies are employed in the IDE, wherein patients learn to discriminate between the miserable feelings associated with pathological behavior and the relief that results from behaving adaptively with the therapist. The message (the motivational strategy) to patients becomes clear over time: "If you don't like the negative way you feel, then you must change your behavior!"

Use of Motivational Variables: CT

Beck et al. contend, as I do, that motivation to change is increased whenever aversive emotional states are terminated. Motivating patients to change is discussed throughout the Beck et al. (1979) text. Here is an example:

> The ideal way to motivate the patient to work on his problems is to produce prompt lessening of symptoms through working together on particular problems. Thus, "education" or "reeducation" is preferable to prestige or authoritarian reassurance. (p. 103)

Several techniques are proposed to enhance what I have described earlier as "negative reinforcement effects": working together collaboratively; motivational charting; formulating a specific therapy plan for each session; graded task assignment in which successful performance is highlighted as patients move up the task ladder; *in vivo* "experiments" to overcome motivational blocks; and presenting a clear explanation to beginning patients concerning why they are depressed and how CT will go about resolving their depression.

Use of Motivational Variables: IPT

The word "motivation" is not indexed in the Klerman et al. (1984) text, so it is more difficult to pinpoint specific suggestions by these authors for motivating patients to change their behavior. Specific strategies *are* evident, though, and can be seen in the authors' "integrative case examples." For example, collaboration is obvious as one IPT motivational strategy. Empathic listening keeps patients talking about their problems and reduces isolation and loneliness. IPT therapists seem to rely strongly on suggestions and interpretations to motivate patients to change, as illustrated by the following quote in which an IPT therapist addresses a patient:

> The different ways that you have felt bad—the sadness and crying, being unable to get yourself going, trouble concentrating, not wanting to face other people—are all part of a picture of depression that seems to have hit you as a result of losing many things over the past several years. As you point out, the way you are now is clearly different from the way you were: you've lost your husband; you've lost his companionship even before that; you lost the plans you had for a happy retirement. It's very hard to get over these losses. Part of what we will be doing is trying to help you do this . . . confront what you've lost and help you manage it. As we do this I expect that your symptoms will improve. (p. 157)

Another example of a motivational strategy is pointing out logical discrepancies in patients' verbal reports. For example, a patient may report thinking that he/she will fail in certain situations yet may consistently say that he/she has been successful in these very areas. The clinician will then point out this discrepancy with the intent of mitigating the negative expectancy concerning performance. Motivating the person to relinquish the negative expectancy would be the goal here.

Further cases of negative reinforcement delivery include those where grieving patients experience happy moments and report feeling guilty because they are not sad. IPT clinicians downplay the negative state (guilt) and highlight and emphasize the experience of felt joy. Encouraging positive affect on such occasions is the way therapists give these patients permission to feel less guilt when experiencing positive emotions.

Clarifying experiences of competing emotions is another device used to assist or motivate individuals to accept equivocal reactions. To use our example of grief again, a person who has lost a spouse may report guilt when discussing a recent and enjoyable date. The therapist assists the individual to accept the fact that he/she is not quite finished with the grieving process, thus helping him/her to accept the ambivalent feelings.

In every case, terminating or resolving emotional, behavioral, or cognitive conflicts that lead to distressing emotional states is a basic IPT motivational strategy. It is not clear, however, how much the distress is actually reduced and whether the therapist helps the person process what led to what. Though CBASP, CT, and IPT all employ negative reinforcement strategies to motivate patients, there are differences in the particular ways each model goes about accomplishing the task.

Distinctions: CBASP versus CT and IPT

If therapists want patients to learn that two elements, such as a specific behavior and the reduction of their distress, are associated, the best way to accomplish this goal is to make certain that such associations are highlighted every time they happen, until patients are able to recognize the contingent events by themselves. CBASP saturates the sessions with this contingency awareness program. In contrast, IPT only alludes to negative reinforcement, as illustrated in the quotation above, when the practitioner tells the patient that if she learns to confront her loss and manage her grief, she will feel better. Beck et al. (1979), on the other hand, say specifically: "When the patient shows an improvement, the therapist should encourage him to pinpoint what methods (if any) contributed to the improvement" (p. 32). My guess is that CT and CBASP differ only in the frequency with which these relief moments are pinpointed and highlighted. I would also speculate that CBASP clinicians are more sensitive to these in-session relief moments, due to the extensive training they undergo in the use of contingency awareness (negative reinforcement) to modify patient behavior. CBASP clinicians are encouraged to stop whatever they are doing when the relief moments occur and help the patient determine what has led to a decrease in misery. They also highlight the relief moments when patients report such events occurring on the outside.

Why does CBASP utilize negative reinforcement to such an extent?

The reasons come from learning research. We know that without rehearsal, short-term memory of the associated elements—in this case, a causal behavior and its effects—is fleeting, and the associations never enter long-term memory (Solso, 1995; Waugh & Norman, 1965). CBASP practitioners want patients exiting therapy knowing that the quality of their behavior is specifically connected to the way they feel. This learning is crucial for preventing relapse after treatment ends. If too much time elapses between the behavior and the distress reduction event, or if clinicians overlook the relief moments during sessions, the probability that patients will make the association between the behavior and the positive consequence is negligible.

Perceptual Focus and Behavior Change Techniques

The way each of us perceives the environment is the "basic connection link" that ties us to the world we live in (Goldfried et al., 1997, 1998; James, 1890; Kiesler, 1999; Wright & Thase, 1992). Perceptual cognitive-emotional processes represent our gateway to the environment and, conversely, the environment's access route to us. All psychotherapy systems make contact with patients at this perceptual gate. CBASP, CT, and IPT behavior change techniques may be distinguished from one another by examining carefully how each therapy system manipulates the perceptual focus of its patients.

Perceptual Focus and Behavior Change: CBASP

Chronically depressed patients are taught to focus on the consequences of their behavior within discrete situational contexts. The goal of these exercises is to strengthen the perceived connection between individuals and the world they live in. Primary psychopathology in CBASP is defined as the perceived disengagement of individuals from their environment. Thus, as long as the perceived disengagement remains in place, enduring behavioral change is impossible, and the person remains trapped in the withdrawal phase of the depressive experience. Every technique in the CBASP arsenal directs the perceptual focus of patients toward behavioral consequences.

Perceptual Focus and Behavior Change: CT

In contrast, Beck's model defines the primary psychopathology of depressed patients as being the distorted manner in which they view themselves, their ongoing experiences, and the future. Further manifestation of pathology is evident in the particular way individuals process information (overgeneralization, catastrophizing, all-or-none thinking, etc.). CT techniques guide the perceptual focus of patients toward an examination of their distorted thinking and of the effects these distortions have on their emotions and behavior. The ultimate goal of CT is to realign the individual's *thinking* with reality and, in so doing, to change the depressive behavior.

Perceptual Focus and Behavior Change: IPT

IPT views the primary psychopathology of major depressive patients as involving social maladjustment in current interpersonal conflicts. The perceptual focus of IPT is directed towards the usual four areas of problematical functioning: grief, role dispute, role transition, and interpersonal deficit. Once patients contract with IPT therapists about which of these interpersonal conflict domains treatment will address, techniques are administered that perceptually focus the attention of patients on the problem spheres. IPT strategies are designed to remediate the interpersonal conflict problems and, in so doing, to improve social adjustment and decrease depressive symptomatology.

Distinctions: CBASP versus CT and IPT

As noted above, the major technique distinctions among CBASP, CT, and IPT arise out of their contrasting views of the primary pathology of depression. Since depression is defined differently by each model, it follows that treatment focuses the patient's attention on different aspects of phenomenological and psychosocial functioning. CBASP focuses attention on the "person × environment" interaction; CT requires that attention be focused on cognitive content and its congruence (or lack thereof) with reality; IPT highlights problematical interpersonal domains as they pertain to role expectations and enactment. CBASP techniques help patients concentrate on discrete temporal events in order to demonstrate to them the fact that they are functionally related to the world they live in. In so doing, patients learn to perceive themselves and others in formal operations terms and hence to revise their preoperational view of the world. CT, on the other hand, relies on techniques that expose and refute unrealistic thinking, all the while showing the individual that cognitive distortions potentiate and maintain depression. Since IPT conceptualizes interpersonal role conflicts as precursors of major depression, IPT techniques highlight the importance of addressing problematical relationship areas and then teach patients to resolve their role conflicts.

CONCLUSION

Significant differences exist among CBASP, CT, and IPT. The uniqueness of CBASP cannot be understood apart from the idiosyncratic pathology of the chronically depressed adult. Since habitual and treatment-resistant patterns of behavior must be modified, therapists deal not only with patients' current problems in living, but also with negative interpersonal patterns that come from the patients' developmental histories of maltreatment. Not infrequently, these interpersonal behaviors adversely affect the dyadic relationship. The degree to which therapists successfully inhibit the patient's pulls for dominance and hostility; the extent to which transference issues are successfully addressed in the moment and revised; the way clinicians manage motivational problems with individuals who feel chronically helpless and hopeless; and the way they deal with their own frustration, hostility, and/or fatigue (which all too often accompany working with this challenging population) lead to many of CBASP's unique features.

CHAPTER THIRTEEN

Resolving Common Patient Problems and Crises

> The same conditions that bring about depression (helplessness) in reverse serve frequently the restitution from depression.
>
> —E. BIBRING (1953, p. 43)

In suggesting ways to manage several problem areas and crisis events with chronically depressed patients, I will rely upon the "person × environment" behavioral model (Chapter 2) as the underlying principle for intervention. During emergency periods, clinicians must help patients focus attention on their connection to the environment. In most instances, this means that practitioners must accentuate their role as "the environment" and "consequate" the behavior of patients in some obvious manner. The assumption underlying the consequation strategy is that when individuals perceive the immediate effects of their behavior, they will be more likely to confront the stress than to avoid it.

Most of the problems and crises discussed in this chapter erupt during stressful events in which individuals feel helpless—meaning that they fail to perceive the consequences of their own behavior. The use of disciplined personal involvement by CBASP psychotherapists, whereby they utilize their reactions to patients as behavioral consequences, potentiates their effectiveness. For example, halting a patient's slide into a major depressive episode or defusing the affect driving a threat of suicide can often be accomplished by revealing the immediate consequences these behaviors produce in the clinician. Accentuating the "person × environment" connection is also useful during "acting-out" periods, when treatment becomes problematical because of a lack of improvement or when therapists are faced with hostile-obsessive or passive-dependent individuals. In cases where therapists overintellectualize treatment, particularly in instances of SA when they become overly concerned about patients' performing all the steps perfectly, refocusing on behavioral consequences will restore the proper therapeutic perspective. And, finally, highlighting behavioral consequences in the patient-therapist relationship is often an effective means of modifying refractory cognitive-emotional reactions.

HALTING A SLIDE INTO A MAJOR DEPRESSIVE EPISODE

All of us have seen patients teetering on the brink of a major depressive episode; such events happen frequently in sessions with these patients. I like to use a metaphor to describe the situation: Slipping into a major depressive episode is like sliding down a steep hill where there are no footholds or barriers to stop the slide. In order for therapists to serve as a "brake" on the slide, short of hospitalization or increasing medication dosage, they must personally move into the path of the slide. Following is one way to use the "person × environment" type of interaction to serve as a brake.

One outpatient reported a severe argument with her daughter that resulted in extremely cutting and hurtful comments from the adolescent girl. The patient, "Sally," had been improving steadily until then: Her weekly BDI scores up to this point had been in the middle teens, down from a screening BDI score of 32. In this 10th session, when she came in and told me about the crisis, her BDI score was 35 and her general appearance was disheveled: She wore no makeup (she usually did), her hair was uncombed, and she looked as if she had just gotten out of bed—a stark contrast to her usual neat appearance.

THERAPIST: Sally, why didn't you take the time to fix yourself up before you came to the session?

SALLY: Nothing matters any more. It doesn't matter how I look. Everything I try to do with my daughter is wrong. We'll never get along.

THERAPIST: It matters to me how you look.

SALLY: Huh?

THERAPIST: I said, it matters to me how you look. I have a suggestion. Why don't you go to the bathroom and take a moment and fix yourself up. Then, come back and we'll begin again.

When Sally returned, her first comment was "God, I looked awful." My next remark was designed to strengthen the earlier statement that it mattered to me how she looked when she came to therapy.

THERAPIST: I bet my comments about the way you looked surprised you.

SALLY: They did. I didn't think it would matter.

THERAPIST: It matters to me how you look and how things are going in your life. Now, are you ready to tackle the problem with your daughter? How you handle this crisis is important to me.

This scenario can take many forms and be played out in many different ways. The crucial tactic is deciding the best way to interrupt the patient's felt helplessness and then demonstrating the effects his/her behavior is having upon the therapist. This tactic will often buy enough time so that the clinician and patient will have an opportunity to plan out a strategy to deal with the stress event that originally precipitated the patient's withdrawal maneuver (see Figure 2.1). Clinicians are in an optimal position to make environmental effects obvious. In my experience, it is difficult for patients to continue their unimpeded slide into major depression once they perceive the effects they are having on their therapists. This is true even though difficult problems remain to be solved.

STANDING BETWEEN THE PATIENT AND SUICIDE

The most dangerous symptoms of depression are suicidal ideation and attempts. In a review of 17 studies on the course and outcome of depressive disorders, Guze and Robins (1970) reported that approximately 15% of patients with depression lasting more than one month committed suicide. It is crucial that psychotherapists remain vigilant for the omnipresent threat of suicide. When suicide is an ongoing issue, I recommend that it be treated immediately and vigorously with both medication and psychotherapy.

Several caveats must be mentioned before I proceed. First and foremost, the technique to be described must never be attempted unless a clinician is highly confident that the *therapeutic alliance* is rock solid. In addition, several clinical "markers," if present, argue against using this intervention. The markers are as follows: (1) the presence of a formal plan/proposed method (time, place, how) for suicide; (2) severe anxiety; (3) ongoing panic attacks; (4) severe insomnia; (5) alcohol abuse/dependence; and (6) a severe loss of interest and pleasure (anhedonia) in activities or people (Clark & Fawcett, 1992; Fawcett et al., 1990).

It is well known that suicidal patients feel extremely helpless. Interpersonally, however, they are not helpless at all; they actually wield incredible power. A suicidal individual can mobilize an entire family, a circle of friends, and the mental health community into action, including 24-hour surveillance and supervision. The problem is that suicidal patients are not aware of the environmental impact they are having. One reason they pose a danger to themselves is because of their extreme perceptual disengagement from the environment. How can therapists consequate their behavior during such crises?: By "personalizing" the effects of a suicide on the life of the therapist. I'll use a verbatim example taken from one of my sessions with a male patient to illustrate the point.

PATIENT: I don't want to live any more. It wouldn't matter to anyone if I died. No one cares.

THERAPIST: What effect do you think you would have on me if you took your own life?

PATIENT: Aw, you'd be upset for a while, but you'd get over it. Pretty quick, I imagine.

THERAPIST: You surely don't think much of me.

PATIENT: What do you mean?

THERAPIST: We've worked together for two months. You have no idea of the effect you would have on me if you killed yourself. You blow off my personal reaction to you like we are perfect strangers.

PATIENT: You've been trained to turn off your feelings in such situations.

THERAPIST: Let me ask you again. You never really answered my question. You just blew off any serious reaction I would have to your death. What effect do you really think you would have on me if you took your own life?

PATIENT: I really don't know—I have no idea.

THERAPIST: Let me tell you what some of the effects would be. First off, you would ram me in the gut with a two-by-four and push me into real emotional turmoil and anguish. Not only would I be angry at myself for not being able to help you through this, but I would be mad as hell with you for jumping overboard on me during this crisis. I've got to know something, and I'm very serious about this. Why would you want to do this to me? I want an answer, because you're talking about doing something that would hurt me in the worst way.

PATIENT: I never thought about it this way.

THERAPIST: Why would you want to treat me like this?

PATIENT: I never thought I mattered to anyone. I didn't think it would really make a damn what the hell I did. You make it sound so damn personal!

THERAPIST: It *is* personal—it's between you and me right now. I'm not talking about anyone else. I'm talking about the effects you have just had on me. Based on my reaction to you, what effects would you say you have just had on me? Let's talk about this.

This tactic is extreme, and I don't use it often. Moreover, if this consequation of the patient's behavior doesn't mitigate the crisis, then hospitalization is clearly the next step. Most of the time, though, I find that reacting in this way mitigates the affect driving the suicidal threat and lessens some of the pressure to take action. My anger as well as that of the patient is made public in this exchange, because I have played out the consequences of the hostile suicidal threat. But I'm also not play-acting. My stated feelings are genuine and they are felt intensely in the moment. In requiring this person to look at the effects he would have on me and then asking why he would want to hurt me this way, I moved the patient into the position of having to "stare down the barrel" of the consequences of the behavior he is threatening. In such moments, this is the safest place to be with the suicidal patient. Again, I must state that without a stable dyadic alliance solidly in place, this strategy should never be attempted.

INHIBITING "ACTING OUT" BEHAVIOR

Patients who constantly bring crises into psychotherapy avoid having to talk seriously about their problems. In such cases, treatment becomes an arena in which clinicians have to put out one brush fire after another. It's not surprising that patient and clinician never have sufficient time to deal with the underlying issues fueling the crises. In the face of the constant external sturm und drang, the clinician is unable to arrange contingencies to affect the behavior of the patient. The usual comment from therapists who work with these patients is, "I can't get anything done in the session!"

A practitioner must direct such a patient's focus to the therapy relationship and refuse to deal with any external crises. If the patient does not comply with the therapist's effort to redirect his/her attention, the therapy will remain ineffective. Once the clinician has firmly established the boundaries of the in-session focus, the next step is to conduct SAs addressing interpersonal events that occur during the session. When SAs are focused solely on events that occur between the therapist and patient, the interpersonal encounter will intensify. *More often than not, the same behavioral difficulties producing trouble on the outside become problematical in the session.* Once the shift in focus has been achieved and the individual is now concentrating on the in-session relationship and actively resolving the problems, the frequency and intensity of the outside crises often subside.

The efficacy of this shift in focus lies in the fact that now the patient has to talk about cognitive interpretations, behaviors, and AOs and DOs that all involve the therapist. The immediacy of processing what goes on *in the current interaction* places the therapist in an optimal position either to confirm or to disconfirm the patient's perceptions of the situation and to help the individual remedy the behaviors that are producing the interpersonal chaos.

Once the external crises have diminished to manageable levels, the focus in therapy can be shifted back to interpersonal situations that involve significant people in the individual's life. An example will show how one therapy session began and how the therapist structured the in-session focus for the patient:

THERAPIST: What kind of week have you had? ["Phillip," a 25-year-old male double depressive, reported weekly on hostile interpersonal crises involving his father, two brothers, and a younger teenaged sister. The encounters were severe, and the previous five sessions had been spent talking about the crises. Nothing that was discussed in sessions appeared to have any effect on Phillip's behavior when he was with his family.]

PHILLIP: I got into another vicious argument with my father last night. He made a stupid comment about President Clinton, and I told him off. He got mad, and we yelled at each other for 15 minutes. I stormed out of the house, slammed the front door, squealed my tires taking off, and then drove around fuming most of the night. It was after four in the morning when I got back to my apartment.

THERAPIST: Phillip, we've got to change some in-session ground rules for you and me.

PHILLIP: What do you mean?

THERAPIST: I mean that you and I are getting nowhere fast. From now on I want us to concentrate on what is going on between the two of us—either in the present session or during the last session. We can save some time at the end of the session if you want, in order to talk about what is going on with your family. But for the next few sessions, I want your situational analyses to reflect what goes on between us.

PHILLIP: How is this going to help me deal with my family?

THERAPIST: I think it will in the long run, but for right now, spending your time in here talking about the family is clearly not helping. Let's change the focus. Pick an event that happened last week between you and me, and let's do an SA on it.

It turned out that Phillip had disagreed with several comments the clinician had made during previous sessions, but he had never mentioned his disagreement. Once the disagreements were addressed in SA, Phillip learned how to express his differences of opinion without hostilely confronting the therapist. The SA exercises also led to more conversational give-and-take during the sessions. Phillip started asking the therapist what he thought about his ideas and whether he found them relevant and important. Phillip was learning to be empathic by using language to understand and be understood. Not surprisingly, his family crises diminished in frequency and intensity.

STRATEGY FOR DEALING WITH LACK OF IMPROVEMENT

Most SAs involve encounters that have occurred between the patient and others on the outside. This is as it should be. In some instances, the intensity of the depression remains unchanged over time, and the individual continues to report problematical situations on the outside in which similar problems crop up repeatedly. In short, there is no evidence that the person is making any progress. The absence of behavioral change signals the need for a change in strategy for the clinician. What can be done to loosen the logjam?

Nine times out of ten, the specific interpersonal problems (with persons on the outside) implicated in the SAs are being manifested in the sessions between therapist and patient—a phenomenon called "parallel process" (Gerson, 1996). Earlier I have noted that the cognitive-emotional and behavioral rigidity of chronic patients makes their behavior quite predictable, whatever the setting. The best way to loosen the logjam on the outside is to refocus the patient's attention on in-session events by asking the patient to construct SAs involving the therapist (similar to the strategy above). This tactic should remain in place until the interpersonal issue is resolved and progress is evident. Then attention can be shifted back to the outside arena. Let me illustrate the strategy with an example.

One patient of mine, a sales clerk in a large department store, kept reporting difficulties with her manager. Having been told by the manager to alter the dress displays on the floor, "Margaret" would go to the manager and explain why altering the displays his way was not wise. She would explain and elaborate her reasons until the manager became angry and ordered her to do it his way. She would leave his office angry and depressed, comply with his wishes, and then pout for several days.

I had explained the SA procedure to Margaret during the third session. She came in for the fourth session and began telling me how she thought the information could be gathered in a more effective way. After listening for some time, I then simply requested that she adhere to the SA format. Margaret did so, albeit reluctantly, over the next five sessions. The SA content involved her run-ins with the manager and other coworkers. Therapy progress was at a standstill. During the eighth session, I asked Margaret to select a situation that had occurred between the two of us during the previous session. The event that was analyzed involved an exchange in which another verbal disagreement had occurred between Margaret and me.

THERAPIST: How did the exchange come out for you?

MARGARET: We got into another argument.

THERAPIST: How did you want the event to come out for you?

MARGARET: I wanted us to be able to talk together without arguing [this was a DO she didn't know how to produce].

THERAPIST: Did you get what you wanted here?

MARGARET: No!

THERAPIST: Why?

MARGARET: Because I couldn't stop trying to explain my side of the story.

During the remediation phase of SA, two action interpretations were added to help move Margaret closer to attaining the DO: (1) "I've got to listen to what Dr. McCullough is saying," and (2) "I've got to ask Dr. McCullough if he understands what I'm saying." The behaviors needed were "listening to Dr. McCullough" and "inquiring whether he has listened to me" (this was an *empathy* strategy). What transpired over the next few sessions was teaching the patient to listen to me as well as to inquire whether she had been heard—and then to arrive at a decision. Once it became obvious that Margaret had added the listening component in therapy, we returned the SA focus to her encounters with others. She began to make progress in therapy and reported having less conflict with her manager and coworkers.

MANAGING HOSTILE-OBSESSIVE PATIENTS

Among the most difficult chronically depressed individuals to work with are the hostile-obsessive patients who can be described as persons "living without an interpersonal environment." These individuals enter therapy entrapped by their own rituals, routines, and reflexive anger. They complain bitterly that others, such as spouses and colleagues, are incompetent nincompoops because they don't behave according to their (these patients') wishes. Listening to endless tirades in which these patients claim despairingly that they just cannot understand why others don't see the utter stupidity of their ways and do things the patients' ways, wise therapists know that in a short time, they too will join the band of incompetent nincompoops. The strong interpersonal pull from these individuals is to counteraggress and tell them that they are full of baloney.

The upper part of Figure 13.1 illustrates the implacable entrapment of the hostile-obsessive patient (capital "P") by depicting the person "boxed in" behind a barrier of reflexive anger that deflects (deflecting

The hostile-obsessive patient who functions without an interpersonal environment by deflecting behavioral consequences with hostility.

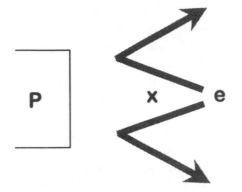

The passive-dependent patient who is dominated and overwhelmed by the interpersonal environment and who copes via excessive compliance.

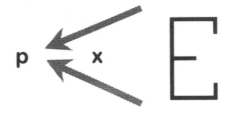

FIGURE 13.1. Contrasting interpersonal styles of hostile-obsessive and passive-dependent patients.

arrows) environmental consequences. Other people (the environment, symbolized by an "e" in lower-case to indicate an absence of influence) cannot penetrate the interpersonal barrier and thus have no formative influence on the individual's behavior. (The passive-dependent, depicted in the lower portion of Figure 13.1, is discussed in the following section.)

One way to approach this problem is to figure out how to penetrate the interpersonal barrier so that the practitioner can become an active player in the patient's life. This can be done by using a ploy called "becoming a problem for the patient." The individual's focus must be directed to the interpersonal impact he/she is having on the clinician; the SA assignment must again require the patient to construct scenarios based on in-session events that have occurred between the practitioner and the individual. Becoming a problem for a patient is also accomplished by repeatedly feeding back the effects of the patient's behavior—pointing out the hostile comments, demeaning innuendos, and nonverbal gestures that lead to negative interpersonal impacts on the clinician.

For example, one practitioner frequently asked her patient why he wanted to treat her so hostilely. She wanted to know what she had done to deserve this treatment. At first, her questions elicited angry outbursts and verbal tantrums, but she didn't let the patient avoid her questions; in short, she assumed the role of an in-session problem for the patient. Gradually he began telling her why he got so mad, and after a number of sessions, he admitted that his outbursts were rude and hurtful. By the end of treatment, the patient had gained some control over his outbursts; more importantly, he was able to communicate with the therapist in genuine dialogue. The clinician's disciplined personal involvement and candid feedback about the hurtful effects of this hostile-obsessive patient modified the patient's behavior.

Another effective therapist I observed administering this technique did it by using a "naive demeanor" (a naive style mimiking Peter Falk in his *Columbo* role) that communicated a total lack of understanding why anyone would want to treat him so rudely. The practitioner just kept asking the patient why he continued to treat him like a punching bag. One such inquiry was as follows:

"You just insinuated that I don't know what I'm doing. Why do you want to treat me this way? I really want to know."

Finally, after several sessions of continual feedback, the patient made an astounding comment: "Do you think I treat others this way?" The breakthrough had finally happened! The environment had broken through the interpersonal barrier. The therapist's persistent consequation strategy had finally broken through the reflexive barrier of anger, and now the clinician could become an active player in the person's life. Environmental consequences could now begin to influence behavior!

MANAGING PASSIVE-DEPENDENT PATIENTS

The passive-dependent chronic patient presents another type of difficult interpersonal problem that can easily escalate to crisis levels if managed improperly. With a passive-dependent individual, a therapist feels a strong interpersonal pull to assume a dominant, take-charge role. As stated throughout this book, CBASP clinicians are discouraged from assuming a dominant role with any chronically depressed patient. Nevertheless, this kind of behavior makes it particularly difficult for a therapist to resist assuming a dominant role.

The passive-dependent patient's interpersonal style is shown in the lower portion of Figure 13.1. The lower-case "p" interacting with the capital "E" is intended to suggest that others (E) always override (one-way arrows) the patient's (p) wishes, opinions, decisions, feelings, and concerns. Such individuals reflexively expect people to tell them what to do, and they are rarely disappointed. They have little or no self-confidence, and at the first sign of interpersonal difficulty, they look to others for help and direction. Passive-dependent individuals spend considerable time being lectured at and preached to by spouses, relatives, friends, ministers, doctors, and (sadly) some psychotherapists. Nothing seems to modify their reliance upon others. The refractory behavior stems from the fact that as long as they can remain in the submissive role, they can avoid the responsibility of actively participating in encounters with others.

The issue in therapy with a passive-dependent individual is this: How can the practitioner facilitate the emergence of assertive behavior so that the patient becomes a proactive player with the environment? The first rule of thumb is to assume a task-focused role (see the "optimal" therapist IMI profiles in Figures 8.2 and 8.3) and rely totally on the SA methodology to demonstrate the consequences of submissive behavior. Behavioral consequences for submission are often unpleasant and disturbing. Given that despite these consequences, the person continues to behave this way, helping him/her see that the misery is produced by his/her passive-dependent style is essential.

THERAPIST: You said that the DO you wanted was for your wife to quit telling you what to do. How the situation came out for you was that you got another lecture. Why didn't you get what you wanted here?

PATIENT: Because I just sat there and said nothing.

THERAPIST: Let's go back through the situation and see what has to be changed in order for you to obtain your desired outcome.

Everyone told this man what to do. The result was that he was usually immobilized and said nothing. Over sessions, he began to see alternatives to his passive behavior. Patiently waiting for him to articulate what he wanted, the therapist refused to tell him what to do or to do the work of SA for him. When he made decisions, the clinician carefully avoided suggesting ways to improve the plans. Gradually the patient became bolder and learned to say what he wanted directly and forcefully. Not surprisingly, he reported that others behaved toward him in a less dominant manner. By the end of treatment, he had become more assertive.

Helping passive-dependent patients to "even up the score" with the environment is the best strategy. In terms of Figure 13.1, this means helping "p × E" individuals to transform the p into P—in other words, to feel empowered to assert their opinions, wishes, feelings, and concerns to others with a greater degree of confidence. The consequences of the behavior change will be accompanied by SAs that describe situations where others behave in a less dominant fashion and where patients begin to achieve their DOs. As the person becomes more of an environmental player, the in-session pulls for dominance also diminish.

INHIBITING OVERINTELLECTUALIZED THERAPY ADMINISTRATION

The danger in conducting any type of cognitive behavioral psychotherapy is the possibility of turning treatment into an intellectual exercise and doing the work for the patient. What I mean by this in relation to CBASP is that therapists can easily become more concerned with how patients are thinking or behaving than they are with the environmental consequences produced by these behaviors. In such instances, clinicians compromise the utility of the "person × environment" behavioral model. Cognitions and behaviors are crucially important, but only *because* of the interpersonal consequences they produce. Whenever therapists lose this focus, CBASP techniques are transformed into intellectual exercises. I have become increasingly aware of this tendency to cerebralize CBASP therapy while supervising clinicians in the B-MS study (see Chapters 8, 9, and 10).

SA is a highly structured procedure, with rules guiding each step in both the elicitation and remediation phases. The danger for therapists in administering SA is that they will follow the "letter of the law" but lose the "spirit" of the SA procedure. *The spirit of SA is consequating behavior.* When therapists intellectualize CBASP, they overemphasize administering the method "correctly" or having patients do each SA step "just right." Any time a therapist concentrates solely on making sure a patient does each step perfectly, overintellectualization of the method has occurred and the consequation goals of the exercise are eclipsed.

I have found that one way to inhibit this tendency is to help clinicians remain focused on the consequation components of SA. More specifically, this means keeping an eye fixed on the AO-versus-DO comparison. The major issue for each patient in each SA must continue to be *whether or not the DO was obtained.* One example of overshadowing the consequation emphasis occurs when a therapist begins trying to repair the cognitive errors during the remediation phase but neglects the cognitive linkages to the AO. The SA method is thereby transformed into a "revision-of-thinking" exercise, and the patient's perceptual connection with the environment is compromised.

In CBASP, *the motivational variable necessary for behavior change is the attainment of the DO,* and not correct thinking. Therapists cannot help patients change their behavior by training them to think with impeccable logic. Behavior is changed when the goal is desirable enough to motivate the person to alter his/her thinking and behavior to obtain it. An example of intellectualizing SA will illustrate the point.

One patient found it difficult to assert herself with others; she simply couldn't tell others what she wanted. During one session I observed on videotape, the SA involved an exchange between the patient and her mother wherein the mother had made several demeaning remarks. The patient had said nothing to her mother about her inappropriate behavior, and the conversation had ended with the patient's becoming enraged, then depressed. The DO involved telling the mother to stop talking rudely. The clinician spent a great deal of time revising the woman's interpretations, in essence splitting intellectual hairs on the nuances of each phrase. The revision process almost turned into a grammatical parsing lesson. The conclusion I drew while observing this session was that the clinician was assuming that if the patient could just find the most "correct" wording for her interpretations, then her behavior with her mother would change. No, it wouldn't! Another example (revising an interpretation during the remediation phase) will illustrate the point:

PATIENT: I can't quit saying "no" to anyone who asks me for something.

THERAPIST: You've inserted the wrong verb in your sentence.

PATIENT: What do you mean?

THERAPIST: The verb "can't" means that extraneous factors prevent you from changing your behavior.

PATIENT: Well, I'm not sure what they are, but I just can't.

THERAPIST: Why don't you substitute the verb "won't" for the word "can't" and restate your sentence?

PATIENT: I won't quit saying "no" to anyone who asks me for something. Yeah, I see what you are getting at, but I just can't make myself do it.

THERAPIST: I don't think you're seeing the volitional implications that differentiate the two verbs from each other. "Can't" implies you don't have a volitional choice. "Won't" implies you are making a choice by not saying "no."

PATIENT: What you're saying sounds good, but I just can't do it.

The practitioner in this case overintellectualized the remediation process and overlooked the fact that consequences, not substitute verbs, modify the behavior of chronically depressed adults. The supervisor gave feedback and helped the therapist to see how he had lost sight of the DO target in putting an overintellectualized strategy designed to modify behavior with logic.

Consequences modify cognitions and behavior. Situational interpretations and behaviors are important only to the degree that patients recognize their relevance to both AOs and DOs. If the patient in the dialogue above wanted to start saying "no," then she would first need to be motivated to terminate the misery resulting from saying "yes." Because she perceived no connection between feeling miserable and saying "yes," the patient was right: She cannot say "no!"

MODIFYING REFRACTORY
COGNITIVE-EMOTIVE RESPONSES

Chronically depressed patients sometimes present entrenched cognitive-emotive reactions that they readily admit they cannot change. For example, one patient disclosed that he felt guilty over having committed a past misdeed and then stated unequivocally, "I can never forgive myself for what I have done." A second type of refractory cognitive-emotive response involves negative reactions toward the self that appear to operate independently of any precipitating stimulus event. Examples might be, "I hate myself and I always will," "I'm no damn good," and "I'm always angry with myself."

In normal cognitive-emotional functioning, specific spatio-temporal events exert influence on the person (Cicchetti et al., 1995; Lazarus, 1966, 1990; Schachter, 1964; Schachter & Singer, 1962). It follows that in order to modify negative and refractory cognitive-emotional reactions, one must highlight the situational context implicated in these reactions. In the first case, where a perceived misdeed led to enduring feelings of guilt, the therapist would need *to change the situation* in order to modify the guilt. In the second instance, where there is no apparent situational stimulus, the therapist would have *to construct a situation*, link the old global emotional reaction to the newly created situation, and work from there. To refer back to the "person × environment" behavioral model, another way to describe this therapeutic approach is to say that a refractory emotional response must be linked to a tangible environmental parameter before it can be modified (see Figure 13.2).

Consider what two therapists did when they were faced with the above two problems. Strategies similar to those described earlier will be evident. In the case of the unforgivable misdeed, the patient cannot perceptually sever his reflexive negative reaction to the original event. The second example involves a cognitive-emotive reaction in which the original learning situation has been lost and all that remains is a negative reaction toward the self. Conceptualizing these situations from the "person × environment" perspective, the environment is changed for one patient and a new environment is created for the second.

The first patient needed to encounter a new situational context for the old response. The encounter with the therapist becomes that new situation (see Figure 13.2), as demonstrated in the following dialogue.

THERAPIST: You have stated, once again, that you are experiencing guilt over the affair you had years ago. Are you feeling the guilt right now, here with me?

PATIENT: Yes, I feel it really strongly.

THERAPIST: What is my reaction to you, now that I know what you have done?

PATIENT: You have never made much of it. You don't seem to think it was that terrible.

THERAPIST: Obviously my reaction has not influenced your emotional reaction. What I want you to do right now is to tell me why I don't think you need to be punished. How can I possibly feel differently about you than you feel about yourself?

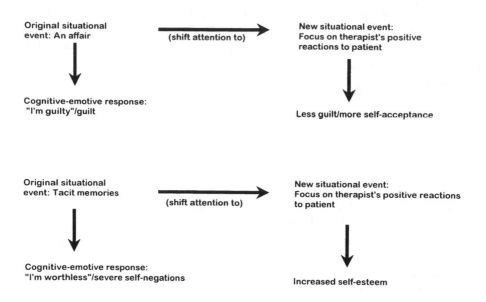

FIGURE 13.2. Procedure for modifying refractory cognitive-emotive patterns.

PATIENT: I'm not sure. Maybe you have different moral values.

THERAPIST: I'm not talking about moral values. I'm referring to my feelings that I don't want to punish you for the affair.

PATIENT: Maybe you can accept me even though I did it.

THERAPIST: Are you able to experience my acceptance of you right now?

PATIENT: I'm not sure, but it would certainly be nice to think that someone could still like me, knowing what I did.

THERAPIST: Do you feel that I like you?

PATIENT: I've always felt you did, even from the first time we met.

THERAPIST: How is that possible, given what you have done?

PATIENT: I'm not sure, but I feel you do.

THERAPIST: How strong is the guilt reaction right now?

PATIENT: Well, it's still there, but it's not as strong as it was.

THERAPIST: Hmm. Wonder why?

PATIENT: Maybe it has to do with my feeling that I'm not a total outcast—that someone else could care for me in spite of this.

The clinician has changed the situational context for the old cognitive-emotional reaction (guilt) by connecting it to the therapist's positive responses to the patient. To put it another way, the old situational condition is infiltrated by the presence of the therapist, who seeks to link the negative reactions to a new and accepting response. The patient is faced with a *new situation* in relation to the *old feeling*.

The second instance can be addressed in a similar manner. Where cognitive-emotive reactions seem to occur independently of situational events, the therapist is in an optimal position to *create* a situational context for the negative patterns (see Figure 13.2). Tacit early learning stemming from interactions with significant others is usually the culprit in this kind of pattern. All that remain from the earlier maltreatment encounters are the negative reactions toward the self. The specific stimulus events have long since been forgotten. Highlighting the negative self-comments (without the identifiable precursor), the clinician then focuses the patient's attention on the current dyadic relationship. For example:

THERAPIST: You make these awful comments about yourself being worthless. You are also unable to identify where these feelings come from. What reaction do you think I have when you make these remarks about yourself?

PATIENT: It's the way I feel.

THERAPIST: What effects do you think these comments have on me?

PATIENT: Why should it matter?

THERAPIST: Because you are not alone when you make these statements about yourself.

PATIENT: You mean because you are here with me?

THERAPIST: That's right. Now, what effects do you think they have upon me?

PATIENT: I guess you think they sound sort of silly.

THERAPIST: They don't sound silly to me at all. They sound damning, utterly rejecting. They make me cringe every time you say them. I feel like you think you deserve the worst of everything—like maybe I ought to feel that way about you too.

PATIENT: I'd be surprised if you don't.

THERAPIST: I feel quite differently about you—very positively, in fact. Bet you never thought about my feelings toward you in this way.

PATIENT: Frankly, I haven't. I don't see how you can feel that way about me.

THERAPIST: Maybe we ought to focus on my feelings toward you and see where they are coming from.

PATIENT: I think that's a good idea.

Gradually, in this manner, the practitioner creates a situational "person × environment" framework for the negative statements. Pointing out the interpersonal effects of the patient's remarks and then focusing attention on the clinician's actual feelings toward the patient increasingly anchors the negative self-image to the therapist-patient relationship, where it can be modified. A new and specific environment has been created as a context for the patient's reaction by the clinician's linking of his response to the patient to those deriving from earlier maltreatment interactions. Now the environment can begin to exert a modifying influence over the refractory patterns.

FINAL THOUGHTS

I've thought a long time about my DO for ending this book. I have decided that my DO is to end the book on a word of hope.

Patients who have lived with chronic despair discover the real meaning of "existential hope" when they push the dark clouds of depression away and the sun comes out. A CBASP supervisor whom I supervised in the national B-MS study faxed me a letter written by one of his successfully treated patients (depressed for 24 years). One paragraph in that letter is infused with hope:

> I have hope now, and I believe in myself. I no longer feel that my life is out of control. I'm connected to people, and I've learned just how much they mean to me. I used to feel that nothing I did mattered. No more! Everything I do matters. I think it always did, but I never saw things that way before. When I get into situations now, I start thinking about what I want. I'm concerned about my goals now. Goals, goals, goals! My life has direction, and I plan on working hard to keep it this way. Thanks for your help—you and I have really accomplished a marvelous thing here.

Did my AO = DO? Yes!

APPENDICES

APPENDIX A

Therapist Prompts for Administering Situational Analysis (PASA)

Patient _____   Therapist _____

Session # _____   Date of Therapy Session _____

ELICITATION PHASE OF SITUATIONAL ANALYSIS

Obtaining a Situational Description

Goal: The patient learns to be a situational observer.

Step 1.   "Describe *what* happened:" ("Tell me, in your own words, what happened.")

Elicitation Phase Review. "So, what I hear you saying is ... Have I retold your
story right?" Encourage the person to avoid attributing motives,
meanings, emotions, or the like to characters in the story. The situational description should be like a silent movie: "This happened,
then that, then this." Use the patient's words in retelling of the story
(*don't paraphrase*).

Remediation Phase. No revisions necessary if guidelines above are adhered to.

Obtaining the Situational Interpretations

Goal: While in the situation, the patient learns to construct
interpretations that are anchored to the ongoing flow of
events (relevant interpretations) and that reflect correctly
what is transpiring (accurate interpretations). Appropriate
action interpretation(s) is/are inserted when necessary.

Step 2.   "Describe your *interpretation* of what happened:" ("Tell me, what did
the situation *mean* to you?" or "How did you *read* the situation?" or
"How did you *size up* the situation?") Avoid obtaining more than
three or four interpretations, and allow only one sentence per interpretation ("It meant that ... ").

Interpretation 1.

(Revision #1.)

Interpretation 2.

(Revision #2.)

Interpretation 3.

(Revision #3.)

Elicitation Phase Review. After each interpretation, feed back what you heard:
"So it meant ... is that correct?" or "Have I understood you correctly?"

Remediation Phase. (a) Is the interpretation *relevant/connected* to the specific situation being analyzed? (b) Is it *accurate* in describing what is going

on between the patient and the other person? (c) Does it contribute
to the attainment of the DO (either by keeping the person on task
until the DO can be attained or by directly contributing to attainment of the DO)? Revise each interpretation accordingly.

Describing Situational Behavior

Goal: The patient is able to communicate clearly what he/she did
or how he/she behaved in the situation, and can focus on
the important behaviors while excluding unnecessary
explanations or rationalizations.

Step 3.   "Describe what you *did* during the situation. Be as explicit as you
can:" ("Tell me what you said, how you said it, and what gestures
you used, or give me other information about your behavior in general in the situation. Let's see if we can paint a picture of what you
did while interacting with . . .").

Elicitation Phase Review. After the description, feed back what you heard: "So,
if I understand you correctly, you did..."

Remediation Phase. "Now that we have revised your interpretations in the situation, what behaviors are needed to help you obtain the DO?" *Also,
target behaviors (e.g., assertive behavior, etc.) that need to be shaped up
and practiced after the SA is completed.*

Pinpointing the Actual Outcome

Goal: The patient learns to pinpoint the most salient/important
situational outcome. The AO is stated in one declarative
sentence and constructed in behavioral terms.

Step 4.   "Describe *how* the event came out for you. That is, what was the *actual outcome?*"

Elicitation Phase Review. Feed back what you have heard: "So, if I understand you, this is your AO . . ." The AO must be constructed in behavioral terms. If more than one AO is given, have the patient rank the most important and work *only* with the first-ranked AO. Make certain that the AO restates or describes the "endpoint" or "exit point" in the situational description above. Descriptions of emotional reactions may accompany the AO sentence, but focus only on the behavioral AO.

Remediation Phase. None required if conditions above are adhered to.

Pinpointing the Desired Outcome

Goal: The patient learns to construct one DO using a declarative sentence and stating the DO in behavioral terms. The DO must be *attainable* (the environment can deliver it) and *realistic* (the individual can produce it). A secondary goal is for the patient to learn to construct the DO either before or during the situation to enhance goal-directed behavior.

Step 5.   "Describe how you would have *wanted* the event to come out for you. That is, what is your *desired outcome?*"

Desired Outcome 1.

(Revision #1).

Elicitation Phase. A one-sentence DO must be constructed in behavioral terms. It is acceptable if patients suggest how they want to feel, but *never* accept a DO that is constructed in emotional terms (e.g., "I want to finish the conversation feeling confident and satisfied"). If more than one DO is given, have patients rank the most important and work *only* with the first-ranked DO.

Note: If a patient cannot think of a DO at first, then ask him/her to focus on the AO and try to think of a DO in light of the just-constructed AO. One useful prompt is this: "In the best of all possible worlds, how would you want this situation to come out for you?"

Remediation Phase. The DO must be (a) *realistic* (i.e., the patient has the capacity to produce the DO) and (b) *attainable* (i.e., the environment can produce or deliver it). The DO must be revised whenever it is exposed to be *unrealistic* or *unattainable*. If revision of the DO is necessary, it will usually happen early in the revision of the interpretations.

Comparing the Actual Outcome to the Desired Outcome

> **Goal**: The patient learns to evaluate his/her failure to obtain the DO *or* his/her successful attainment of the DO.

Step 6.   "Did you get what you wanted in the situation?"

Yes _____   versus   No _____

Elicitation Phase Review. Encourage the patient to answer with either "yes" or "no" responses. Avoid obsessive elaboration, general explanations, or statements to the effect that the DO was not really important or that it was attained later. Either the DO was attained at the time of the event or it was not.

Determining Why the Desired Outcome Was Not Obtained

> **Goal**: The patient learns to pinpoint accurately the reasons why attainment of the DO was not accomplished, if this was the case.

Step 6a.   "Wonder why you didn't get what you wanted here?"

Elicitation Phase Review. A brief reply is all that is needed here, not a lengthy explanation. The main purpose is to see what sense the patient can make of his/her failure to achieve the DO. Note the individual's reason and move on to the remediation phase.

REMEDIATION PHASE OF SITUATIONAL ANALYSIS

Note: If the AO = DO (meaning that the DO was obtained), then go back through the SA to *highlight* and *reinforce* the correct cognitive and behavioral maneuvers! Don't allow patients to overlook their accomplishments! Do not spend time correcting small mistakes. Celebrate the big picture—the DO has been achieved!

Revising the Situational Interpretations

Goal: The patient learns to self-correct his/her interpretation errors.

Step 1.   "Now, let's go back and look at what you put into this situation to see if we can determine what might have prevented you from getting what you wanted. First we'll begin by looking at your interpretations and see how they helped or hindered your attainment of the DO. Let's begin with your first interpretation and see what it contributed to your getting what you wanted here." ("Based on this interpretation, how would it have been possible for you to get what you wanted here?")

Remediation Phase Review. All interpretations are revised until the interpretations anchor the person to the situation (relevancy), correctly reflect what has actually transpired (accuracy), and/or denote what action the person must take to achieve the DO (action interpretation).

Note: The first time it becomes obvious that there are problems with the DO (it is either *unrealistic* or *unattainable*), the DO will have to be revised. Then go back and examine the original interpretations in light of the revised DO.

Revising Situational Behaviors

Goal: The patient learns to self-correct problematic behaviors and pinpoint necessary behaviors that will lead to attainment of the DO.

Step 2. "We've completed revising your reads in the situation. Now, based on these new interpretations, what specific behaviors would have helped you attain the DO?"

Remediation Phase Review. The patient learns to pinpoint the requisite behaviors that are needed for achievement of the DO. As noted above under Step 3 of elicitation, the clinician will be able to determine what behavioral deficits are present and what behaviors must be taught and practiced following the completion of the SA.

Wrap-Up and Summary of SA

Goal: The patient learns how to recognize the step errors he/she made in the situation and to understand what revisions are needed to attain the DO.

Step 3. "Now let's review what you've learned in this SA. As best you can, describe what went wrong. Then review how you corrected the problems and summarize what you've learned."

Remediation Phase Review. Wait until the patient has reviewed the learning. If
there are any further points that have been overlooked, mention
them at this time.

Generalization and Transfer of Learning

Goal: The patient learns how to generalize and transfer the
insights gained in the current SA to discrete problem
situations in other areas of his/her life.

Step 4.   "How does what you have learned in this situation apply to other
problem situations in your life? Be as specific as you can. Try to
think of similar problem situations in your life, and consider how the
solutions you found in this SA apply to these other situations."

Remediation Phase Review. Help the patient pinpoint other specific problem situations. Avoid talking about situations *in general* and describing how
this SA learning will help the patient "deal better with life problems" or the like. The most effective generalization occurs when the
person can describe how learning in this event would apply *specifically* to cognitive or behavioral trouble spots in another (specific)
problematical event.

Behavioral Skill Training and Practice Following SA

Use the remaining time in the session to work on behavioral deficits
that have become apparent in the SA exercise.

APPENDIX B

Rating Scales for Adherence Monitoring and for Evaluating the Quality of the Interpersonal Relationship

Therapist _____   Session Date/# _____

Patient _____   Rater _____

Date of Rating _____

PART ONE: RATING SCALE FOR SUPERVISORS EVALUATING ADHERENCE AND COMPETENCY OF THERAPISTS ADMINISTERING CBASP

Instructions: **Rate the therapist by circling one of the choices.**

I.   Elicitation of the situational description.

    1 = Does not use CBASP procedure.

    2 = Attempts to use CBASP procedure but strays from routine; clearly needs supervisory assistance.

3 = Utilizes CBASP procedure adequately but may need some supervisory assistance.

4 = Utilizes CBASP procedure adequately.

5 = Excellent use of CBASP procedure.

II. Elicitation of the patient's interpretations.

1 = Does not use CBASP procedure.

2 = Attempts to use CBASP procedure but strays from the routine, clearly needs supervisory assistance.

3 = Uutilizes CBASP procedure adequately but may need some supervisory assistance.

4 = Utilizes CBASP procedure adequately.

5 = Excellent use of CBASP procedure.

III. Elicitation of the patient's situational behaviors.

1 = Does not use CBASP procedure.

2 = Attempts to use CBASP procedure but strays from the routine; clearly needs supervisory assistance.

3 = Utilizes CBASP procedure adequately but may need some supervisory assistance.

4 = Utilizes CBASP procedure adequately.

5 = Excellent use of CBASP procedure.

IV. Elicitation of the actual outcome (AO).

1 = Does not use CBASP procedure.

2 = Attempts to use CBASP procedure but strays from the routine; clearly needs supervisory assistance.

3 = Utilizes CBASP procedure adequately but may need some supervisory assistance.

4 = Utilizes CBASP procedure adequately.

5 = Excellent use of CBASP procedure.

V. Elicitation of the desired outcome (DO).

1 = Does not use CBASP procedure.

2 = Attempts to use CBASP procedure but strays from the routine; clearly needs supervisory assistance.

3 = Utilizes CBASP procedure adequately but may need some supervisory assistance.

4 = Utilizes CBASP procedure adequately.

5 = Excellent use of CBASP procedure.

VI. Elicitation of the AO-versus-DO comparison and ascertaining "why" the DO was not/was attained.

1 = Does not use CBASP procedure.
2 = Attempts to use CBASP procedure but strays from the routine; clearly needs supervisory assistance.
3 = Utilizes CBASP procedure adequately but may need some supervisory assistance.
4 = Utilizes CBASP procedure adequately.
5 = Excellent use of CBASP procedure.

Please provide written comments describing the therapist's ability to adhere to the elicitation steps above. Include specific suggestions for improvement and/or reasons why there is a need for further supervision.

VII. Remediation of interpretation errors.

1 = Does not use CBASP procedure.
2 = Attempts to use CBASP procedure but strays from the routine; clearly needs supervisory assistance.
3 = Utilizes CBASP procedure adequately but may need some supervisory assistance.
4 = Utilizes CBASP procedure adequately.
5 = Excellent use of CBASP procedure.

VIII. Remediation of situational behaviors.

    1 = Does not use CBASP procedure.

    2 = Attempts to use CBASP procedure but strays from the routine; clearly needs supervisory assistance.

    3 = Utilizes CBASP procedure adequately but may need some supervisory assistance.

    4 = Utilizes CBASP procedure adequately.

    5 = Excellent use of CBASP procedure.

IX. Wrap-up and summary of SA.

    1 = Does not use CBASP procedure.

    2 = Attempts to use CBASP procedure but strays from the routine; clearly needs supervisory assistance.

    3 = Utilizes CBASP procedure adequately but may need some supervisory assistance.

    4 = Utilizes CBASP procedure adequately.

    5 = Excellent use of CBASP procedure.

X. Generalization and transfer of SA learning.

    1 = Does not use CBASP procedure.

    2 = Attempts to use CBASP procedure but strays from the routine; clearly needs supervisory assistance.

    3 = Utilizes CBASP procedure adequately but may need some supervisory assistance.

    4 = Utilizes CBASP procedure adequately.

    5 = Excellent use of CBASP procedure.

Please provide written comments describing the therapist's ability to adhere to the remediation steps above. Include specific suggestions for improvement and/or reasons why there is a need for further supervision.

PART TWO: RATING SCALE FOR SUPERVISORS ASSESSING THE QUALITY OF THE INTERPERSONAL RELATIONSHIP

Instructions: **Rate the therapist by circling one of the choices.**

I.   Collaborative rapport.

   1 = Inadequate collaborative rapport present.
   2 = Some positive aspects of collaborative rapport present; clearly needs supervisory assistance.
   3 = Adequate collaborative rapport present but may need some supervisory assistance.
   4 = Adequate collaborative rapport present.
   5 = Excellent collaborative rapport present.

II. Therapeutic empathy extended to patient.

   1 = Inadequate empathy extended to patient.
   2 = Some empathy extended; clearly needs supervisory assistance.
   3 = Adequate empathy extended but may need some supervisory assistance.
   4 = Adequate empathy extended.
   5 = Excellent empathy extended.

III. Effective listening.

   1 = Inadequate listening to patient.
   2 = Some positive aspects of listening present; clearly needs supervisory assistance.
   3 = Adequate listening present but may need some supervisory assistance.
   4 = Adequate listening present.
   5 = Excellent listening present.

IV. Therapist is appropriately controlling the session.

   1 = Inadequate control of the session.
   2 = Some control utilized; clearly needs supervisory assistance.
   3 = Adequate control utilized but may need some supervisory assistance.
   4 = Adequate utilization of control.
   5 = Excellent utilization of control.

V.   Tolerance of patient's negative affect.

   1 = Inadequate tolerance of patient's negative affect.
   2 = Some tolerance of patient's negative affect present; clearly needs supervisory assistance.

3 = Adequate tolerance of patient's negative affect but may need supervisory assistance.

4 = Adequate tolerance of patient's negative affect.

5 = Excellent tolerance of patient's negative affect.

VI. Therapist administers Interpersonal Discrimination Exercise (IDE) when the situation warrants it.

a = No opportunity in session to use the IDE.

1 = Therapist does not try to administer the IDE when the situation warrants it.

2 = Some attempt made to administer IDE; clearly needs supervisory assistance.

3 = Adequate administration of IDE but may need supervisory assistance.

4 = Adequate administration of IDE.

5 = Excellent administration of IDE.

VII. Effective use of disciplined personal involvement with patient.

1 = Therapist does not try to use disciplined personal involvement with patient when the situation warrants it.

2 = Some attempt made to use disciplined personal involvement; clearly needs supervisory assistance.

3 = Adequate use of disciplined personal involvement but may need supervisory assistance.

4 = Adequate use of disciplined personal involvement.

5 = Excellent use of disciplined personal involvement.

Please provide written comments describing the quality of the interpersonal relationship. Include specific suggestions for improvement and/or reasons why there is a need for further supervision.

APPENDIX C

Rating the Presence of Optimal CBASP Therapist Qualities and Abilities

Target Therapist _____   Date _____

Instructions: Rate the degree to which each optimal quality is present in the target therapist, based on your impressions and observations of his/her therapy administrations. Rating of 1 = "therapist weak on this quality/ability"; rating of 5 = "therapist satisfactory on this quality/ability"; rating of 10 = "therapist excellent on this quality/ability." Do *not* rate a quality item if you have had no opportunity to observe it.

A.   Possesses a stable self-identity.

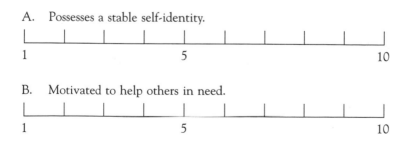

1   5   10

B.   Motivated to help others in need.

1   5   10

C.   Sensitive to the verbal/nonverbal emotional expressions of others.

|___|___|___|___|___|___|___|___|___|
1   5   10

D.   Exhibits a supportive interpersonal demeanor.

|___|___|___|___|___|___|___|___|___|
1   5   10

E.   Willing to adhere to a structured therapy plan over time.

|___|___|___|___|___|___|___|___|___|
1   5   10

F.   Emotionally open to himself/herself and others; that is, the individual
     can interact empathically.

|___|___|___|___|___|___|___|___|___|
1   5   10

G.   Able to "track" the moment-to-moment emotional reactions
     of another person.

|___|___|___|___|___|___|___|___|___|
1   5   10

H.   Able to "track" his/her own moment-to-moment emotional reactions
     and to use his/her emotions in facilitative ways.

|___|___|___|___|___|___|___|___|___|
1   5   10

I.   Able to tolerate periods of moderate-to-severe negative affect in
     himself/herself and others.

|___|___|___|___|___|___|___|___|___|
1   5   10

J.   Able to conceptualize an interpersonal relationship from a historical-
     process perspective.

|___|___|___|___|___|___|___|___|___|
1   5   10

K.   Willing and able to set interpersonal limits on patients.

|___|___|___|___|___|___|___|___|___|
1   5   10

L.   Able to arrange in-session contingencies to modify behavior.

|____|____|____|____|____|____|____|____|____|____|
1   5   10

M.   Willing and able to use empirical measurement to monitor patient
     learning and change.

|____|____|____|____|____|____|____|____|____|____|
1   5   10

References

Akiskal, H. S. (1983). Dysthymic disorder: Psychopathology of proposed chronic depressive subtypes. *American Journal of Psychiatry, 140*, 11–20.

Akiskal, H. S. (1995). Toward a temperament-based approach to depression: Implications for neurobiological research. *Advances in Biochemical Psychopharmacology, 49*, 99–112.

Akiskal, H. S., & McKinney, W. T. (1973). Depressive disorders: Toward a unified hypothesis. *Science, 182*, 20–28.

Akiskal, H. S., & McKinney, W. T. (1975). Overview of recent research in depression: Integration of ten conceptual models into a comprehensive clinical picture. *Archives of General Psychiatry, 32*, 285–305.

Akiskal, H. S., Rosenthal, T. L., Haykal, R. F., Lemmi, H., Rosenthal, R. H., & Scott-Strauss, A. (1980). Characterological depressions: Clinical and sleep EEG findings separating "subaffective dysthymias" from "character spectrum disorders." *Archives of General Psychiatry, 37*, 777–783.

Alexander, F. (1950). *Psychosomatic Medicine: Its Principles and Applications*. New York: Norton.

Alnaes, R., & Torgensen, S. (1991). Personality and personality disorders among patients with various affective disorders. *Journal of Personality Disorders, 5*, 107–121.

American Psychiatric Association (APA). (1952). *Diagnostic and Statistical Manual of Mental Disorders* (1st ed.). Washington, DC: Author.

American Psychiatric Association (APA). (1968). *Diagnostic and Statistical Manual of Mental Disorders* (2nd ed.). Washington, DC: Author.

American Psychiatric Association (APA). (1980). *Diagnostic and Statistical Manual of Mental Disorders* (3rd ed.). Washington, DC: Author.

American Psychiatric Association (APA). (1987). *Diagnostic and Statistical Manual of Mental Disorders* (3rd ed. rev). Washington, DC: Author.

American Psychiatric Association (APA). (1993). Practice guideline for major depressive disorder in adults. *American Journal of Psychiatry, 150*(suppl), 1–26.

295

American Psychiatric Association (APA). (1994). *Diagnostic and Statistical Manual of Mental Disorders* (4th ed.). Washington, DC: Author.

Anchin, J. C., & Kiesler, D. J. (1982). *Handbook of Interpersonal Psychotherapy.* Elmsford, NY: Pergamon Press.

Andrews, J. D. W. (1991). *The Active Self in Psychotherapy: An Integration of Therapeutic Styles.* New York: Gardner Press.

Bandura, A. (1961). Psychotherapy as a learning process. *Psychological Bulletin, 58,* 143–159.

Bandura, A. (1977a). Self-efficacy: Toward a unifying theory of behavior change. *Psychological Review, 84,* 191–215.

Bandura, A. (1977b). *Social Learning Theory.* Englewood Cliffs, NJ. Prentice-Hall.

Bandura, A. (1982). Self-efficacy mechanisms in human agency. *American Psychologist, 37,* 122–147.

Bandura, A. (1986). *Social Foundations of Thought and Action: A Social Cognitive Theory.* Englewood Cliffs, NJ: Prentice-Hall.

Barchas, J., & Freedman, D. (1963). Brain amines: Response to physiological stress. *Biochemical Pharmacology, 12,* 1232–1235.

Baron, A., Kaufman, A., & Stauber, K. A. (1969). Effects of instructions and reinforcement-feedback on human operant behavior maintained by fixed-interval reinforcement. *Jounal of the Experimental Analysis of Behavior, 12,* 701–712.

Baron, R. M., & Kenny, D. A. (1986). The moderator-mediator variable distinction in social psychological research: Conceptual, strategic, and statistical considerations. *Journal of Personality and Social Psychology, 51,* 1173–1182.

Beck, A. T. (1963). Thinking and depression: I. Idiosyncratic content and cognitive distortions. *Archives of General Psychiatry, 9,* 324–333.

Beck, A. T. (1964). Thinking and depression: II. Theory and therapy. *Archives of General Psychiatry, 10,* 561–571.

Beck, A. T. (1967). *Depression: Clinical, Experimental and Theoretical Aspects.* New York: Hoeber.

Beck, A. T. (1976). *Cognitive Therapy and the Emotional Disorders.* New York: International Universities Press.

Beck, A. T., Rush, A. J., Shaw, B. F., & Emery, G. (1979). *Cognitive Therapy of Depression.* New York: Guilford Press.

Beeghly, M., & Cicchetti, D. (1994). Child maltreatment, attachment, and the self system: Emergence of an internal state lexicon in toddlers at high social risk. *Development and Psychopathology, 6,* 5–30.

Bibring, E. (1953). The mechanism of depression. In P. Greenacre (Ed.), *Affective Disorders* (pp.13–48). New York: International Universities Press.

Blackburn, I. M., Bishop, S., Glen, A. I. M., Whalley, L. J., & Christie, J. E. (1981). The efficacy of cognitive therapy in depression: A treatment trial using cognitive therapy and pharmacotherapy, each alone and in combination. *British Journal of Psychiatry, 139,* 181–189.

Blanchard, E. B. (1977). Behavioral medicine: A perspective. In R. B. Williams & W. D. Gentry (Eds.), *Behavioral Approaches to Medical Treatment* (pp. 1–13). Cambridge, MA: Ballinger.

Bland, R. C. (1997). Epidemiology of affective disorders: A review. *Canadian Journal of Psychiatry, 42,* 367–377.

Blatt, S. J. (1991). A cognitive morphology of psychopathology. *Journal of Nervous and Mental Disease, 179,* 449–458.

Bliss, E., & Zwanziger, J. (1966). Brain amines and emotional stress. *Journal of Psychiatric Research, 4,* 189–198.

Bremner, J. D., & Narayan, M. (1998). The effects of stress on memory and hippocampus throughout the life cycle: Implications for childhood development and aging. *Development and Psychopathology, 10,* 871–885.

Bremner, J. D., Randall, P. R., Capelli, S., Scott, T., McCarthy, G., & Charney, D. S. (1995). Deficits in short-term memory in adult survivors of childhood abuse. *Psychiatry Research, 59,* 97–107.

Breslow, L., & Cowan, P. A. (1984). Structural and functional perspectives on classification and seriation in psychotic and normal children. *Child Development, 55,* 226–235.

Bristol-Myers Squibb Company, (1996, May 13). *Protocol: A Prospective Multi-Center Study Comparing the Safety and Efficacy of Nefazodone HCl to Cognitive Behavioral Analysis System of Psychotherapy (CBASP) and Combined Nefazodone and CBASP for the Acute, Continuation and Maintenance Treatment of Chronic Forms of Depression.* Plainsboro, NJ: Author.

Cannon, W. B. (1929). *Bodily Changes in Pain, Hunger, Fear and Rage.* New York: Appleton-Century-Crofts.

Cannon, W. B. (1932) *The Wisdom of the Body.* New York: Norton.

Cashdan, S. (1973). *Interactional Psychotherapy: Stages and Strategies in Behavioral Change.* New York: Grune & Stratton.

Caspi, A., Moffitt, T. E., Newman, D. L., & Silva, P. A. (1966). Behavioral observations at age 3 years predict adult psychiatric disorders. *Archives of General Psychiatry, 23,* 1033–1039.

Chambless, D. L., Baker, M. J., Baucom, D. H., Beutler, L. E., Calhoun, K. S., Crits-Christoph, P., Daiuto, A., DeRubeis, R., Detweiler, J., Haaga, D. A. F., Johnson, S. B., McCurry, S., Mueser, K. T., Pope, K. S., Sanderson, W. C., Shoham, V., Stickle, T., Williams, D. A. & Woody, S. R. (1998). An update on empirically validated therapies, II. *The Clinical Psychologist, 51,* 3–16.

Cicchetti, D. (1991). Fractures in the crystal: Developmental psychopathology and the emergence of the self. *Developmental Review, 11,* 271–287.

Cicchetti, D. (1993). Developmental psychopathology: Reactions, reflections, projections. *Developmental Review, 13,* 471–502.

Cicchetti, D., Ackerman, B. P., & Izard, C. E. (1995). Emotions and emotion regulation in developmental psychopathology. *Development and Psychopathology, 7,* 1–10.

Cicchetti, D., & Barnett, D. (1991). Attachment organization in maltreated preschoolers. *Development and Psychopathology, 3,* 397–411.

Clark, D. C., & Fawcett, J. (1992). Review of empirical risk factors for evaluation of the suicidal patient. In B. Bongar (Ed.), *Suicide: Guidelines for Assessment, Management, and Treatment* (pp. 16–48). New York: Oxford University Press.

Cohen, R. L. (1960). A coefficient of agreement for nominal scales. *Education and Psychological Measurement, 20,* 37–46.

Conte, H. R., Plutchik, R., Wild, K. V., & Karasu, T. B. (1986). Combined psychotherapy and pharmacotherapy for depression: A systematic analysis for the evidence. *Archives of General Psychiatry, 43,* 471–479.

Conway, J. B. (1987). A clinical interpersonal perspective for personality and psychotherapy: Some research examples. Paper presented to the Department of Psychology, University of British Columbia, Vancouver, British Columbia, Canada.

Costa, P. T. & McCrae, R. R. (1992). Normal personality assessment in clinical practice: The NEO Inventory. Psychological Assessment, 4, 5–13.

Cowan, P. A. (1978). Piaget with Feeling: Cognitive, Social, and Emotional Dimensions. New York: Holt, Rinehart & Winston.

Coyne, J. C. (1976). Toward an interactional description of depression. Psychiatry, 39, 3–13.

Coyne, J. C., & Gotlib, I. (1986). Studying the role of cognition in depression: Well-trodden paths and cul-de-sacs. Cognitive Therapy and Research, 10, 695–705.

Cramer, B., Manzano, J., Palacio, F., & Torrado, M. (1984). Problems in diagnostic assessment of young children. Acta Paedopsychiatrica, 50, 283–290.

de Jong, R., Treiber, R., & Henrich, G. (1986). Effectiveness of two psychological treatments for inpatients with severe and chronic depressions. Cognitive Therapy and Research, 10, 645–663.

Derogatis, L. R. (1983). SCL-90-R: Administration, Scoring and Procedures Manual. Towson, MD: Clinical Psychometric Research.

Dodge, K. A. (1990). Developmental psychopathology in children of depressed mothers. Developmental Psychology, 26, 3–6.

Dodge, K. A. (1993). Social-cognitive mechanisms in the development of conduct disorder and depression. Annual Review of Psychology, 44, 559–584.

Drotar, D., & Sturm, L. (1991). Psychosocial influences in the etiology, diagnosis, and prognosis of nonorganic failure to thrive. In H. E. Fitzgerald, B. M. Lester, & M. W. Yogman (Eds.), Theory and Research in Behavioral Pediatrics (pp. 19–59). New York: Plenum Press.

D'Zurilla, T. J., & Goldfried, M. R. (1971). Problem-solving and behavior modification. Journal of Abnormal Psychology, 78, 107–126.

D'Zurilla, T. J., & Maydeu-Olivares, A. (1995). Conceptual and methodological issues in social problem-solving assessment. Behavior Therapy. 26, 409–432.

Elkin, I., Shea, M. T., Watkins, J. T., Imber, S. D., Sotsky, S. M., Collins, J. F., Glass, D. R., Pilkonis, P. A., Leber, W. R., Docherty, J. P., Fiester, S. J., & Parloff, M. B. (1989). National Institute of Mental Health Treatment of Depression Collaborative Research Program: General effectiveness of treatments. Archives of General Psychiatry, 46, 971–982.

Engel, G. L. (1977). The need for a new medical model: A challenge to biomedicine. Science, 196, 129–136.

Ericsson, K. A., & Simon, H. A. (1980). Verbal reports as data. Psychological Review, 87, 215–251.

Eysenck, H. J., & Eysenck, S. B. G. (1968). Eysenck Personality Inventory: Manual. San Diego, CA: Educational and Industrial Testing Service.

Farmer, R., & Nelson-Gray, R. O. (1990). Personality disorders and depression: Hypothetical relations, empirical findings, and methodological considerations. Clinical Psychology Review, 10, 453–476.

Fawcett, J., Scheftner, W. A., Fogg, L., Clark, D. C., Young, M. A., Hedeker, D., & Gibbons, R. (1990). Time-related predictors of suicide in major affective disorder. American Journal of Psychiatry, 147, 1189–1194.

Fennell, M. J. V., & Teasdale, J. D. (1982). Cognitive therapy with chronic, drug refractory depressed outpatients: A note of caution. *Cognitive Therapy and Research, 6,* 455–460.

Ferster, C. H. (1973). A functional analysis of depression. *American Psychologist, 28,* 857–870.

Festinger, L. (1957). *A Theory of Cognitive Dissonance.* Evanston, Il: Row, Peterson.

Folkman, S., & Lazarus, R. S. (1980). An analysis of coping in a middle-aged community sample. *Journal of Health and Social Behavior, 21,* 219–239.

Folkman, S., & Lazarus, R. S. (1988). *Ways of Coping Questionnaire: Manual, Test Booklet, Scoring Key.* Palo Alto, CA: Mind Garden.

Fox, S. J., Barrnett, R. J., Davies, M., & Bird, H. R. (1990). Psychopathology and developmental delay in homeless children: A pilot study. *Journal of the American Academy of Child and Adolescent Psychiatry, 29,* 732–735.

Frank, E., Kupfer, D. J., Perel, J. M., Cornes, C. L., Jarrett, D. J., Mallinger, A., Thase, M. E., McEachran, A. B., & Grochocinski, V. J. (1990). Three-year outcomes for maintenance therapies in recurrent depression. *Archives of General Psychiatry, 47,* 1093–1099.

Frank, J. (1973). *Persuasion and Healing: A Comparative Study of Psychotherapy.* Baltimore: Johns Hopkins University Press.

Frankl, V. (1959). *Man's Search for Meaning.* Boston: Beacon Press.

Freud, S. (1933). *New Introductory Lectures on Psycho-analysis.* New York: Norton.

Freud, S. (1950). Mourning and Melancholia. In S. Freud, *Collected Papers* (Vol 4, pp. 152–172). London: Hogarth Press. (Original work published 1917)

Freud, S. (1960). *A General Introduction to Psychoanalysis.* New York: Washington Square Press. (Original work published 1916–1917)

Freud, S. (1963). *Character and Culture.* New York: Collier Books.

Garamoni, G. L., Reynolds, C. F., Thase, M. E., Frank, E., & Fasiczka, A. L. (1992). Shifts in affective balance during cognitive therapy of major depression. *Journal of Consulting and Clinical Psychiatry, 60,* 260–266.

Gardner, H. (1983). *Frames of Mind: The Theory of Multiple Intelligences.* New York: Basic Books.

Gentry, W. D. (1984). Behavioral medicine: A new research paradigm. In W. D. Gentry (Ed.), *Handbook of Behavioral Medicine,* (pp. 1–12). New York: Guilford Press.

Gerson, M. J. (1996). *The Embedded Self: A Psychoanalytic Guide to Family Therapy.* Hillsdale, NJ: The Analytic Press.

Goldfried, M. R. (1980). Toward the delineation of therapeutic change principles. *American Psychologist, 35,* 991–999.

Goldfried, M. R., Castonguay, L. G., Hayes, A. M., Drozd, J. F., & Shapiro, D. A. (1997). A comparative analysis of the therapeutic focus in cognitive-behavioral and psychodynamic-interpersonal sessions. *Journal of Consulting and Clinical Psychology, 65,* 740–748.

Goldfried, M. R. & Davison, G. C. (1976). *Clinical Behavior Therapy.* New York: Holt, Rinehart & Winston.

Goldfried, M. R., Raue, P. J., & Castonguay, L. G. (1998). The therapeutic focus in significant sessions of master therapists: A comparison of cognitive-behavioral and psychodynamic-interpersonal interventions. *Journal of Consulting and Clinical Psychology, 66,* 803–810.

Gordon, D. E. (1988). Formal operations and interpersonal and affective disturbances in adolescents. In E. D. Nannis & P. A. Cowan (Eds.), *Developmental Psychopathology and Its Treatment*, (pp. 51–73). San Francisco: Jossey-Bass.

Guidano, V. F. (1987). *Complexity of the Self: A Developmental Approach to Psychopathology and Therapy*. New York: Guilford Press.

Guidano, V. F., & Liotti, G. (1983). *Cognitive Processes and Emotional Disorders*. New York: Guilford Press.

Gurtman, M. B. (1994). The circumplex as a tool for studying normal and abnormal personality: A methodological primer. In S. Strack & M. Lorr (Eds.), *Differentiating Normal and Abnormal Personality* (pp. 243–263). New York: Springer.

Guze, S. B., & Robins, E. (1970). Suicide and primary affective disorders. *British Journal of Psychiatry, 117*, 437–438.

Haaga, D. A., Dyck, M. J., & Ernst, D. (1991). Empirical status of cognitive theory of depression. *Psychological Bulletin, 110*, 215–236.

Hamilton, M. (1967). Development of a rating scale of primary depressive illness. *British Journal of Social and Clinical Psychology, 6*, 278–296.

Hammen, C. (1992). Cognitive, life stress, and interpersonal approaches to a developmental model of depression. *Development and Psychopathology, 4*, 189–206.

Hammen, C., Burge, D., & Adrian, C. (1991). The timing of mother and child depression in a longitudinal study of children at risk. *Journal of Consulting and Clinical Psychology, 59*, 341–345.

Hammen, C. L., Burge, D., Daley, S. E., Davila, J., Paley, B., & Rudolph, K. D. (1995). Interpersonal attachment cognitions and prediction of symptomatic responses to interpersonal stress. *Journal of Abnormal Psychology, 104*, 436–443.

Harpin, R. E., Liberman, R. P., Marks, I., Stern, R., & Bohannon, W. E. (1982). Cognitive-behavior therapy for chronically depressed patients: A controlled pilot study. *Journal of Nervous and Mental Disease, 170*, 295–301.

Harrison, W. M., & Stewart, J. W. (1993). Pharmacotherapy of dysthymia. *Psychiatric Annals, 23*, 638–648.

Hoberman, H. M., Lewinsohn, P. M., & Tilson, M. (1988). Group treatment of depression: Individual predictors of outcome. *Journal of Consulting and Clinical Psychology, 56*, 393–398.

Hollon, S. D. (1990). Cognitive therapy and pharmacotherapy for depression. *Psychiatric Annals, 20*, 249–258.

Holmbeck, G. N. (1997). Toward terminological, conceptual, and statistical clarity in the study of mediators and moderators: Examples from the child-clinical and pediatric psychology literatures. *Journal of Consulting and Clinical Psychology, 65*, 599–610.

Howland, R. H. (1993a). Chronic depression. *Hospital and Community Psychiatry, 44*, 633–639.

Howland, R. H. (1993b). General health, health care utilization, and medical comorbidity. *International Journal of Psychiatry Medicine, 23*, 211–238.

Howland, R. H. (1996). Psychosocial therapies for dysthymia. In J. Lonsdale (Ed.), *The Hatherleigh Guide to Managing Depression* (pp. 225–241). New York: Hatherleigh Press.

Inhelder, B., & Piaget, J. (1958). *The Growth of Logical Thinking from Childhood to Adolescence*. New York: Basic Books. (Original work published 1955)

Izard, C. E. (1993). Four systems for emotional activation: Cognitive and non-cognitive processes. *Psychological Review, 100*, 68–90.

James, W. (1890). *The Principles of Psychology*. New York: Holt.

Kasnetz, M. D., McCullough, J. P., & Kaye, A. L. (1995). *Patient Manual for Cognitive Behavioral Analysis System of Psychotherapy (CBASP)*. Richmond: Virginia Commonwealth University.

Kaufman, A., Baron, A., & Kopp, R. E. (1966). Some effects of instructions on human operant behavior. *Psychonomic Monograph Supplements, 1*, 243–250.

Kaye, A. L., McCullough, J. P., Roberts, W. C., McCune, K. J., Hampton, C., & Kornstein, S. G. (1994). Differentiating affective and characterologic DSM-III-R psychopathology in non-treatment, community unipolar depressives. *Depression, 2*, 80–88.

Keitner, G. I., Ryan, C. E., Miller, I. W., Kohn, R., & Epstein, N. B. (1991). Twelve-month outcome of patients with major depression and comorbid psychiatric or medical illness (compound depression). *American Journal of Psychiatry, 148*, 345–350.

Keller, M. B. (1988). Diagnostic issues and clinical course of unipolar illness. In A. J. Frances & R. E. Hales (Eds.), *Review of Psychiatry* (Vol. 7, pp. 188–212). Washington, DC: American Psychiatric Press.

Keller, M. B. (1990). Diagnostic and course-of-illness variables pertinent to refractory depression. In A. Tasman, S. M. Goldfinger, & C. A. Kaufman, (Eds.), *Review of Psychiatry* (Vol. 9, pp. 10–32). Washington, DC: American Psychiatric Press.

Keller, M. B., Gelenberg, A. J., Hirschfeld, R. M. A., Rush, A. J., Thase, M. E., Kocsis, J. H., Markowitz, J. C., Fawcett, J. A., Koran, L. M., Klein, D. N., Russell, J. M., Kornstein, S. G., McCullough, J. P., Davis, S. M., & Harrison, W. M. (1998). The treatment of chronic depression: Part 2. A double-blind, randomized trial of sertraline and imipramine. *Journal of Clinical Psychiatry, 59*, 598–607.

Keller, M. B., & Hanks, D. L. (1994). The natural history and heterogeneity of depressive disorders. *Journal of Clinical Psychiatry, 56*, 22–29.

Keller, M. B., Harrison, W., Fawcett, J. A., Gelenberg, A., Hirschfeld, R. M. A., Klein, D. N., Kocsis, J. H., McCullough, J. P., Rush, A. J., Schatzberg, A., & Thase, M. E. (1995). Treatment of chronic depression with sertraline or imipramine: Preliminary blinded response rates and high rates of undertreatment in the community. *Psychopharmacology Bulletin, 31*, 205–212.

Keller, M. B., Klein, D. N., Hirschfeld, R. M. A., Kocsis, J. H., McCullough, J. P., Miller, I., First, M. B., Holzer, C. P., III, Keitner, G. I., Marin, D. B. & Shea, T. (1995). Results of the DSM-IV Mood Disorders Field Trial. *American Journal of Psychiatry, 152*, 843–849.

Keller, M. B., Lavori, P. W., Klerman, G. L., Andreasen, N. C., Endicott, J., Coryell, W., Fawcett, J., Rice, J. P., & Hirschfeld, R. M. A. (1986). Low levels and lack of predictors of somatotherapy and psychotherapy received by depressed patients. *Archives of General Psychiatry, 43*, 458–466.

Keller, M. B., Lavori, P. W., Endicott, J., Coryell, W., & Klerman, G. (1983). Double depression: A two year follow-up. *American Journal of Psychiatry, 140*, 680–694.

Keller, M. B., Lavori, P. W., Lewis, C. E., & Klerman, G. (1983). Predictors of relapse in major depressive disorder. *Journal of the American Medical Association, 250*, 3299–3304.

Keller, M. B., Lavori, P. W., Mueller, T. I., Endicott, J., Coryell, W., Hirschfeld, R. M. A., & Shea, M. (1992). Time to recovery, chronicity, and levels of psychopathology in major depression. *Archives of General Psychiatry, 49,* 809–816.

Keller, M. B., Lavori, P. W., Rice, J., Coryell, W., & Hirschfeld, R. M. A. (1986). The persistent risk of chronicity in recurrent episodes of nonbipolar major depressive disorder: A prospective follow-up. *American Journal of Psychiatry, 143,* 24–28.

Keller, M. B., McCullough, J. P., Rush, A. J., Klein, D. N., Schatzberg, A. F., Gelenberg, A. J., & Thase, M. E. (1999, May 19). *Nefazodone HCl, Cognitive Behavioral Analysis System of Psychotherapy and combination therapy for the acute treatment of chronic depression.* Paper presented at the 152nd Annual Convention of the American Psychiatric Association, Washington, DC.

Keller, M. B., McCullough, J. P., Klein, D. N., Arnow, B. A., Dunner, D. L., Gelenberg, A. J., Markowitz, J. C., Nemeroff, C. B., Russell, J. M., Thase, M. E., Trivedi, M. H., Zajecka, J. (2000). The acute treatment of chronic forms of major depression: A comparison of nefazodone, Cognitive Behavioral Analysis System of Psychotherapy, and their combination. *New England Journal of Medicine, 342,* 1462–1470.

Keller, M. B., & Shapiro, R. W. (1984). Double depression, major depression, and dysthymia: Distinct entities or different phases of a single disorder? *Psychopharmacology Bulletin, 20,* 399–402.

Keller, M. B., & Shapiro, R. W. (1982). "Double depression": Superimposition of acute depressive episodes on chronic depressive disorders. *American Journal of Psychiatry, 139,* 438–442.

Keller, M. B., Shapiro, R. W., Lavori, P. W., & Wolfe, N. (1982a). Recovery in major depressive disorder. *Archives of General Psychiatry, 38,* 905–910.

Keller, M. B., Shapiro, R. W., Lavori, P. W., & Wolfe, N. (1982b). Relapse in major depressive disorder. *Archives of General Psychiatry, 39,* 911–915.

Kendall, R. E. (1986). What are mental disorders? In A. M. Freedman, R. Brotman, I. Silverman, & D. Hutson (Eds.), *Issues in Psychiatric Classification: Science, Practice and Social Policy* (pp. 23–45). New York: Human Sciences Press.

Kessler, R. C., McGonagle, K. A., Zhao, S., Nelson, C. B., Hughes, M., Eshleman, S., Hans-Ulrich, W., & Kendler, K. S. (1994). Lifetime and 12-month prevalence of DSM-III-R psychiatric disorders in the United States. *Archives of General Psychiatry, 51,* 8–19.

Kiesler, D. J. (1982). Confronting the client-therapist relationship in psychotherapy. In J. C. Anchin & D. J. Kiesler (Eds.), *Handbook of Interpersonal Psychotherapy* (pp. 274–295). Elmsford, NY: Pergamon Press.

Kiesler, D. J. (1983). The 1982 Interpersonal Circle: A taxonomy for complementarity in human transactions. *Psychological Review, 90,* 185–214.

Kiesler, D. J. (1986a). Interpersonal methods of diagnosis and treatment. In R. Michels, & J. O. Cavenar (Eds.), *Psychiatry* (Vol. 1, pp. 1–23). Philadelphia: Lippincott.

Kiesler, D. J. (1986b). The 1982 Interpersonal Circle: An analysis of DSM-III personality disorders. In T. Millon & G. L. Klerman (Eds.), *Contemporary Directions in Pscyhopathology: Toward the DSM-IV* (pp. 571–597). New York: Guilford Press.

Kiesler, D. J. (1987). *Research Manual for The Impact Message Inventory.* Palo Alto, CA: Consulting Psychologists Press.

Kiesler, D. J. (1988). *Therapeutic Metacommunication: Therapist Impact Disclosure as Feedback in Psychotherapy*. Palo Alto, CA: Consulting Psychologists Press.

Kiesler, D. J. (1991). Interpersonal methods of asessment and diagnosis. In C. R. Snyder & D. R. Forsyth (Eds.), *Handbook of Social and Clinical Psychology: The Health Perspective* (pp. 438–468). Elmsford, NY: Pergamon Press.

Kiesler, D. J. (1996). *Contemporary Interpersonal Theory and Research: Personality, Psychopathology, and Psychotherapy*. New York: Wiley.

Kiesler, D. J. (1999). *Beyond the Disease Model of Mental Disorders*. Westport, CT: Praeger.

Kiesler, D. J., & Schmidt, J. A. (1993). *The Impact Message Inventory: Form IIA Octant Scale Version*. Redwood City, CA: Mind Garden.

Kiresuk, T. J., & Sherman, R. (1968). Goal Attainment Scaling: A general method for evaluating comprehensive community mental health programs. *Community Mental Health Journal, 4*, 443–453.

Klein, D. N., Clark, D. C., Dansky, L., & Margolis, E. T. (1988). Dysthymia in the offspring of parents with primary unipolar affective disorder. *Journal of Abnormal Psychology, 97*, 265–274.

Klein, D. N., Norden, K. A., Ferro, T., Leader, J. B., Kasch, K. L., Klein, L. M., Schwartz, J. E., & Aronson, T. A. (1998). Thirty-month naturalistic follow-up study of early-onset dysthymic disorder: Course, diagnostic stability, and prediction of outcome. *Journal of Abnormal Psychology, 107*, 338–348.

Klein, D. N., Schatzberg, A. F., McCullough, J. P., Keller, M. B., Dowling, F., Goodman, D., Howland, R. H., Markowitz, J. C., Smith, C., Miceli, R., & Harrison, W. M. (1999). Early- versus late-onset dysthymic disorder: Comparison in outpatients with superimposed major depressive episodes. *Journal of Affective Disorders, 52*, 187–196.

Klein, D. N., Taylor, E. B., Dickstein, S., & Harding, K. (1988a). The early-late onset distinction in DSM-III-R dysthymia. *Journal of Affective Disorders, 14*, 25–33.

Klein, D. N., Taylor, E. B., Dickstein, S., & Harding, K. (1988b). Primary early-onset dysthymia: Comparison with primary nonbipolar nonchronic major depression on demographic, clinical, familial, personality, and socioenvironmental characteristics and short-term outcome. *Journal of Abnormal Psychology, 97*, 387–398.

Klein, D. N., Taylor, E. B., Harding, K., & Dickstein, S. (1988). Double depression and episodic major depression: Demographic, clinical familial, personality, and socioenvironmental characteristics and short-term outcome. *American Journal of Psychiatry, 145*, 1226–1231.

Klerman, G. L., & Weissman, M. M. (Eds.). (1993). *New Applications of Interpersonal Psychotherapy*. Washington, DC: American Psychiatric Press.

Klerman, G. L., Weissman, M. M., Rounsaville, B. J., & Chevron, E. S. (1984). *Interpersonal Psychotherapy of Depression*. New York: Basic Books.

Kocsis, J. H. (1993). DSM-IV "major depression": Are more stringent criteria needed? *Depression, 1*, 24–28.

Kocsis, J. H. & Frances, A. J. (1987). A critical discussion of DSM-III dysthymic disorder. *American Journal of Psychiatry, 144*, 1534–1542.

Kolenberg, R. J. & Tsai, M. (1991). *Functional Analytic Psychotherapy: Creating Intense and Curative Therapeutic Relationships*. New York: Plenum Press.

Lambert, M. (Ed.). (1983). *Psychotherapy and Patient Relationships*. Homewood, IL: Dorsey.

Landis, J. R., & Koch, G. G. (1977). The measurement of observer agreement for categorical data. *Biometrics, 33,* 159–174.

Lane, R. D., & Schwartz, G. E. (1987). Levels of emotional awareness: A cognitive-developmental theory and its application to psychopathology. *American Journal of Psychiatry, 144,* 133–143.

Lazarus, R. S. (1966). *Psychological Stress And The Coping Process.* New York: McGraw-Hill.

Lazarus, R. S. (1984). On the primacy of cognition. *American Psychologist, 39,* 124–129.

Lazarus, R. S. (1990). Theory-based stress management. *Psychological Inquiry, 1,* 3–13.

Lazarus, R. S., & Alfert, E (1964). Short-circuiting of threat by experimentally altering cognitive appraisal. *Journal of Abnormal and Social Psychology, 69,* 195 205.

Lazarus, R. S., Opton, E. M., Markellos, S., Nomikos, M. S., & Rankin, N. O. (1965). The principle of short-circuiting of threat: Further evidence. *Journal of Personality, 33,* 622–635.

Lefcourt, H. M. (1976). *Locus of Control: Current Trends in Theory and Research.* Hillsdale, NJ: Lawrence Erlbaum.

Linehan, M. M. (1993). *Cognitive-Behavioral Treatment of Borderline Personality Disorder.* New York: Guilford Press.

Lipsett, D. R. (1970). Medical and psychological characteristics of "crocks." *Psychiatric Medicine, 1,* 15–25.

Lizardi, H., Klein, D. N., Quimette, P. C., Riso, L. P., Anderson, R. L., & Donaldson, S. K. (1995). Reports of the childhood home environment in early-onset dysthymia and episodic major depression. *Journal of Abnormal Psychology, 104,* 132–139.

Logan, G. D. (1988). Toward an instance theory of automatization. *Psychological Review, 95,* 492–527.

Mahoney, M. J. (1991). *Human Change Processes: The Scientific Foundations of Psychotherapy.* New York: Basic Books.

Manning, D. W., Markowitz, J. C., & Frances, A. J. (1992). A review of combined psychotherapy and pharmacotherapy in the treatment of depression. *Journal of Psychotherapy: Practice and Research, 1,* 103–116.

Markowitz, J. C. (1993a, May). *Dysthymia: Psychosocial treatment strategies.* Paper presented at the 146th Annual Convention of the American Psychiatric Association, San Francisco.

Markowitz, J. C. (1993b). Psychotherapy of the post-dysthymic patient. *Journal of Psychotherapy: Practice and Research, 2,* 157–163.

Markowitz, J. C. (1994). Psychotherapy of dysthymia. *American Journal of Psychiatry, 151,* 1114–1121.

Markowitz, J. C. (1995). Comorbidity of dysthymic disorder. In J. H. Kocsis & D. N. Klein (Eds.), *Diagnosis and Treatment of Chronic Depression* (pp. 41–57). New York: Guilford Press.

Markowitz, J. C., Moran, M. E., Kocsis, J. H., & Frances, A. J. (1992). Prevalence and comorbidity of dysthymic disorder among psychiatric outpatients. *Journal of Affective Disorders, 24,* 63–71.

Mason, B. J., Markowitz, J. C., & Klerman, G. L. (1993). Interpersonal psychotherapy for dysthymic disorders. In G. L. Klerman & M. M. Weissman (Eds.), *New Applications of Interpersonal Psychotherapy* (pp. 225–264). Washington, DC: American Psychiatric Press.

May, R. (1960). Contributions of existential psychotherapy. In R. May (Ed.), *Existence: A New Dimension in Psychiatry and Psychology* (pp. 37–91). New York: Basic Books.

Mayer, J. D., & Salovey, P. (1993). The intelligence of emotional intelligence. *Intelligence, 17*, 433–442.

McCullough, J. P. (1980a). *Cognitive Behavioral Analysis System of Psychotherapy: Methodological perspective (II)*. Unpublished manuscript. Richmond, VA: Virginia Commonwealth University.

McCullough, J. P. (1980b). How to help depressed patients gain control over their lives using a situational analysis procedure. *Behavioral Medicine, 7*, 33–34.

McCullough, J. P. (1984a). Cognitive-behavioral analysis system of psychotherapy: An interactional treatment approach for dysthymic disorder. *Psychiatry, 47*, 234–250.

McCullough, J. P. (1984b). Single-case investigative research and its relevance for the nonoperant clinician. *Psychotherapy: Theory, Research, and Practice, 21*, 382–388.

McCullough, J. P. (1984c). The need for new single-case design structure in applied cognitive psychology. *Psychotherapy: Theory, Research, and Practice, 21*, 389–400.

McCullough, J. P. (1991). Psychotherapy for dysthymia: Naturalistic study of ten cases. *Journal of Nervous and Mental Disease, 179*, 734–740.

McCullough, J. P. (1995a). *Rating Scales for Evaluating Competency of the Therapist Administering CBASP Procedures and for Evaluation of the Management of the Interpersonal Relationship*. Unpublished rating scales. Richmond, VA: Virginia Commonwealth University.

McCullough, J. P. (1995b). *Therapist Manual for Cognitive Behavioral Analysis System of Psychotherapy (CBASP)*. Richmond: Virginia Commonwealth University.

McCullough, J. P. (1996a). The importance of diagnosing comorbid personality disorder with patients who are chronically depressed. *Depressive Disorders: Index and Reviews, 1*(1), 16–17.

McCullough, J. P. (1996b, October 3). *Treating the patient who is chronically depressed with Cognitive-Behavior Therapy for the Chronic Depressions (CBT-CD)*. Paper presented at the Twenty-Sixth Congress of the European Association for Behavior and Cognitive Therapy, Budapest, Hungary.

McCullough, J. P., Braith, J. A., Chapman, R. C., Kasnetz, M. D., Carr, K. F., Cones, J. H., Fielo, J., Shoemaker, O. S., & Roberts, W. C. (1990). Comparison of early and late onset dysthymia. *Journal of Nervous and Mental Disease, 78*, 577–581.

McCullough, J. P., & Carr, K. F. (1987). Stage process design: A predictive confirmation structure for the single case. *Psychotherapy: Theory, Research, and Practice, 24*, 759–768.

McCullough, J. P., Kasnetz, M. D., Braith, J. A., Carr, K. F., Cones, J. H., Fielo, J., & Martelli, M. F. (1988). A longitudinal study of an untreated sample of predominantly late onset characterological dysthymia. *Journal of Nervous and Mental Disease, 176*, 658–667.

McCullough, J. P., & Kaye, A. L. (1993, May 26). Differential diagnosis of chronic depressive disorders. Paper presented at the 146th Annual Convention of the American Psychiatric Association, San Francisco.

McCullough, J. P., Keller, M. B., Hirschfeld, R. M. A., Russell, J. M., Dunner, D. L., Thase, M. E., & Kocsis, J. H. (1997, June 26). *Collaborative study of nefazodone and CBT-CD in chronically depressed patients*. Poster presented at the Sixth World Congress of Biological Psychiatry, Nice, France.

McCullough, J. P., Klein, D. N., Keller, M. B., Holzer, C. E., Davis, S. M., Kornstein, S. G., Howland, R. H., Thase, M. E., & Harrison, W. M. (in press). Comparison of DSM-III-R chronic major depression and major depression superimposed on dysthymia (double depression): Validity of the distinction. *Journal of Abnormal Psychology*.

McCullough, J. P., Klein, D. N., Shea, T., Miller, I., & Kaye, A. L. (1992, August 17). *DSM-IV field trials for major depression, dysthymia and minor depressions*. Paper presented at the 100th Annual Convention of the American Psychological Association, Washington, DC.

McCullough, J. P., Kornstein, S. G., Klein, D. N., Kocsis, J. H., Dunner, D. L., & Koran, L. M. (1997, May 15). *Cognitive Behavior Therapy for the Chronic Depressions (CBT-CD): Combined collaborative national study*. Poster presented at the annual convention of the Society of Biological Psychiatry, San Diego, CA.

McCullough, J. P., Kornstein, S. G., McCullough, J. P., Belyea-Caldwell, S., Kaye, A. L., Roberts, W. C., Plybon, J. K., & Kruus, L. K. (1996). Differential diagnosis of chronic depressive disorders. *Psychiatric Clinics of North America, 19*, 55–71.

McCullough, J. P., McCune, K. J., Kaye, A. L., Braith, J. A., Friend, R., Roberts, W. C., Belyea-Caldwell, S., Norris, S. L. W., & Hampton, C. (1994a). One-year prospective replication study of an untreated sample of community dysthymia subjects. *Journal of Nervous and Mental Disease, 182*, 396–401.

McCullough, J. P., McCune, K. J., Kaye, A. L., Braith, J. A., Friend, R., Roberts, W. C., Belyea-Caldwell, S., Norris, S. L. W., & Hampton, C. (1994b). Comparison of a community dysthymia sample at screening with a matched group of nondepressed community controls. *Journal of Nervous and Mental Disease, 182*, 402–407.

McCullough, J. P., Roberts, W. C., McCune, K. J., Kaye, A. L., Hampton, C., Caldwell, S. B., Norris, S. L. W., & Kornstein, S. G. (1994). Social adjustment, coping style, and clinical course among DSM-III-R community unipolar depressives. *Depression, 2*, 36–42.

McKechnie, J. L. (Ed.). (1979). *Webster's New Universal Unabridged Dictionary* (2nd ed.). New York: Dorset & Baber.

Merikangas, K. R., Prusoff, B. A., & Weissman, M. M. (1988). Parental concordance for affective disorders: Psychopathology in offspring. *Journal of Affective Disorders, 15*, 279–290.

Miller, G. A. (1981). Trend and debates in cognitive psychology. *Cognition, 10*, 215–225.

Miller, I. W. (1997). Combined treatment for depressive disorders. *Depressive Disorders: Index and Reviews, 2*(3), 16–17.

Mischel, W. (1973). Toward a cognitive social learning reconceptualization of personality. *Psychological Review, 80*, 252–283.

Money, J. (1992). *The Kaspar Hauser Syndrome of "Psychosocial Dwarfism": Deficient Structural, Intellectual and Social Growth Induced by Child Abuse*. Buffalo, NY: Prometheus Books.

Money, J., Annecillo, C., & Hutchinson, J. W. (1985). Forensic and family psychiatry in abuse dwarfism: Munchausen's syndrome by proxy, atonement, and addiction to abuse. *Journal of Sex and Marital Therapy, 11,* 30–40.

Nannis, E. D. (1988). Cognitive-developmental differences in emotional understanding. In E. D. Nannis & P. A. Cowan (Eds.), *Developmental Psychopathology and Its Treatment (pp. 31–49). San Francisco: Jossey-Bass.*

Nisbett, R. E. & Wilson, T. D. (1977). Telling more than we can know: Verbal reports on mental processes. *Psychological Review, 84,* 231–259.

Noam, G. G. (1988). A constructivist approach to developmental psychopathology. In E. D. Nannis & P. A. Cowan (Eds.), *Developmental Psychopathology and Its Treatment* (pp. 91–121). San Francisco: Jossey-Bass.

Noam, G. G., & Cicchetti, D. (1996). Reply. *Human Development, 39,* 49–56.

Parsons, T. (1951). Illness and the role of the physician: A sociological perspective. *American Journal of Orthopsychiatry, 21,* 452–460.

Pepper, C. M., Klein, D. N., Anderson, R. L., Riso, L. P., Quimette, P. C., & Lizardi, H. (1995). DSM-III-R Axis II comorbidity in dysthymia and major depression. *American Journal of Psychiatry, 152,* 239–247.

Peterson, C., Semmel, A., Von Baeyer, C., Abramson, L. Y., Metalsky, G. I., & Seligman, M. E. P. (1982). The Attributional Style Questionnaire. *Cognitive Therapy and Research, 6,* 287–299.

Piaget, J. (1926). *The Language and Thought of the Child.* New York: Harcourt, Brace. (Original work published 1923)

Piaget, J. (1967). *Six Psychological Studies* (D. Elkind, Ed.). New York: Random House. (Original work published 1964)

Piaget, J. (1981). *Intelligence and Affectivity: Their Relationship during Child Development.* Palo Alto, CA: Annual Reviews. (Original work published 1954)

Platt, J. J., Siegel, J. M., & Spivack, G. (1975). Do psychiatric patients and normals see the same solutions as effective in solving interpersonal problems? *Journal of Consulting and Clinical Psychology, 43,* 279.

Platt, J. J., & Spivack, G. (1972). Problem-solving thinking of psychiatric patients. *Journal of Consulting and Clinical Psychology, 39,* 148–151.

Platt, J. J., & Spivack, G. (1974). Means of solving real-life problems: I. Psychiatric patients vs. controls and cross-cultural comparisons of normal females. *Journal of Community Psychology, 2,* 45–48.

Platt, J. J., & Spivack, G. (1975). Unidimensionality of the means-ends problem-solving (MEPS) procedure. *Journal of Clinical Psychology, 31,* 15–16.

Polanyi, M. (1966). *The Tacit Dimension.* Garden City, NY: Doubleday.

Polanyi, M. (1968). Logic and psychology. *American Psychologist, 23,* 27–43.

Reid, D. W., & Ware, E. E. (1974). Multidimensionality of internal versus external control: Addition of a third dimension and non-distinction of self versus others. *Canadian Journal of Behavioural Science, 6,* 131–142.

Riso, L. P., Klein, D. N., Ferro, T., Kasch, K. L., Pepper, C. M., Schwartz, J. E., & Aronson, T. A. (1996). Understanding the comorbidity between early-onset dysthymia and Cluster B personality disorders: A family study. *American Journal of Psychiatry, 153,* 900–906.

Rogers, C. R. (1942). *Counseling and Psychotherapy.* Boston: Houghton Mifflin.

Rogers, C. R. (1957). The necessary and sufficient conditions of therapeutic personal change. *Journal of Counseling Psychology, 21,* 93–103.

Rogers, C. R. (1959). A theory of therapy, personality, and interpersonal relationships, as developed in the client-centered framework. In S. Koch (Ed.), *Psychology: A Study of A Science* (Vol. 3, pp. 184–256). New York: McGraw-Hill.

Rohde, P., Lewinsohn, P. M., & Seeley, J. R. (1991). Comorbidity of unipolar depression: II. Comorbidity with other mental disorders in adolescents and adults. *Journal of Abnormal Psychology, 100*, 214–222.

Roth, A., Fonagy, P., Parry, G., Target, M., & Woods, R. M. (1996). *What Works for Whom?: A Critical Review of Psychotherapy Research.* New York: Guilford Press.

Rotter, J. B. (1954). *Social Learning and Clinical Psychology.* Englewood Cliffs, NJ: Prentice-Hall.

Rotter, J. B. (1966). Generalized expectancies for internal versus external control of reinforcements. *Psychological Monographs, 80* (1, Whole no. 609).

Rotter, J. B. (1978). Generalized expectancies for problem-solving and psychotherapy. *Cognitive Therapy and Research, 2*, 1–10.

Rotter, J. B. (1990). Internal versus external control of reinforcement: A case history of a variable. *American Psychologist, 45*, 489–493.

Rubin, K. H., Coplan, R. J., Fox, N. A., & Calkins, S. D. (1995). Emotionality, emotional regulation, and preschoolers' social adaptation. *Development and Psychopathology, 7*, 49–62.

Rush, A. J., Beck, A. T., Kovacs, M., & Hollon, S. D. (1977). Comparative efficacy of cognitive therapy and pharmacotherapy in the treatment of depressed outpatients. *Cognitive Therapy and Research, 1*, 17–37.

Rush, A. J., & Thase, M. E. (1999). Psychotherapies for depressive-disorders: A review. In M. Madge and N. Satorius (Eds.). *WPA Series Evidence and Experience in Psychiatry: Vol. 1. Depressive Disorders* (pp. 161–206). Chichester, UK: Wiley.

Rutter, M., & Quinton, P. (1984). Parental psychiatric disorder: Effects on children. *Psychological Medicine, 14*, 853–880.

Safran, J. D. (1990a). Towards a refinement of cognitive therapy in light of interpersonal theory: I. Theory. *Clinical Psychology Review, 10*, 87–105.

Safran, J. D. (1990b). Towards a refinement of cognitive therapy in light of interpersonal theory: II. Practice. *Clinical Psychology Review, 10*, 107–121.

Safran, J. D., & Segal, Z. V. (1990). *Interpersonal Process in Cognitive Therapy.* New York: Basic Books.

Sanderson, W. C., Wetzler, S., Beck, A. T., & Betz, F. (1992). Prevalence of personality disorders in patients with major depression and dysthymia. *Psychiatry Research, 42*, 93–99.

Sartre, J.-P. (1961). *No Exit and Three Other Plays.* New York: Vintage Books.

Schachter, S. (1964). The interaction of cognitive and physiological determinants of emotional state. In L. Berkowitz (Ed.), *Advances in Experimental Social Psychology.* New York: Academic Press.

Schachter, S., & Singer, J. E. (1962). Cognitive, social, and physiological determinants of emotional state. *Psychological Review, 69*, 379–399.

Scheier, M. F., & Carver, C. S. (1987). Dispositional optimism and physical well-being: The influence of general outcome expectancies on health. *Journal of Personality, 55*, 169–210.

Scheier, M. F., & Carver, C. S. (1992). Effects of optimism on psychological and physical well-being: Theoretical overview and empirical update. *Cognitive Therapy and Research, 16,* 201–228.

Selye, H. (1976). *The Stress of Life.* New York: McGraw-Hill.

Shapiro, P. A., Lidagoster, L., & Glassman, A. H. (1997). Depression and heart disease. *Psychiatric Annals, 27,* 347–352.

Shrout, P. E., & Fleiss, J. L. (1979). Intraclass correlations: Uses in assessing rater reliability. *Psychological Bulletin, 86,* 420–428.

Sidman, M. (1960). *Tactics of Scientific Research.* New York: Basic Books.

Siegler, R. S., & Ellis, S. (1996). Piaget on childhood. *Psychological Science, 7,* 211–215.

Simons, A. D., Garfield, S. L., & Murphy, C. E. (1984). The process of change in cognitive therapy and pharmacotherapy for depression. *Archives of General Psychiatry, 41,* 45–51.

Simons, A. D., & Thase, M. E. (1990). Mood disorders. In M. E. Thase, B. A. Edelstein, & M. Hersen (Eds.), *Handbook of Outpatient Treatment of Adults: Nonpsychotic Mental Disorders* (pp. 91–138). New York: Plenum Press.

Skinner, B. F. (1953). *Science and Human Behavior.* New York: Macmillan.

Skinner, B. F. (1956). A case history in scientific method. *American Psychologist, 11,* 221–233.

Skinner, B. F. (1968). *The Technology of Teaching.* New York: Appleton-Century-Crofts.

Skinner, B. F. (1969). *Contingencies of Reinforcement: A Theoretical Analysis.* New York: Appleton-Century-Crofts.

Solso, R. L. (1995). *Cognitive Psychology.* Needham Heights, MA: Allyn & Bacon.

Sotsky, S. M., Glass, D. R., Shea, M. T., Pilkonis, P. A., Collins, J. F., Elkin, I., Watkins, J. T., Imber, S. D., Leber, W. R., Moyer, J., & Oliveri, M. E. (1991). Patient predictors of response to psychotherapy and pharmacotherapy: Findings in the NIMH Treatment of Depression Collaborative Research Program. *American Journal of Psychiatry, 148,* 997–1008.

Spitz, R. (1946). Hospitalism: A follow-up report on investigation described in Volume I, 1945. *Psychoanalytic Study of the Child, 2,* 113–117.

Spitzer, R. L., Williams, J. B. W., Gibbon, M., & First, M. B. (1990). *Structured Clinical Interview for DSM-III-R: Patient Edition (with Psychotic Screen).* Washington, DC: American Psychiatric Press.

Strupp, H. & Bergen, A. E. (1969). Some empirical and conceptual bases for coordinated research in psychotherapy. *International Journal of Psychiatry, 7,* 17–90.

Thase, M. E. (1992). Long-term treatments of recurrent depressive disorders. *Journal of Clinical Psychiatry, 53,* 32–44.

Thase, M. E., & Kupfer, D. J. (1996). Recent developments in the pharmacotherapy of mood disorders. *Journal of Consulting and Clinical Psychology, 64,* 646–659.

Thase, M. E., Reynolds, C. F., Frank, E., Simmons, A. D., Garamoni, G. D., McGeary, J., Harden, T., Fasiczka, A. L., & Cahalane, J. F. (1994). Response to cognitive-behavioral therapy in chronic depression. *Psychiatry Research, 3,* 204–214.

Thase, M. E., Simons, A. D., McGeary, J., Cahalane, J. F., Hughes, C., Harden, T., & Friedman, E. (1992). Relapse following cognitive behavior therapy for depression: Potential implications for longer forms of treatment? *American Journal of Psychiatry, 149,* 1046–1052.

Wachtel, P. L. (1973). Psychodynamics, behavior therapy and the implacable experimenter: An inquiry into the consistency of personality. *Journal of Abnormal Psychology, 82,* 324–334.

Wachtel, P. L. (1977). *Psychoanalysis and Behavior Therapy.* New York: Basic Books.

Wakefield, J. C. (1992a). Disorder as harmful dysfunction: A conceptual critique of DSM-III-R's definition of mental disorder. *Psychological Review, 99,* 232–247.

Wakefield, J. C. (1992b). The concept of mental disorder: On the boundry between biological facts and social values. *American Psychologist, 47,* 373–388.

Waugh, N. C., & Norman, D. A. (1965). Primary memory. *Psychological Review, 72,* 89–104.

Weiss, P. (1961). Deformities as cues to understanding development of form *Perspectives in Biology and Medicine, 4,* 133–151.

Weiss, P. (1969). The living system: Determinism stratified. In A. Koestler & J. Smythies (Eds.), *Beyond Reductionism* (pp. 3–55). Boston: Beacon Press.

Weissman, M. M. (1975). The assessment of social adjustment: A review of techniques. *Archives of General Psychiatry, 32,* 357–356.

Weissman, M. M., & Akiskal, H. S. (1984). The role of psychotherapy in chronic depressions: A proposal. *Comprehensive Psychiatry, 25,* 23–31.

Weissman, M. M., & Bothwell, S. (1976). Assessment of social adjustment by patient self-report. *Archives of General Psychiatry, 33,* 1111–1115.

Weissman, M. M., & Markowitz, J. C. (1994). Interpersonal psychotherapy: Current status. *Archives of General Psychiatry, 51,* 599–606.

Welch, B., & Welch, A. (1968). Differential activation by restraint stress of a mechanism to conserve brain catecholamines and serotonin in mice differing in excitability. *Nature, 218,* 575–577.

Wells, K. B., Burnam, M. A., Rogers, W., Hays, R., & Camp, P. (1992). The course of depression in adult outpatients: Results from the Medical Outcomes Study. *Archives of General Psychiatry, 49,* 788–794.

Whisman, M. A. (1993). Mediators and moderators of change in cognitive therapy of depression. *Psychological Bulletin, 114,* 248–265.

White, P. (1980). Limitations on verbal reports of internal events: A refutation of Nisbett and Wilson and of Bem. *Psychological Review, 87,* 105–112.

Whybrow, P. C., Akiskal, H. S., & McKinney, W. T. (1985). *Mood Disorders: Toward a New Psychobiology.* New York: Plenum Press.

Wilkinson, G. (1989). Research report: The General Practice Research Unit at the Institute of Psychiatry. *Psychological Medicine, 19,* 789–790.

Wright, J. H., & Thase, M. E. (1992). Cognitive and biological therapies: A synthesis. *Psychiatric Annals, 22,* 451–458.

Author Index

Note: t indicates a table and f indicates a figure.

311

Subject Index

Note: *t* indicates a table and *f* indicates a figure.